T0215125

Acute Brain and Spinal Cord Injury

ACUTE BRAIN AND SPINAL CORD INJURY

EVOLVING PARADIGMS AND MANAGEMENT

Edited by

Anish Bhardwaj
Oregon Health & Science University
Portland, Oregon, USA

Dilantha B. Ellegala
Oregon Health & Science University
Portland, Oregon, USA

Jeffrey R. Kirsch
Oregon Health & Science University
Portland, Oregon, USA

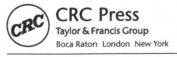

CRC Press
Taylor & Francis Group
Boca Raton London New York

CRC Press is an imprint of the
Taylor & Francis Group, an **informa** business

CRC Press
Taylor & Francis Group
6000 Broken Sound Parkway NW, Suite 300
Boca Raton, FL 33487-2742

First issued in paperback 2019

© 2010 by Taylor & Francis Group, LLC
CRC Press is an imprint of Taylor & Francis Group, an Informa business

No claim to original U.S. Government works

ISBN-13: 978-1-4200-4794-3 (hbk)
ISBN-13: 978-1-138-38138-4 (pbk)

A CIP record for this book is available from the British Library.

Library of Congress Cataloging-in-Publication Data available on application

Visit the Taylor & Francis Web site at
http://www.taylorandfrancis.com

and the CRC Press Web site at
http://www.crcpress.com

*To my daughter Lara, and Richard J. Traystman, a great mentor, teacher, and a dear friend. – **Anish Bhardwaj***

*To my parents, whose self sacrifice have made this and all else possible. They are the American dream realized. – **Dilantha B. Ellegala***

*To my loving wife, Robin, and my wonderful children Jodi, Alan, and Ricki. – **Jeffrey R. Kirsch***

Foreword

All over the world, acute brain and spinal cord injury represents one of the most important public health problems that society faces. This is true in both the most progressive and sophisticated areas of the world and in developing areas where advanced medical care is often lacking. This welcome volume addresses the issues of the diagnosis and management of head and spinal cord injury in an up-to-date and comprehensive fashion. Appropriately, it includes some areas of controversy in concepts and in practical management. In doing so the stage is set for better outcomes and future investigative work in this important field of endeavor.

Understanding of the pathophysiology of brain and spinal cord injuries has led to important interventions such as decompressive craniectomy, cerebral protection, hypothermia, and reversal of vasospasm. New methods of monitoring patients have led to early recognition of potentially reversible injuries, alterations in homeostasis, and a better understanding of the epiphenomena of brain and spinal cord trauma.

The different sections of the book each focus on a part of the spectrum of brain and spinal cord injury. Brain and spinal cord trauma; vascular insults to the brain and spinal cord from stroke, ischemia, and subarachnoid hemorrhage; intracranial and spinal hemorrhagic lesions; and metabolic derangements are all covered in an expert and comprehensive fashion.

The systematic review presented in this book provides a basis for new paradigms in the effective management of CNS trauma. The result is an inspiration for clinical and basic neuroscientists to continue to make further advances in this clinical, investigative, and neuroscientifically essential field critical to global public health.

Edward R. Laws, MD, FACS
Professor of Neurosurgery
Stanford University Medical Center
Stanford, California, U.S.A.

Preface

The clinical management of patients with acute brain and spinal cord injury has evolved significantly with the advent of new diagnostic and therapeutic modalities. Our understanding of the pathophysiology of brain injury of diverse etiologies, from ischemic stroke and intracerebral and subarachnoid hemorrhage to traumatic brain and spinal cord injury, continues to grow from laboratory-based experimental work and clinical trials. The care of such patients by a trained team of neurointensivists, neurosurgeons, anesthesiologists, and nurses, coupled with the advent of newer monitoring techniques in a dedicated neuro-ICU, has evolved in patients with acute brain and spinal cord injury. It is believed that these advances have contributed to improved outcomes. However, considerable uncertainty persists regarding key areas of clinical management in this subset of patients. While numerous textbooks are available on each of the injury paradigms, none has focused on selected controversies and the evolving paradigms in clinical management of each of these disorders.

This textbook is divided into five sections, which cover the state-of-the-art management that exists in the clinical management of patients with traumatic brain injury, ischemic stroke, intracerebral hemorrhage, subarachnoid hemorrhage, and spinal cord injury. Our intent is to present a comprehensive review on the subject from published data and to provide clinicians, neuroscientists, and clinician scientists with a guide for bedside management, as well as foster clinical and translational research in these important areas. We anticipate that the rigorous evaluation and implementation of such data will provide a basis for improvement in short- and long-term outcomes in these injury paradigms. We hope that this book will achieve this goal.

We, the editors, are indebted to the authors for their valuable contributions. Special thanks are due to Tzipora Sofare for her editorial assistance. Her never-ending quest for accuracy and consistency has greatly enhanced the quality of this volume. We also recognize and thank Debbie Bird for her efforts in coordinating the development of this book. We would also like to particularly express our thanks to a number of funding sources, such as the American Heart Association, the National Stroke Association, and the National Institutes of Health extramural programs, which have supported our investigative work in neurosciences critical care.

Anish Bhardwaj, MD, FAHA, FCCM
Dilantha B. Ellegala, MD
Jeffrey R. Kirsch, MD

Contents

Contributors

Alfred Aschoff, MD, PhD, Associate Professor   Department of Neurosurgery, University of Heidelberg, Heidelberg, Germany

Emun Abdu, MD, Senior Resident   Department of Neurological Surgery, Oregon Health & Science University, Portland, Oregon, U.S.A.

P. David Adelson, MD, FACS, FAAP, Professor[a] and Vice Chairman[b]
A. Leland Albright Professor of [a]Neurological Surgery and [b]Pediatric Neurosurgery, Children's Hospital of Pittsburgh, University of Pittsburgh School of Medicine, Pittsburgh, Pennsylvania, U.S.A.

Issam Awad, MD, Professor   Department of Neurological Surgery, Northwestern University Feinberg School of Medicine, Chicago, Illinois, U.S.A.

Yekaterina Axelrod, MD, Assistant Professor[a,b]   Department of [a]Neurology, [b]Neurosurgery, Washington University School of Medicine, St. Louis, Missouri, U.S.A.

Stanley L. Barnwell, MD, Associate Professor   Department of Radiology, Oregon Health & Science University, Portland, Oregon, U.S.A.

H. Hunt Batjer, MD, Professor and Chairman   Department of Neurological Surgery, Northwestern University Feinberg School of Medicine, Chicago, Illinois, U.S.A.

Anish Bhardwaj, MD, FAHA, FCCM, Professor[a] and Director[b]
[a]Neurology, Neurological Surgery, Anesthesiology & Peri-Operative Medicine, [b]Neurosciences Critical Care Program, Oregon Health & Science University, Portland, Oregon, U.S.A.

Thomas P. Bleck, MD, FCCM, Ruth Cain Ruggles Chairman[a], Vice Chairman[b], and Professor[c] [a]Department of Neurology, Evanston Northwestern Healthcare, [b]Department of Neurology, [c]Departments of Neurology, Neurosurgery, and Medicine, Northwestern University Feinberg School of Medicine, Chicago, Illinois, U.S.A.

Ansgar Brambrink, MD, PhD, Professor Department of Anesthesiology & Peri-Operative Medicine, Oregon Health & Science University, Portland, Oregon, U.S.A.

Steven Casha, MD, PhD, FRCSC, Assistant Professor Department of Clinical Neurosciences, Division of Neurosurgery and University of Calgary Spine Program, Foothills Hospital and Medical Centre, Calgary, Alberta, Canada

Rene Celis, MD, Research Assistant Department of Neurosurgery, Baylor College of Medicine, Houston, Texas, U.S.A.

Carolyn A. Cronin, MD, PhD, Resident Department of Neurology, The Johns Hopkins University School of Medicine, Baltimore, Maryland, U.S.A.

Dawn Dillman, MD, Assistant Professor Department of Anesthesiology & Peri-Operative Medicine, Oregon Health & Science University, Portland, Oregon, U.S.A.

Michael Diringer, MD, FCCM, Professor[a,b,c] and Director[d] Department of [a]Neurology, [b]Neurosurgery, and [c]Anesthesia; [d]Neurology and Neurosurgery Intensive Care Unit, Washington University School of Medicine, St. Louis, Missouri, U.S.A.

Aclan Dogan, MD, Assistant Professor Department of Radiology, Oregon Health & Science University, Portland, Oregon, U.S.A.

Ian F. Dunn, MD, Senior Resident Department of Neurosurgery, Brigham and Women's Hospital, Harvard Medical School, Boston, Massachusetts, U.S.A.

Jonathan A. Edlow, MD, FACEP, Vice Chairman[a] and Associate Professor[b] [a]Department of Emergency Medicine, Beth Israel Deaconess Medical Center, and [b]Department of Medicine, Harvard Medical School, Boston, Massachusetts, U.S.A.

Dilantha B. Ellegala, MD, * Assistant Professor Department of Neurosurgery, Oregon Health & Science University, Portland, Oregon, U.S.A.

Kairash Golshani, MD, Senior Resident Department of Neurological Surgery, Oregon Health & Science University, Portland, Oregon, U.S.A.

Aaron W. Grossman, PhD, Medical Student University of Illinois College of Medicine at Urbana-Champaign, Urbana, Illinois, U.S.A.

Present affiliation: Assistant Professor, Director of Cerebrovascular Program, Department of Neurosurgery, Medical University of South Carolina, Charleston, South Carolina, U.S.A.

Lotfi Hacein-Bey, MD, Professor   Departments of Radiology and Neurological Surgery, Loyola University, Chicago, Illinois, U.S.A.

Tarik Hanane, MD, Fellow   Mayo Clinic College of Medicine, Rochester, Minnesota, U.S.A.

Olga Helena Hernandez, MD, Fellow   Neurocritical Care, Case Medical Center, Case Western Reserve University, Cleveland, Ohio, U.S.A.

Patrick C. Hsieh, MD, Resident   Department of Neurological Surgery, Northwestern University Feinberg School of Medicine, Chicago, Illinois, U.S.A.

R. John Hurlbert, MD, PhD, FRCSC, FACS, Associate Professor Department of Clinical Neurosciences, Division of Neurosurgery and University of Calgary Spine Program, Foothills Hospital and Medical Centre, Calgary, Alberta, Canada

Pascal M. Jabbour, MD, Chief Resident   Department of Neurological Surgery, Thomas Jefferson University, Jefferson Hospital for Neuroscience, Philadelphia, Pennsylvania, U.S.A.

Brian Jankowitz, MD, Resident   Department of Neurosurgery, University of Pittsburgh School of Medicine, Pittsburgh, Pennsylvania, U.S.A.

Eric Jüttler, MD   Department of Neurology, University of Heidelberg, Heidelberg, Germany

Salah Keyrouz, MD*, Fellow   Neurology and Neurosurgery Intensive Care Unit, Washington University School of Medicine, St. Louis, Missouri, U.S.A.

Dong H. Kim,** MD, Assistant Professor   Department of Neurosurgery, Brigham and Women's Hospital, Harvard Medical School, Boston, Massachusetts, U.S.A.

Shivanand P. Lad, MD, PhD, Resident   Department of Neurosurgery, Stanford University School of Medicine, Palo Alto, California, U.S.A.

Giuseppe Lanzino, MD, Professor   Department of Neurological Surgery, Mayo Clinic College of Medicine, Rochester, Minnesota, U.S.A.

David Lee, MD, Assistant Professor   Department of Radiology, Oregon Health & Science University, Portland, Oregon, U.S.A.

Gordon Li, MD, Resident   Department of Neurosurgery, Stanford University School of Medicine, Palo Alto, California, U.S.A.

**Present affiliation:* Assistant Professor, Department of Neurology, University of Arkansas for Medical Sciences, Little Rock, Arkansas, U.S.A.

***Present affiliation:* Professor and Chairman, Department of Neurosurgery, The University of Texas, and Director, The Mischer Neuroscience Institute, Memorial Hermann Hospital, Houston, Texas, U.S.A.

Zachary N. Litvack, MD, Senior Resident   Department of Neurological Surgery, Oregon Health & Science University, Portland, Oregon, U.S.A.

Gary Nesbit, MD, Associate Professor   Department of Radiology, Oregon Health & Science University, Portland, Oregon, U.S.A.

David O. Okonkwo, MD, PhD, Assistant Professor   Department of Neurosurgery, University of Pittsburgh School of Medicine, Pittsburgh, Pennsylvania, U.S.A.

Bryan Petersen, MD, Associate Professor   Department of Radiology, Oregon Health & Science University, Portland, Oregon, U.S.A.

Adnan I. Qureshi, MD, Professor and Vice Chair of Neurology   Zeenat Qureshi Stroke Research Center, University of Minnesota, Minneapolis, Minnesota, U.S.A.

Claudia S. Robertson, MD, Professor   Department of Neurosurgery, Baylor College of Medicine, Houston, Texas, U.S.A.

Gustavo J. Rodríguez, MD, Fellow   Endovascular Surgical Neuroradiology, Zeenat Qureshi Stroke Research Center, University of Minnesota, Minneapolis, Minnesota, U.S.A.

Robert H. Rosenwasser, MD, FACS, FAHA, Professor and Chairman[a] and Professor[b]   [a]Department of Neurological Surgery, [b]Radiology, Neurovascular Surgery, and Interventional Neuroradiology, Thomas Jefferson University, Jefferson Hospital for Neuroscience, Philadelphia, Pennsylvania, U.S.A.

Stefan Schwab, Professor Doctor, Director   Department of Neurology, University of Erlangen, Erlangen, Germany

Nathan R. Selden, MD, PhD, FACS, FAAP, Associate Professor[a], Vice-Chairman[b], and Head[c]   [a]Mario and Edith Campagna Associate Professor, [b]Education and Program Director, [c]Division of Pediatric Neurosurgery, and Department of Neurological Surgery, Oregon Health & Science University, Portland, Oregon, U.S.A.

Christopher Shaffrey, MD, Professor   Department of Neurological Surgery, University of Virginia, Charlottesville, Virginia, U.S.A.

Qaisar A. Shah, MD, Fellow   Endovascular Surgical Neuroradiology, Zeenat Qureshi Stroke Research Center, University of Minnesota, Minneapolis, Minnesota, U.S.A.

Ganesh M. Shankar, BA, Medical Student   Department of Neurosurgery, Brigham and Women's Hospital, Harvard Medical School, Boston, Massachusetts, U.S.A.

Richard H. Singleton, MD, PhD, Senior Resident   Department of Neurosurgery, University of Pittsburgh School of Medicine, Pittsburgh, Pennsylvania, U.S.A.

Gary K. Steinberg, MD, PhD, Professor[a] and Chairman[b]   [a]Bernard and Ronni Lacroute-William Randolph Hearst Professor of Neurosurgery and the Neurosciences, [b]Department of Neurosurgery, Stanford University School of Medicine, Palo Alto, California, U.S.A.

Jose I. Suarez, MD, Director[a] and Professor[b]   [a]Vascular Neurology and Neurocritical Care, [b]Neurology and Neurosurgery, Baylor College of Medicine, Houston, Texas, U.S.A.

Patrick Sugrue, MD, Resident   Department of Neurological Surgery, Northwestern University Feinberg School of Medicine, Chicago, Illinois, U.S.A.

Roland A. Torres, MD, Clinical Professor   Department of Neurosurgery, Stanford University School of Medicine, Palo Alto, California, U.S.A.

Panayiotis N. Varelas, MD, PhD, Director[a] and Senior Staff[b]   [a]Neuro-ICU, [b]Departments of Neurology and Neurosurgery, Henry Ford Hospital, Detroit, Michigan, U.S.A.

Erol Veznedaroglu, MD, FACS, Associate Professor[a] and Director[b] [a]Department of Neurological Surgery, [b]Division of Neurovascular Surgery and Endovascular Neurosurgery, Thomas Jefferson University, Jefferson Hospital for Neuroscience, Philadelphia, Pennsylvania, U.S.A.

Lindsay Wenger   Department of Radiology, Oregon Health & Science University, Portland, Oregon, U.S.A.

Eelco F. M. Wijdicks, MD, Professor   Mayo Clinic College of Medicine, Rochester, Minnesota, U.S.A.

Robert J. Wityk, MD, FAHA, Associate Professor   Department of Neurology, The Johns Hopkins University School of Medicine and Cerebrovascular Division, The Johns Hopkins Hospital, Baltimore, Maryland, U.S.A.

Anil V. Yallapragada, MD, Resident   Department of Internal Medicine, SUNY Downstate Medical Center, Brooklyn, New York, U.S.A.

NEUROLOGICAL DISEASE AND THERAPY

Advisory Board

Gordon H. Baltuch, M.D., Ph.D.
Department of Neurosurgery
University of Pennsylvania
Philadelphia, Pennsylvania, U.S.A.

Cheryl Bushnell, M.D., M.H.S.
Duke Center for Cerebrovascular Disease
Department of Medicine, Division of Neurology
Duke University Medical Center
Durham, North Carolina, U.S.A.

Louis R. Caplan, M.D.
Professor of Neurology
Harvard University School of Medicine
Beth Israel Deaconess Medical Center
Boston, Massachusetts, U.S.A.

Mark A. Stacy, M.D.
Movement Disorders Center
Duke University Medical Center
Durham, North Carolina, U.S.A.

Mark H. Tuszynski, M.D., Ph.D.
Professor of Neurosciences
Director, Center for Neural Repair
University of California—San Diego
La Jolla, California, U.S.A.

Ajay K. Wakhloo, M.D., Ph.D.
Department of Radiology
University of Massachusetts Medical School
Worcester, Massachusetts, U.S.A.

Decompressive Hemicraniectomy in the Management of Severe Traumatic Brain Injury

Ian F. Dunn, MD, Senior Resident

Department of Neurosurgery, Brigham and Women's Hospital, Harvard Medical School, Boston, Massachusetts, U.S.A.

Dilantha B. Ellegala,* MD, Assistant Professor

Department of Neurosurgery, Oregon Health & Science University, Portland, Oregon, U.S.A.

We have presented our appraisal of the case material, not so much as proof of its superiority over other methods, but rather as provocation for further critical appraisal of its use.

Kjellberg and Prieto, on decompressive craniectomy (1)

INTRODUCTION

Kjellberg's and Prieto's words are no less prophetic today as during the writing of their highly influential paper in 1971, which not only resurrected decompressive craniectomy (DC) but also challenged the field to validate or refute its utility in the management of cerebral edema. We are stuck on their refrain nearly

**Present affiliation*: Assistant Professor, Director of Cerebrovascular Program, Department of Neurosurgery, Medical University of South Carolina, Charleston, South Carolina, U.S.A.

40 years later, as attempts at synthesizing reported outcomes in the intervening years have been confounded by variable surgical technique, dramatic improvements in perioperative care of patients with severe traumatic brain injury (TBI), and a near-total absence of class I data on DC in TBI. As we reach a discomforting therapeutic plateau in the postoperative medical management of the sequelae of severe TBI, the use of DC in these patients has renewed interest. Discussed in this chapter are the rationale for DC in severe TBI; technical considerations in its implementation; the extant evidence regarding its efficacy; and two randomized, controlled trials that are underway, the results of which are eagerly anticipated. Other indications for DC, including malignant cerebral infarction, are discussed in other chapters in this text.

TERMINOLOGY

Two classes of DC are performed by neurosurgeons. *Primary DC* is performed at the time of evacuation of an extra- or intra-axial hematoma to facilitate postoperative management of intracranial pressure (ICP); it is routinely practiced during surgery for evacuation of a unilateral hematoma and involves closing the scalp without replacing the bone flap, or in neurosurgical parlance, leaving the bone flap "off." Little controversy exists surrounding this practice as it is performed in the primary phase of TBI.

Delayed or secondary DC is performed specifically for ICP control in the hours or days after primary injury and is targeted to the management of secondary brain injury. The employment of secondary DC involves considerable variation. *Early* or *ultra-early* secondary DC is performed within the first few hours after injury and when initial medical management fails to bring ICP under control. Many neurosurgeons (the authors included) advocate early DC, within six to eight hours of injury, if acute medical management fails to control ICP. Very little data exist to either support or refute this practice, and the theory is extrapolated from animal spinal cord compression and decompression experiments (2,3). More recent work has shown that earlier decompression in an animal cranial model of compression results in less permanent neuronal damage (4). Delayed secondary DC is performed many hours or even days after the initial injury and when all medical management efforts have been exhausted. The single prospective randomized controlled trial to investigate the efficacy of secondary DC after TBI was conducted in pediatric patients, with a moderate reduction in death and disability recorded in patients undergoing decompressive procedures (5). Data in adult patients consist of retrospective series, small case studies, or prospective nonrandomized trials. Unfortunately, no rigorous evaluations of the precise timing of ultra-early versus delayed secondary DC have been performed. Except where indicated, subsequent discussion focuses on the implementation of secondary DC in the management of patients with TBI.

DECOMPRESSIVE CRANIECTOMY AFTER TBI: PATHOPHYSIOLOGIC RATIONALE

A significant body of literature discusses both purported and objective indications for DC in cases of severe TBI. Primary brain injury and the myriad intracellular and extracellular events that constitute secondary brain injury result in a pathologic triad of brain herniation, cerebral ischemia, and elevated ICP. Following is a review of the data in humans that support the benefit of DC in addressing these three sequelae in severe TBI.

Brain Herniation

An unquestionable benefit of DC is the decompression of vital brain stem structures by permitting outward—rather than centrifugal—movement of swollen brain parenchyma. The basis of this simplistic physical rationale for DC was codified by the Monro–Kellie doctrine. The total volume available for intracranial contents [i.e., cerebral blood volume (CBV), cerebrospinal fluid (CSF), and brain] is constant, and an augmentation in one compartment must be accompanied by a diminution in the other. An uncompensated increase in one or more compartments results in ICP above the normal range of 5 to 15 mmHg. In the absence of a mass lesion, increased ICP in severe TBI results from alterations in CSF flow, CBV, and the development of vasogenic and cytotoxic edema. Resistance to absorption of CSF in traumatic subarachnoid hemorrhage may lead to an increase in overall CSF. A rise in CBV results from the loss of autoregulation in severe TBI, and vasogenic and cytotoxic edema result from a compromised blood-brain barrier and osmotic dysregulation in ischemic cells. Physiologic volume-buffering mechanisms exist and involve alterations of blood and CSF volume and include arteriolar vasoconstriction, increasing cerebral venous outflow and downward CSF displacement through the foramen magnum or into expanded root sleeves. Once these mechanisms are exhausted, ICP rises in an exponential fashion (Fig. 1). In such states, small volumetric changes can lead to rapid and devastating neurologic deterioration. Sustained ICP readings of greater than 20 mmHg are abnormal; ICP readings between 20 and 40 mmHg represent severe intracranial hypertension; and ICP readings greater than 40 mmHg typically presage neurologic death.

The physical consequence of excessive volume is brain herniation. The displacement or herniation of brain through openings in the dura and skull occurs in several patterns: subfalcine herniation, uncal herniation, central downward herniation, tonsillar herniation, and external herniation of brain through an open skull fracture. Of particular importance are uncal herniation and downward herniation. Uncal herniation is produced by medial displacement of the temporal lobe by lateral middle fossa or temporal lobe lesions in which the ipsilateral oculomotor nerve, cerebral peduncle, reticular activating system, and possibly contralateral cerebral peduncle (i.e., Kernohan phenomenon) are compromised.

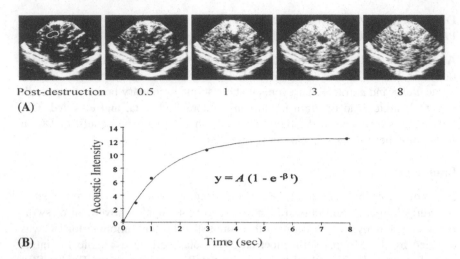

Figure 1 Ultrasound images immediately after high-power destructive pulses in 1 dog (brain). Central nonfilling region is the right and left ventricle, with the third ventricle near the foramen of Monroe. (**A**) A region of interest is shown in the first frame, from which acoustic intensity (AI) was automatically measured in all frames. (**B**) Corresponding time versus acoustic intensity plot fitted to the exponential function: $y = A(1 - e^{-\beta t})$, where y is the acoustic intensity at time t, A is the plateau acoustic intensity reflecting CB_{vol}, and the rate constant β represents the rate of microbubble (or red blood cell) replenishment (CB_{vel}). The product $A \times \beta$ reflects rCBF. *Abbreviation*: AI, acoustic intensity.

The resulting clinical syndrome involves coma, ipsilateral fixed and dilated pupil, and contralateral hemiparesis. Should the contralateral peduncle be compressed against the contralateral tentorial edge, ipsilateral motor function may also be compromised. Central or downward herniation may result from globally increased ICP and is defined by progressive caudal displacement of the brain stem through the foramen magnum. Basilar artery perforators are stretched and may cause hemorrhage (i.e., Duret hemorrhages). The clinical syndrome may include the Cushing triad (i.e., arterial hypertension, bradycardia, and respiratory irregularity), resulting in coma.

Cerebral Ischemia

Cerebral Blood Flow and Brain Tissue Oxygenation

A growing literature has explored the effect of DC on physiologic parameters such as cerebral blood flow (CBF) and brain tissue oxygenation. The preponderance of evidence supports an improvement in these indices of cerebral perfusion after DC in TBI. Early work using single-positron emission CT with [99m]technetium-hexamethyl-propyleneamine oxime (^{99m}Tc-HMPAO) demonstrated an increase in perfusion after DC, which increased further in the week following surgery but attenuated by one month after surgery (6). More recently, CT perfusion has shown perfusion restriction before—and its restoration after—DC (7); while the indication for DC in this study was middle cerebral artery infarction, we look forward to the application of improving CT perfusion technology to the study of vascular sufficiency before and after DC in TBI patients.

Transcranial Doppler studies on patients requiring bifrontal or unilateral DC for elevated ICP demonstrated a general increase in CBF after cranial decompression (8,9); in cases of unilateral decompression, CBF was elevated in both hemispheres. More recent work has not only supported the notion that CBF is enhanced by DC in TBI but has also demonstrated how such monitoring techniques may be practically implemented in a critical care setting.

The utility of contrast-enhanced ultrasonography (CEU), a noninvasive perfusion imaging technique that has been used to evaluate microvascular perfusion in the heart (10), skeletal muscle (11), and kidneys (12,13) has been described. This technique relies on ultrasonic detection of intravenously injected, gas-filled, encapsulated, microbubble contrast agents that possess microvascular rheologic characteristics similar to those of RBCs. To assess perfusion, microbubbles are infused intravenously and reach a steady state within the microcirculation. The microbubbles are then destroyed by a high-power ultrasonographic pulse, and the subsequent rate and extent of microbubble replenishment are used to determine microvascular blood velocity and volume, respectively (Fig. 1). The pilot study, which employed CEU in TBI, involved six patients in whom early secondary DC was performed for refractory ICP. Among a number of provocative results was the finding that over the three-day study period, DC resulted in a nearly fivefold increase in microvascular perfusion as assessed by CEU (14). Moreover, contrast-enhanced ultrasound was able to quantify changes in blood flow produced by DC (Fig. 2), to assess CBF alterations related to patient position and ICP, and to evaluate spatial heterogeneity of flow produced by parenchymal hematoma. Although it is difficult to draw conclusions from a nonrandomized study with few patients, the results from this pilot study support the claim that decompression of the traumatic brain in certain circumstances may result in an increase in CBF (14). Moreover, the ability to quickly assess microvascular perfusion at the bedside may enhance the capacity to limit cerebral ischemia through improved recognition of inadequate blood flow. We await the results of larger studies that investigate this technique's performance and impact on outcomes.

Brain tissue oxygenation (PtiO$_2$) has been used as a surrogate for the direct measure of real-time CBF, with both jugular venous oxygen saturation (SjvO$_2$) and parenchymal oxygen saturation (PbO$_2$). Several studies suggest a significant association between cerebral hypoxia, as measured by brain tissue oxygenation, and poor outcome after TBI (15–20), prompting interest in the effect of DC on measurable indices of oxygenation. Small studies investigating the effect of DC on PtiO$_2$ report substantial improvement in parenchymal oxygenation after late DC (21,22) in patients with TBI, with only minor changes in SjvO$_2$. Pre-DC PtiO$_2$ was at ischemic levels or was lower than post-DC PtiO$_2$ in patients with

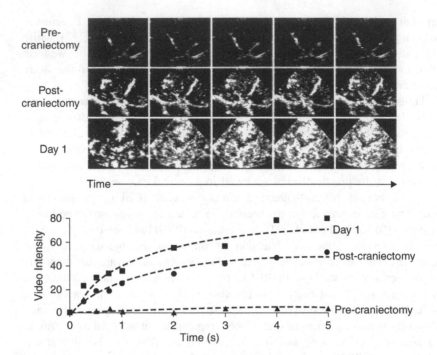

Figure 2 Contrast-enhanced ultrasonographic images obtained in the parasagittal plane after a high-power destructive pulse sequence (*upper*) and graph showing corresponding time versus video-intensity curves in a patient before decompressive craniectomy, immediately after craniectomy, and on postoperative day 1 (*lower*). Perfusion is markedly improved immediately after craniectomy and further improved by day 1, largely because of an increase in microvascular blood volume (plateau VI).

severe TBI. While provocative, these reports remain correlative, as the specific significance of PtiO$_2$ monitoring in TBI—let alone the import of the recovery or elevation of PtiO$_2$ after DC in these patients—is not definitive. Interestingly, the most dramatic increases in PtiO$_2$ after DC appear to be after duraplasty, not craniectomy, supporting expansion of the dural vault as a critical portion of the surgical procedure (22).

Elevated Intracranial Pressure

Nearly 50% of head-injured patients with intracranial mass lesions and 33% of patients with diffuse axonal injury have persistently elevated ICP. Increased ICP also compromises cerebral perfusion. Aside from the fact that increased ICP can decrease cerebral perfusion pressure (CPP), it is also true that drops in CPP can increase ICP. As CPP decreases, pial arterioles vasodilate and accommodate larger CBV, diagrammed in Rosner's vasodilatory cascade (23). This increased

CBV can increase ICP. When CPP is restored, pial arterioles can constrict, and ICP will often decrease.

Medically refractory ICP is the clearest indication for DC today despite the absence of class I data. Yoo et al. were the first to quantify ICP by ventricular catheterization before and after DC and reported on their clinical results in 20 patients, 6 of whom presented with severe TBI. The indications for DC were the appearance of massive unilateral or bilateral brain swelling on CT scans, with clinical deterioration, worsening of Glasgow Coma Scale score and/or dilation of pupils unresponsive to light, midline shift of more than 6 mm, and/or obliteration of perimesencephalic cistern on CT scans (24). Initial ICP readings in patients who underwent DC ranged from 16 to 66 mmHg. Bilateral DC reduced ICP values by approximately 50%, with duraplasty affording even further reductions. Interestingly, rebound ICP to levels of greater than 35 mmHg was associated with 100% mortality (24).

An observational study reported on clinical and physiologic parameters of DC in 26 patients treated as part of a standardized protocol (25). Bifrontal DC was associated with significant 50% reduction in mean ICP from 37 to 18 mmHg, also reducing ICP wave amplitude. While almost 70% of patients were deemed to have had a favorable outcome, it is difficult to assess the effect of ICP reduction by DC on this parameter (25).

Although it is well accepted that DC reduces ICP, whether or not this result improves clinical outcomes remains the subject of debate. Additionally, we anticipate that emerging technologies that can assess the effect of elevated ICP on white matter tracts, such as diffusion tensor imaging, may be able to establish the effect of DC on tractography. While it may not be feasible to perform diffusion tensor imaging routinely in these patients, experimental work that incorporates this technology in outcome studies may enhance our understanding of the effect of DC on cranial anatomy and physiology.

THE LUND CONCEPT: A CAVEAT?

DC is easily rationalized by the Monro–Kellie doctrine and by pressure-centric (CPP, ICP) management protocols that dominate current algorithms for handling TBI patients (26). While most centers have adopted a CPP- and ICP-based paradigm for the perioperative care of TBI patients, the Lund, or volume-centric, concept of management offers a complementary approach that has as its theoretical core the notion that a disrupted blood-brain barrier and a hyperemic brain will accelerate the development of life-threatening cerebral edema in TBI patients (27,28). As such, the four main tenets are (*i*) reduction of capillary hydrostatic pressure, (*ii*) reduction in CBV, (*iii*) maintenance of colloid osmotic pressure and control of fluid balance, and (*iv*) reduction of stress response and cerebral energy metabolism (27,28). As some experimental work suggests that an increase in hyperemia and cerebral edema occurs after DC (29,30), proponents of the Lund concept would favor the implementation of DC, with the caveat that concomitant attention be paid to meticulous nonsurgical control of brain water content (31).

TECHNICAL CONSIDERATIONS

Craniectomy

While a detailed review of surgical techniques is beyond the scope of this chapter, we briefly review the classes of craniectomy and discuss bone flap replacement and complications, as these issues will be encountered by neurosurgeons and neurocritical care specialists alike. Three types of secondary cranial decompression are generally discussed: unilateral, bilateral, and temporal decompression. No experimentally validated criteria exist to guide neurosurgeons in their choice of procedure, but some empirically derived conclusions may be drawn. In patients with medically refractory ICP with a largely unilateral TBI, a large one-sided frontotemporoparietal decompression is often considered; an absolutely critical element of this procedure is adequate temporal release, confirmed by reaching the floor of the middle fossa at surgery and confirming adequate anterior temporal bony decompression (Fig. 3). The lower margin of the craniectomy determines the extent of mesencephalic cisternal decompression (32).

Bilateral injury or diffuse cerebral edema, as in cases of diffuse axonal injury, is managed with bilateral decompression in varying forms. In his seminal work, Kjellberg described the procedure that now bears his name, the most

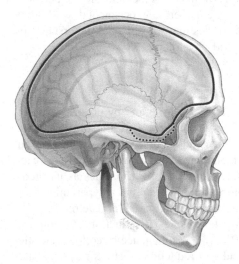

Figure 3 A unilateral hemicraniectomy is shown, with anterior temporal decompression indicated by the dotted line. The cranial cuts are made 1.5 cm lateral to the edge of the sagittal sinus and 1.5 cm above the transverse and sigmoid sinuses.

important feature of which is bifrontal decompression with adequate temporal extension. Considerations include the extent of temporal decompression and whether or not the sagittal sinus is left protected by a thin strip of bone. Some surgeons ligate and transect the anterior sagittal sinus and the falx in an attempt to avoid falcine injury to the outwardly herniating brain and to allow for full expansion of the edematous brain. However, some contend that sinus sacrifice simply eliminates a conduit for fluid egress, increasing venous pressure and exacerbating cerebral edema (33). Bitemporal craniectomies have been described but are not widely practiced, owing to the small degree of cranial decompression offered. The limiting factors in the size of the DC are the dural venous sinuses (i.e., sagittal, transverse, sigmoid). Trepidation of injuring these structures often results in a relatively small DC with subsequent constriction at the bony margins of the expanding brain, which can lead to further brain injury. Therefore, it is imperative to perform an adequately large craniectomy.

An essential element to any chosen decompressive procedure is the expansion of the dural vault. Most neurosurgeons would empirically agree with the conclusions drawn by groups such as Yoo et al. who quantified the additional ICP reduction gained by performing an expansion of the dural vault combined with craniectomy. In their study of TBI and stroke patients in which ICP was measured by ventricular catheter and cranial decompression accomplished by a modified bifrontal approach, dural expansion achieved an additional 35% reduction in ICP to add to a 50% reduction in ICP achieved by craniectomy (24). This conclusion cannot be understated: dural expansion, or duraplasty—by dural substitute or otherwise—is a core element of the DC.

Cranioplasty

How a bone flap is handled once it is removed and replaced varies among institutions. Unless concern exists for contamination, surgeons may either store a removed bone flap in a designated freezer or create a subcutaneous abdominal pocket in the patient for temporary storage. The benefits of interring the bone flap in a patient are weighed against the risk of an additional incision and risk of infection. Usually, bone flaps are replaced no earlier than eight weeks after initial decompression to allow sufficient time for cerebral edema to resolve.

Also meriting consideration is a poorly understood "postcraniectomy syndrome" or "syndrome of the trephined," with symptoms including fatigue, headache, and progressive neurologic deficits (34,35). Ascribed to fluid disequilibrium, or potentially to microvascular cerebral perfusion changes, these symptoms may prompt earlier cranioplasty.

Complications/Sequelae

Neurocritical care specialists should be aware of the range of complications that may develop after DC, aside from bleeding and infection. Epidural collections from leaking CSF are not uncommon, with one report declaring a 20% rate of epidural hygroma (33). Such a collection may simply indicate an imperfect dural closure or may ominously herald the presence of hydrocephalus, with a reported incidence of between 5% and 30% (33,36,37).

EVIDENCE OF EFFICACY

Adult Patients

No class I data exist to support the use of DC in adult patients with TBI for ICP control or improved outcome, a finding that is supported by an independent Cochrane review published recently (38). However, the results of several non-randomized studies were provocative enough to have merited two large, randomized, controlled trials to investigate the effect of DC on the control of refractory ICP after TBI compared to optimal medical management. The design of the RESCUEicp (Randomized Evaluation of Surgery with Craniectomy for Uncontrollable Elevation of intracranial pressure) and DECRA (DEcompressive CRAniectomy) trials is discussed in later sections.

The group at the University of Virginia published a series of 35 patients in whom bifrontal DC was performed in medically refractory ICP, comparing these results with historical controls from the Traumatic Coma Databank (36). The important results were moderately improved outcome in patients with DC compared to control, improved outcome in pediatric patients when compared to adult patients, and worse outcome if ICP reached levels of 40 mmHg or if surgery was performed after 48 hours. The Wurzburg group published an early retrospective analysis that detailed the outcome by Glasgow Outcome Scale (GOS) score in 28 patients with severe TBI in whom DC was performed an average of 68 hours after trauma. ICP levels uniformly diminished (< 25 mmHg), while a good outcome (GOS, 4, 5) was reported in 56% of patients at one year (39). A similar rate of favorable outcomes (58%) was reported in 57 patients who underwent either unilateral or bilateral DC (33). More recently, the Shock Trauma group in Baltimore reported a 40% favorable outcome (GOS, 4, 5) among 50 patients who had undergone unilateral or bilateral DC. Other groups evaluating the use of DC report favorable outcome rates of 38% (40,41), 66% (42), and 68% (43).

While these and other studies report reasonable rates of favorable outcomes, most early studies (before 1980) and some more recent investigations report less sanguine results. One study reported no clear improvement in outcome in 49 patients who underwent DC (32), another group reported good outcomes in only 29% of 62 patients who underwent DC in their retrospective study (44), and a third reported only a 16% favorable outcome rate (45).

Analysis of all these findings highlights the astounding absence of clarity. The lack of consensus in the utility of DC in improving outcome in adult patients with severe TBI in whom alternative nonsurgical treatment options are exhausted is likely because of several variables, not the least of which are profound differences in study designs. From timing of injury to DC, to indications for DC, to level of prehospital and in-hospital neurocritical care, and to the manner in which patients are decompressed, the confounding variables are significant enough to preclude clear recommendations for DC.

It is worth mentioning the attempts of the Addenbrooke group to address these issues by inclusion of DC as part of a rigid treatment algorithm (46). With DC part of a protocol-driven approach to the care of patients with TBI, 61% had a favorable outcome. These encouraging data are strengthened by their prospective recording.

Pediatric Patients

In contrast to the adult literature, data from pediatric patients more consistently support the use of DC in the management of patients who are younger than 18 years with refractory intracranial hypertension after TBI (5). In what constitutes the only prospective randomized controlled trial in the adult and pediatric DC literature, researchers at the Royal Children's Hospital in Melbourne randomized 27 patients over a seven-year period; 14 patients were randomized to medical care alone, and 13 received medical management and DC. The salient conclusions were significant ICP reduction, fewer dangerous ICP spikes, and favorable outcomes in 54% of patients in the DC arm compared with 14% of patients in the nonsurgical arm, though this did not reach significance (5).

Though this study represents the only class I data that support the use of DC, it, too, bears features that have hampered consensus in the field. For instance, decompression was performed in a bitemporal fashion, with relatively conservative 3–4-cm sections of bone removed and the dura sometimes left intact. Looking ahead, it would dramatically simplify cross-study comparisons if similar approaches were used and if duraplasty was included in all the procedures.

ONGOING TRIALS

Taken together, current data support the use of DC in patients who are younger than 18 years with medically refractory intracranial hypertension. Even these conclusions, however, are not without caveats. Differences such as timing of surgery, type of decompression, and approach to medical management have led to wide variance in clinical outcomes and preclude a solid foundation on which to base clinical decision making. Another concern harbored by neurosurgeons and neurointensivists alike is the concept that DC may simply be shifting patients from impending death to severe permanent vegetative state (47).

To generate class I data with which to answer these questions and others, two multicentered trials are underway that seek to compare optimal medical management to delayed DC in the management of refractory ICP following brain trauma. These trials should help to resolve the ambiguity surrounding the use of delayed DC in head injury management and establish the range of complications expected during the routine use of DC. At the core of these trials is one question:

Does DC improve outcome in patients with medically refractory intracranial hypertension? We review the designs of these two trials in turn.

RESCUE ICP

The RESCUE ICP trial is a large, multicentered trial run collaboratively between the University of Cambridge and the European Brain Injury Consortium. Fifty patients were randomized in the pilot phase to assess the feasibility of randomization. For the primary study, 600 patients will be randomized to optimal medical management or DC. Importantly, patients may have had surgery for evacuation of a mass lesion. More specifically, the inclusion criteria will be patients who are aged 10 to 65 years with head injury and an abnormal CT scan who require ICP monitoring with raised ICP (>25 mmHg for >1–12 hours) refractory to initial medical treatment measures (48). Criteria meriting exclusion from the study are patients with bilateral fixed and dilated pupils, bleeding diathesis, and devastating injury who are not expected to survive for 24 hours. Interestingly, the architects of the study are also excluding patients treated by the Lund protocol, as the Lund and Brain Trauma Foundation/AANS guidelines are in some cases orthogonal.

The primary study end points are GOS at discharge and at six months, with secondary end points including outcome by SF-36 questionnaire, efficacy of ICP control, and duration of stay in the ICU. These are tractable questions whose answers derived in this fashion will have a profound impact on the future of DC.

DECRA

Fewer details of this study are currently available. The DECRA study is also a multicentered, randomized trial that involves centers in New Zealand and Australia and is based at the Alfred Hospital in Melbourne (42). This study aims to enroll fewer patients—200—but has similar primary end points as the RESCUEicp trial. The secondary end points, including ICP control, are similar but also include measurement of brain metabolites in patients treated at the Alfred Hospital.

CONCLUSION AND FUTURE DIRECTIONS

We have reviewed the rationale, technique, and evidence regarding the use of DC in patients with TBI, the future of which rests with the results of ongoing clinical trials. While the RESCUEicp and DECRA trials are ongoing, we also hope that further work such as that recently published by Heppner et al. (14) will continue to provide definitive answers as to what physiologic alterations occur as a result of DC.

The results of these much-needed trials are eagerly awaited in the neuro-critical care community and may clarify decades of speculation on the effectiveness, or lack thereof, of delayed DC in the management of patients with severe TBI. As many neurosurgeons would claim, DC seems to "make sense;" in expanding the physical space to be occupied by edematous brain corralled by the skull's resistive forces, we imagine DC to be a logical maneuver when less invasive means to control brain pressure fail. We long ago passed the era in medicine when procedural indications constituted compilations of case studies and empirical hunches. The field has published these data, and our knowledge of when and why to decompress in delayed fashion has, without doubt, reached an impasse. We hope that DC will be validated as a life-saving and outcome-improving measure so that the current therapeutic plateau may be breached.

REFERENCES

1. Kjellberg RN, Prieto A Jr. Bifrontal decompressive craniotomy for massive cerebral edema. J Neurosurg 1971; 34(4):488–493.
2. Dimar JR, II, Glassman SD, Raque GH, et al. The influence of spinal canal narrowing and timing of decompression on neurologic recovery after spinal cord contusion in a rat model. Spine 1999; 24(16):1623–1633.
3. Shields CB, Zhang YP, Shields LB, et al. The therapeutic window for spinal cord decompression in a rat spinal cord injury model. J Neurosurg Spine 2005; 3(4):302–307.
4. Chen JR, Wang YJ, Tseng GF. The effects of decompression and exogenous NGF on compressed cerebral cortex. J Neurotrauma 2004; 21(11):1640–1651.
5. Taylor A, Butt W, Rosenfeld J, et al. A randomized trial of very early decompressive craniectomy in children with traumatic brain injury and sustained intracranial hypertension. Childs Nerv Syst 2001; 17(3):154–162.
6. Yamakami I, Yamaura A. Effects of decompressive craniectomy on regional cerebral blood flow in severe head trauma patients. Neurol Med Chir 1993; 33(9):616–620.
7. Bendszus M, Mullges W, Goldbrunner R, et al. Hemodynamic effects of decompressive craniotomy in MCA infarction: evaluation with perfusion CT. Eur Radiology 2003; 13(8):1895–1898.
8. Bor-Seng-Shu E, Hirsch R, Teixeira MJ, et al. Cerebral hemodynamic changes gauged by transcranial Doppler ultrasonography in patients with posttraumatic brain swelling treated by surgical decompression. J Neurosurg 2006; 104(1):93–100.
9. Bor-Seng-Shu E, Teixeira MJ, Hirsch R, et al. Transcranial Doppler sonography in two patients who underwent decompressive craniectomy for traumatic brain swelling: report of two cases. Arq Neuropsiquiatr 2004; 62(3A):715–721.
10. Vogel R, Indermuhle A, Reinhardt J, et al. The quantification of absolute myocardial perfusion in humans by contrast echocardiography: algorithm and validation. J Am Coll Cardiol 2005; 45(5):754–762.
11. Dawson D, Vincent MA, Barrett EJ, et al. Vascular recruitment in skeletal muscle during exercise and hyperinsulinemia assessed by contrast ultrasound. Am J Physiol 2002; 282(3):E714–E720.
12. Wei K, Jayaweera AR, Firoozan S, et al. Quantification of myocardial blood flow with ultrasound-induced destruction of microbubbles administered as a constant venous infusion. Circulation 1998; 97(5):473–483.
13. Wei K, Le E, Bin JP, et al. Quantification of renal blood flow with contrast-enhanced ultrasound. J Am Coll Cardiol 2001; 37(4):1135–1140.

14. Heppner P, Ellegala DB, Durieux M, et al. Contrast ultrasonographic assessment of cerebral perfusion in patients undergoing decompressive craniectomy for traumatic brain injury. J Neurosurg 2006; 104(5):738–745.

15. Maas AI, Fleckenstein W, de Jong DA, et al. Monitoring cerebral oxygenation: experimental studies and preliminary clinical results of continuous monitoring of cerebrospinal fluid and brain tissue oxygen tension. Acta Neurochir 1993; 59:50–57.

16. Sarrafzadeh AS, Kiening KL, Callsen TA, et al. Metabolic changes during impending and manifest cerebral hypoxia in traumatic brain injury. Br J Neurosurg 2003; 17(4):340–346.

17. Valadka AB, Gopinath SP, Contant CF, et al. Relationship of brain tissue PO_2 to outcome after severe head injury. Criti Care Med 1998; 26(9):1576–1581.

18. van Santbrink H, van den Brink WA, Steyerberg EW, et al. Brain tissue oxygen response in severe traumatic brain injury. Acta Neurochir (Wien) 2003; 145(6): 429–438 (discussion 438).

19. van den Brink WA, van Santbrink H, Steyerberg EW, et al. Brain oxygen tension in severe head injury. Neurosurgery 2000; 46(4):868–876 (discussion 876–868).

20. van Santbrink H, Maas AI, Avezaat CJ. Continuous monitoring of partial pressure of brain tissue oxygen in patients with severe head injury. Neurosurgery 1996; 38(1):21–31.

21. Stiefel MF, Heuer GG, Smith MJ, et al. Cerebral oxygenation following decompressive hemicraniectomy for the treatment of refractory intracranial hypertension. J Neurosurg 2004; 101(2):241–247.

22. Reithmeier T, Lohr M, Pakos P, et al. Relevance of ICP and PtiO2 for indication and timing of decompressive craniectomy in patients with malignant brain edema. Acta Neurochir (Wien) 2005; 147(9):947–952.

23. Rosner MJ. Introduction to cerebral perfusion pressure management. Neurosurg Clin N Am 1995; 6(4):761–773.

24. Yoo DS, Kim DS, Cho KS, et al. Ventricular pressure monitoring during bilateral decompression with dural expansion. J Neurosurg 1999; 91(6):953–959.

25. Whitfield PC, Patel H, Hutchinson PJ, et al. Bifrontal decompressive craniectomy in the management of posttraumatic intracranial hypertension. British J Neurosurg 2001; 15(6):500–507.

26. The Brain Trauma Foundation. The American Association of Neurological Surgeons. The Joint Section on Neurotrauma and Critical Care. Trauma Systems. J Neurotrauma 2000; 17(6–7):457–462.

27. Asgeirsson B, Grande PO, Nordstrom CH. A new therapy of post-trauma brain oedema based on haemodynamic principles for brain volume regulation. Intensive Care Med 1994; 20(4):260–267.

28. De Luca GP, Volpin L, Fornezza U, et al. The role of decompressive craniectomy in the treatment of uncontrollable post-traumatic intracranial hypertension. Acta Neurochir Suppl 2000; 76:401–404.

29. Moody RA, Ruamsuke S, Mullan SF. An evaluation of decompression in experimental head injury. J Neurosurg 1968; 29(6):586–590.

30. Cooper PR, Hagler H, Clark WK, et al. Enhancement of experimental cerebral edema after decompressive craniectomy: implications for the management of severe head injuries. Neurosurgery 1979; 4(4):296–300.

31. Grande PO, Asgeirsson B, Nordstrom CH. Volume-targeted therapy of increased intracranial pressure: the Lund Concept unifies surgical and non-surgical treatments. Acta Anaesthesiol Scand 2002; 46(8):929–941.

32. Munch E, Horn P, Schurer L, et al. Management of severe traumatic brain injury by decompressive craniectomy. Neurosurgery 2000; 47(2):315–322 (discussion 322–313).
33. Guerra WK, Gaab MR, Dietz H, et al. Surgical decompression for traumatic brain swelling: indications and results. J Neurosurg 1999; 90(2):187–196.
34. Dujovny M, Aviles A, Agner C, et al. Cranioplasty: cosmetic or therapeutic? Surg Neurol 1997; 47(3):238–241.
35. Schiffer J, Gur R, Nisim U, et al. Symptomatic patients after craniectomy. Surg Neurol 1997; 47(3):231–237.
36. Polin RS, Shaffrey ME, Bogaev CA, et al. Decompressive bifrontal craniectomy in the treatment of severe refractory posttraumatic cerebral edema. Neurosurgery 1997; 41(1):84–92 (discussion 92–84).
37. Yang XJ, Hong GL, Su SB, et al. Complications induced by decompressive craniectomies after traumatic brain injury. Chin J Traumatol—Zhonghua chuang shang za zhi 2003; 6(2):99–103.
38. Sahuquillo J, Arikan F. Decompressive craniectomy for the treatment of refractory high intracranial pressure in traumatic brain injury. Cochrane Database 2006; (1): CD003983.
39. Kunze E, Meixensberger J, Janka M, et al. Decompressive craniectomy in patients with uncontrollable intracranial hypertension. Acta Neurochir Suppl 1998; 71:16–18.
40. Albanese J, Leone M, Alliez JR, et al. Decompressive craniectomy for severe traumatic brain injury: evaluation of the effects at one year. Crit Care Med 2003; 31 (10):2535–2538.
41. Csokay A, Egyud L, Nagy L, et al. Vascular tunnel creation to improve the efficacy of decompressive craniotomy in post-traumatic cerebral edema and ischemic stroke. Surg Neurol 2002; 57(2):126–129.
42. Kontopoulos V, Foroglou N, Patsalas J, et al. Decompressive craniectomy for the management of patients with refractory hypertension: should it be reconsidered? Acta Neurochir (Wien) 2002; 144(8):791–796.
43. Skoglund TS, Eriksson-Ritzen C, Jensen C, et al. Aspects on decompressive craniectomy in patients with traumatic head injuries. J Neurotrauma 2006; 23(10):1502–1509.
44. Schneider GH, Bardt T, Lanksch WR, et al. Decompressive craniectomy following traumatic brain injury: ICP, CPP, and neurological outcome. Acta Neurochir Suppl 2002; 81:77–79.
45. Ucar T, Akyuz M, Kazan S, et al. Role of decompressive surgery in the management of severe head injuries: prognostic factors and patient selection. J Neurotrauma 2005; 22(11):1311–1318.
46. Timofeev I, Kirkpatrick PJ, Corteen E, et al. Decompressive craniectomy in traumatic brain injury: outcome following protocol-driven therapy. Acta Neurochir Suppl 2006; 96:11–16.
47. Hutchinson PJ, Menon DK, Kirkpatrick PJ. Decompressive craniectomy in traumatic brain injury–time for randomised trials? Acta Neurochir (Wien) 2005; 147(1):1–3.
48. Hutchinson PJ, Corteen E, Czosnyka M, et al. Decompressive craniectomy in traumatic brain injury: the randomized multicenter RESCUEICP study (Www.Rescueicp.Com). Acta Neurochir Suppl 2006; 96:17–20.

2

Cerebroprotective Strategies in Bedside Management of Traumatic Brain Injury

Ganesh M. Shankar, BA, Medical Student
Ian F. Dunn, MD, Senior Resident
Dong H. Kim,* MD, Assistant Professor
Department of Neurosurgery, Brigham and Women's Hospital,
Harvard Medical School, Boston, Massachusetts, U.S.A.

Traumatic brain injury (TBI) is responsible for nearly 2 million emergency room admissions in the United States and affects 2% of the population per year. Approximately 250,000 of these patients require hospitalization; nearly 50% of those admitted will undergo surgical evacuation of a hematoma (1). Mortality is 20%, and another 35% have significant long-term neurologic deficits (2,3). Given these demographics, efforts have been organized with the International Data Bank and the Traumatic Coma Data Bank (TCDB) to standardize assessment and care of the head-injured patient. This standardization has required a significant effort to define the assessment of coma and identify the critical variables that affect outcome (4,5). Attempts to systematize the care of patients with severe TBI have culminated in evidence-based guidelines issued by a joint task force of the Brain Trauma Foundation and the American Association of Neurological Surgeons (AANS) (6,7). The result of such collaborative efforts is increased focus on managing both the primary injury, which occurs as a direct result of the initial traumatic insult, and secondary injuries, which represent pathophysiologic events that occur minutes, hours, and days after the primary insult. In this chapter, the important considerations in the nonsurgical management

---
**Present affiliation*: Professor and Chairman, Department of Neurosurgery, The University of Texas, and Director, The Mischer Neuroscience Institute, Memorial Hermann Hospital, Houston, Texas, U.S.A.

of patients with severe TBI are reviewed. The classifications and assessment of severe TBI, appropriate management strategies to avoid intracranial hypertension and cerebral ischemia, and overall medical optimization and possibilities for novel neuroprotective strategies are discussed.

INITIAL NEUROLOGIC ASSESSMENT

Glasgow Coma Scale Score

The examination begins with a careful assessment for external head trauma. The neurologic examination is characterized by the Glasgow Coma Scale (GCS) score (Table 1). Developed in 1974 by Jennett and Teasdale, the GCS is the most widely used method of determining the severity of TBI. Included in the assessment are eye opening, verbal response, and motor response, which provide a general gauge of the level of consciousness (8). A well-documented prehospital GCS score is helpful, but situations that arise outside a health care setting can complicate the GCS calculation. Examples include pharmacologic paralysis required for intubation as well as significant facial trauma that precludes accurate eye-opening assessment. Any physiologic derangements at the time of assessment must also be considered. Conditions such as hypotension and hypoxia significantly impair neural response to stimulation, leading to a GCS

Table 1 Glasgow Coma Scale

Eye Opening (E)	Score
Spontaneous	4
To speech	3
To pain	2
Not open	1
Verbal Response (V)	
Conversant	5
Confused	4
Nonsense	3
Sounds	2
Silence	1
Intubated	1T
Motor Response (M)	
To command	6
To pain:	
Localizing	5
Withdrawal	4
Arm flexion	3
Arm extension	2
No response	1
GCS = E + V + M (range 3 or 3T–15)	

Source: From Ref. 8.

score that may not reflect the true extent of injury. When a patient has an endotracheal or tracheostomy tube in place and cannot give a verbal response, a GCS score of "1" is given for that section, followed by a "T" to indicate the intubated status.

GCS scores from 3 to 8 indicate severe TBI and correlate significantly with outcome; the motor score is the most reproducible and carries the most prognostic information (9). Nearly 80% of patients with an initial hospital GCS score 3 to 5 have an eventual outcome of death, severe disability, or vegetative state; patients with an initial GCS score 3 have a 65% mortality rate (9–11). Additionally, patients with a GCS score decline by 2 points or more between the field and the emergency room are more likely to require surgical intervention (12). A recent study found that outcomes were better predicted when the GCS was combined with anatomic measures of injury severity as gauged by the head abbreviated injury score and injury severity score, especially for patients younger than 48 years (13).

Pupillary Examination

The pupillary examination is critical; a dilated pupil that fails to respond to light is evidence of ipsilateral uncal herniation until proven otherwise. Bilaterally dilated pupils may result from hypoxia, hypotension, bilateral nerve dysfunction, or severe irreversible brain stem injury. A change in the pupillary examination is the most reliable indicator in determining the side of a mass lesion and carries an 80% positive predictive value. Recommended standard parameters in the papillary examination include documenting duration of papillary dilation, indicating a pupil size of more than 4 mm as dilated, defining a fixed pupil as nonresponsive to bright light, distinguishing between right and left in cases of asymmetry, and correcting for hypotension and hypoxia prior to examining the pupils (14).

Motor Examination

Hemiparesis is also useful but can be confusing due to the Kernohan's notch phenomenon—a mass lesion may manifest with *ipsilateral* hemiparesis from compromise of the contralateral cerebral peduncle that is pushed against the contralateral tentorial edge.

PRIMARY AND SECONDARY TBI

Primary Brain Injury

Significant morbidity and mortality results not only from the original injury sustained with TBI, but also from ensuing pathophysiologic processes that evolve over a period of hours to days (15,16), prompting the differentiation between what has been termed "primary" and "secondary" brain injury. *Primary*

Table 2 Types of Structural Primary Brain Injury

Focal
  Hematoma
    Epidural
    Subdural
    Intracerebral
  Contusion
  Concussion
  Lacerations
Diffuse
  Concussion
  Multifocal contusion
  Diffuse axonal injury

---

brain injury, referring to the clinical sequelae that result directly from the initial injury, can be broadly divided into focal and diffuse injuries (Table 2). Focal injuries include traumatic intracranial hematomas and contusions. Diffuse injuries comprise the clinical spectrum from concussion to posttraumatic coma or diffuse axonal injury. The particular injury depends on the nature of the force during injury (contact or inertial loading), the type of injury (rotational, translational, or angular acceleration), and the magnitude and duration of impact. While diffuse injuries are more common and account for nearly 60% of severe TBI in the TCDB, mortality rates are higher in focal injuries when compared with diffuse injuries (39% vs. 24%) (17). Because emergent surgical intervention may be required, the first critical step in the management of primary brain injury is determining the presence of a mass lesion by CT scan (see Chap. 1). Furthermore, patients determined by CT imaging to have (by TCDB classification) diffuse injury I–II have better outcomes at 12 months than those with diffuse injury IV or focal injury (18).

Secondary Brain Injury

While primary brain injury refers to a particular traumatic insult, *secondary brain injury* refers to cellular processes that unfold hours to days after the initial brain injury, ultimately compounding the effects of the initial injury. Secondary brain injury results not only from the delayed effects of primary brain injury, but also from aggravating factors such as hypotension, hypoxia, inadequate cerebral perfusion pressure (CPP), and intracranial hypertension (19). Untreated, they ultimately result in cerebral ischemia, which significantly exacerbates the effects of the initial injury. Knowledge of the pathophysiologic basis, indications for monitoring, and available treatments for cerebral ischemia and intracranial hypertension are of paramount importance to the neurosurgeon caring for patients with severe TBI.

CEREBRAL ISCHEMIA

Pathophysiology

Nearly 80% of patients who die after severe TBI have ischemic damage on gross autopsy (20). Cerebral ischemia is defined as cerebral blood flow (CBF) that is inadequate to meet metabolic demands of the brain. While the brain constitutes only 2% to 3% of the body's weight, it consumes 25% of its oxygen and receives approximately 20% of its cardiac output. The brain is almost totally reliant on adequate blood flow; nearly 95% of the brain's metabolism is oxidative, and the brain has limited glucose and glycogen reserves and no significant oxygen storage capacity. As such, a discrete metabolic autoregulatory mechanism exists that couples CBF (in units of mL/100 g/min) with the cerebral metabolic rate of oxygen ($CMRO_2$, measured in mL/100 g/min), so that adequate perfusion exists to support local metabolic needs. This relationship is codified by the Fick equation:

$$CMRO_2 = CBF \times AVDO_2$$

where $AVDO_2$ (mL/dL) is the arteriovenous difference in oxygen and is measured by subtracting the jugular venous oxygen content ($SjvO_2$) from the systemic arterial oxygen content. $CMRO_2$ in comatose patients is typically reduced from a normal value of 3.3 to 2.1 mL/100 g/min (21). Under physiologic conditions, changes in $CMRO_2$ are paralleled by changes in CBF, maintaining a constant $AVDO_2$. However, in cases of decreased CBF, as with systemic hypotension or deranged cerebral pressure autoregulation, $AVDO_2$ increases as the brain increases extraction of oxygen to avoid ischemia, and this change can be tracked by the $SjvO_2$ measurement. Normal oxidative cerebral metabolism is altered in patients with $SjvO_2$ less than 50%, and neurologic deterioration and irreversible ischemic injury are correlated with values less than 20% to 30%. A single episode of $SjvO_2$ reduced below 50% has been tied to a twofold increase in poor outcome; two or more episodes carried a 14-fold increase in poor outcome in the same study (22). Conversely, a high $SjvO_2$ (>75%) can be indicative of a decrease in $CMRO_2$, which lends itself to higher probabilities for death or vegetative state (23).

Cerebral Blood Flow and CPP

A central tenet of cerebrovascular physiology is that a constant supply of metabolic substrates is maintained by a constant CBF over a range of CPPs, a concept known as *pressure autoregulation,* which is distinct from metabolic autoregulation. CPP is defined as the difference between mean arterial pressure (MAP) and the intracranial pressure (ICP). Normally, CBF is relatively constant in a range of CPPs between 40 and 150 mmHg. A dynamic system of arterial vasoconstriction and dilation exists to preserve CBF and oxygen delivery. At low perfusion pressures within this range, the arteriolar bed dilates to reduce cerebral vascular resistance and increase blood flow to normal levels. Conversely, at higher perfusion pressures, arteriolar constriction occurs to protect the vascular bed from overperfusion. At perfusion pressures below the autoregulatory threshold, arterioles passively collapse and CBF falls. At pressures above the autoregulatory limits, vessels are maximally dilated and CBF increases.

An important distinction in cerebrovascular physiology exists between CBF and cerebral blood volume (CBV). CBF is the physiologic parameter that governs cerebral perfusion and adequate oxygenation. CBV is the total intra-cranial blood content and is a major determinant of ICP by the Monro–Kellie doctrine. An important consequence of this principle is that CBV can be reduced while an adequate degree of CBF is maintained to control ICP.

Pressure autoregulation is lost in many patients following TBI (24), which may be assessed by perfusion CT (25). In a series of 117 patients, it was reported that autoregulation was lost in 49% of patients with TBI (26). Even when pressure autoregulation was intact, the parameters at which autoregulation occurred were often shifted, imparting significant therapeutic implications. The lower limit of autoregulation may increase from the 40–50 mmHg range to the 70–90 mmHg range (26–28). The consequence of this increase in the lower limit is that perfusion pressures that are normally adequate may cause ischemia in these patients with deranged autoregulation.

Given these findings, the clinician must assume that in patients with severe TBI, CBF has a linear relationship with CPP. Many local processes can affect CBF, including physical compression of vessels by mass lesions or local edema, reduced cerebral metabolism of oxygen, and posttraumatic vasospasm (29,30). Nearly 33% of patients with severe TBI have CBF values near the ischemic threshold (<18 mL/dL), manifesting most often in patients who present with diffuse cerebral edema and acute subdural hematoma (31–33) within the first 24 hours after primary injury (34,35). Many investigators have demonstrated a significantly higher mortality rate and worse outcomes among survivors when CBF was inadequate at any point during the first seven days after injury (24,36–39).

To prevent cerebral ischemia and maximize chances for a positive out-come, CPP must be closely monitored and maintained. Some authors report that a CPP greater than 60 mmHg maintains adequate PO_2 levels in brain tissue of patients with head injury, while others believe that a CPP of 70 mmHg is required to prevent reduction in $SjvO_2$ (40,41). Prospective studies have demonstrated a mean mortality rate of 21% in patients with severe TBI when CPP is maintained above 70 mmHg, as compared with a 40% mortality rate in the TCDB series (28). Others have shown in retrospective analyses that mortality increased by 20% for each 10 mmHg decrement in CPP below 80 mmHg (42). A recent case control study reported that patients with a MAP greater than 80 mmHg within the first four hours of TBI had a significantly higher survival rate than those with a MAP less than 65 mmHg (43). While targets may differ among various authors, there is consensus that CPP less than 60 mmHg is harmful (6,7).

Systemic Contributors to Ischemia: Hypotension and Hypoxia

Adequate cerebral oxygenation is threatened by systemic hypotension and hypoxia, as underscored by several outcome studies. A 150% increased risk of mortality was shown in patients with severe TBI who had at least one episode of hypotension as defined by systolic blood pressure less than 90 mmHg when compared with patients without hypotension (44,45). Another study noted that mortality doubled in TBI patients who had a single hypotensive episode (systolic blood pressure <90 mmHg) (15). Analysis of the International Mission on Prognosis and Analysis of Clinical Trials in TBI (IMPACT) database found that patients with a systolic blood pressure of 135 mmHg and MAP of 90 mmHg had the best outcomes at six months as measured by the Glasgow Outcome Scale (GOS) (46).

Similarly, it was shown that patients with severe TBI who presented with hypoxic episodes prior to intubation had a 77% mortality rate, and 100% of survivors were severely disabled. In contrast, a 14.3% mortality rate and 4.8% severe disability rate were noted among survivors of severe head injury who had no documented hypoxic episodes (47). More alarmingly, poor outcomes have been correlated with the occurrence of just a single hypoxic episode (9,47). Early intubation in patients with GCS score less than 9 was shown to improve outcomes among 1092 patients with severe head injury (48).

Monitoring

CPP calculation is the most routinely used parameter in treatments aimed at avoiding cerebral ischemia. Systemic arterial oxygen saturation and blood hematocrit are monitored as standard practice in all trauma patients. Other techniques available include direct brain tissue PO_2 (monitoring by fiberoptic catheter) and venous oxygenation sampling (by an internal jugular vein catheter directed toward the jugular bulb). Imaging modalities aimed at directly assessing CBF include noninvasive techniques such as transcranial Doppler, xenon CT, and N_2O uptake, as well as several techniques performed intraoperatively with brain exposed, such as laser Doppler flowmetry and laser flow flowmetry (49,50).

Management Principles

The avoidance of cerebral ischemia is a pillar in the modern management of severe head injury. Management principles center on maintaining an adequate CPP and avoiding systemic hypotension, hypoxia, and anemia, so as to ensure adequate CBF and brain tissue oxygenation. The Brain Trauma Foundation currently supports maintaining CPP above 60 mmHg, while other centers advocate a CPP above 70 mmHg (7). For patients with inadequate CPP, systemic causes of hypotension, such as cardiac or spinal cord injury, tension pneumothorax, and bleeding, must be ruled out. Intravascular volume must also be assessed. Vasopressors are often necessary to maintain adequate CPP. The profiles of commonly used pressors are

Table 3 Pressors and Cerebral Hemodynamics

Agent	MAP	CBF	ICP
Dopamine <2 mcg/kg/min	↔	↔	↔/↓
Dopamine 2–6 mcg/kg/min	↑	↔/↑	↑
Dopamine 7–20 mcg/kg/min	↑	↔/↑	↓/↑
Phenylephrine	↑	↔	↔
Norepinephrine	↑	↔	↔
Epinephrine	↑	↔	↔
Dobutamine	↔/↑	↑	↔/↑

The symbol ↑ indicates increase, ↓ decrease, and ↔ no effect.

listed in Table 3. All listed agents are sympathomimetics; phenylephrine is probably the most commonly used (51–54). Treatment with these agents, while clearly necessary, may be associated with complications such as pulmonary edema and/or expansion of preexisting hematomas or contusions (55). Accordingly, vasopressors must be used with caution (see discussion below).

Because anemia may also decrease tissue oxygenation, the hematocrit deserves particular attention in treating a patient with TBI. While an optimal value has not been established, reports suggest that brain tissue oxygen delivery begins to decrease at hematocrit values below 33% (56). Most centers transfuse packed red blood cells in patients with hematocrits below 30%. As with all trauma patients, a hematocrit refractory to blood transfusion should prompt a search for extracranial bleeding sources.

INTRACRANIAL HYPERTENSION

Pathophysiology

Along with avoidance of cerebral ischemia, the other pillar of modern management is attention to intracranial hypertension, a common complication of severe head injury. Nearly 50% of head-injured patients with intracranial mass lesions and 33% of patients with diffuse axonal injury have persistently elevated ICP (57,58). Many studies have confirmed high mortality rates (~70%) for patients with ICP values greater than 25 mmHg (59). ICP is determined by the contents of the intracranial vault, which is codified by the Monro–Kellie doctrine. The total volume available for intracranial contents (CBV, CSF, and brain) is constant, and an augmentation in one compartment must be accompanied by a diminution in the other. An uncompensated increase in one or more compartments results in ICP above the normal range of 5 to 15 mmHg (60,61). In the absence of a mass lesion, elevated ICP in severe TBI results from altered CSF flow or CBV and the development of vasogenic and cytotoxic edema (62,63). The etiology of increased CSF volume stems from elevated resistance for CSF absorption, which results

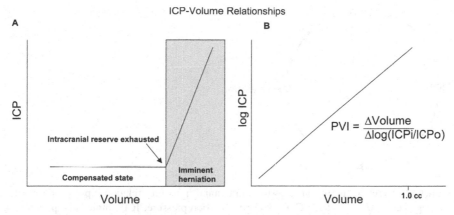

Figure 1 (**A**) Classic pressure-volume curve depicts the exponential rise in ICP once compensatory mechanisms of handling additional intracranial volume are exhausted. In the severely head-injured patient, additional volume may take the form of increased cerebrospinal fluid from poor absorption; increased cerebral blood volume; vasogenic edema from a compromised blood-brain barrier; and cytotoxic edema. (**B**) Change in volume plotted against ICP before (ICPo) and after (ICPi) volume change in a logarithmic fashion. *Abbreviations*: ICP, intracranial pressure; PVI, Pressure-volume index. *Source*: Adapted from Ref. 63.

from traumatic subarachnoid hemorrhage. Increased CBV results from the loss of autoregulation in severe TBI. Vasogenic and cytotoxic edema result from a compromised blood-brain barrier and osmotic dysregulation in ischemic cells. Physiologic volume-buffering mechanisms to adjust blood and CSF volume include arteriolar vasoconstriction, increasing cerebral venous outflow and displacing CSF downward through the foramen magnum or into expanded root sleeves. Once these mechanisms are exhausted, ICP rises exponentially (Fig. 1). In such states, small volume changes can lead to rapid and devastating neurologic deterioration. Another way of conceptualizing ICP and its relationship with volume is Marmarou's linear pressure-volume index in which the ICP and volume are plotted on a semilogarithmic curve, the slope of which is the pressure-volume index, or brain compliance, representing the amount of volume needed to change ICP 10-fold (64,65). Sustained ICP readings of greater than 20 mmHg are abnormal, ICP readings between 20 and 40 mmHg represent moderate intracranial hypertension, and ICP readings of greater than 40 mmHg represent severe preterminal intracranial hypertension (66).

The two principal consequences of elevated ICP are brain herniation and impaired cerebral perfusion (as noted by the formula CPP = MAP – ICP). The displacement or herniation of brain through openings in the dura and skull can occur in various anatomic patterns: subfalcine herniation; uncal herniation; central downward herniation; tonsillar herniation; and external herniation through an open skull fracture. Of particular importance are uncal herniation and downward

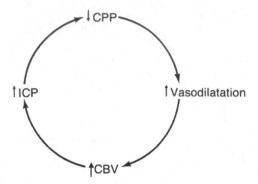

Figure 2 Cerebral perfusion pressure–intracranial pressure relationship in preserved autoregulation. *Abbreviations*: CPP, cerebral perfusion pressure; ICP, intracranial pressure; CBV, cerebral blood volume. *Source*: Adapted from Ref. 28.

herniation. *Uncal herniation* is produced by medial displacement of the temporal lobe by lateral middle fossa or temporal lobe lesions. As a result, the ipsilateral oculomotor nerve, cerebral peduncle, reticular activating system, and possibly, contralateral cerebral peduncle (Kernohan phenomenon) are compromised. The resulting clinical syndrome involves coma, ipsilateral fixed and dilated pupil, and contralateral hemiparesis. Should the contralateral peduncle be compressed against the contralateral tentorial edge (as noted with Kernohan notch phenomenon), ipsilateral motor function may also be compromised. Central or downward herniation may result from globally increased ICP and is defined by progressive caudal displacement of the brain stem through the foramen magnum. Consequently, basilar artery perforators are stretched and can hemorrhage (Duret hemorrhages), which result in coma and possibly Cushing triad (arterial hypertension, bradycardia, and respiratory irregularity).

Increased ICP also compromises cerebral perfusion. Aside from the fact that increased ICP can decrease CPP, it is also true that a drop in CPP can increase ICP. As CPP decreases, pial arterioles vasodilate and accommodate larger blood volumes (CBV) as diagrammed in Rosner's vasodilatory cascade (Fig. 2). This increased intravascular blood volume can increase ICP. When CPP is restored, pial arterioles can constrict and ICP will often decrease (67).

Monitoring

Consensus has emerged regarding indications for placing an ICP monitor in patients with TBI; this is based on the identification of groups at risk for developing intracranial hypertension. At highest risk are patients with GCS scores below 8 and abnormal CT scans; up to 60% of these patients develop elevated ICP readings (68). While patients with GCS scores below 8 with normal-appearing CT scans on admission have a 10% to 15% chance of developing elevated ICPs, a subgroup with a 60% chance of intracranial hypertension does exist: those who present with age over 40 years, systolic blood pressure less than 90 mmHg, and unilateral or bilateral motor posturing (44,68,69). We place ICP-monitoring devices in all patients with GCS scores below 8, unless a coexisting coagulopathy is present. We also consider placement of these devices in some patients with GCS scores above 8 who are undergoing extensive anesthesia for extracranial surgery.

Ventriculostomy: Indications and Technique

Ventriculostomy, permitting CSF drainage and ICP monitoring, is especially indicated in patients with hydrocephalus and intraventricular hemorrhage, or whenever intracranial hypertension is expected to be a significant problem. The risks of placement include a 5% hemorrhage rate (70) and a 5% to 10% infection rate, which can be minimized by appropriate placement and sterile technique. Infection may be further reduced by the use of antibiotic-impregnated catheters (71). Current data do not support prophylactic catheter exchange to reduce infection rates (72).

We favor a right-sided ventriculostomy, avoiding the dominant hemisphere, unless this ventricle is collapsed. With the patient supine, the head is shaved widely and prepared in sterile fashion. Midline is always marked, and careful attention is paid to the position of the ipsilateral midpupillary line, tragus, and medial canthus. A small linear incision is carried down through skin to bone at the spot 10 cm back from the nasion and 3 cm lateral to the midline; this position may also be marked as the spot 1 to 2 cm in front of the coronal suture in the midpupillary line (Fig. 3). A twist drill is used to open the cranium. After the

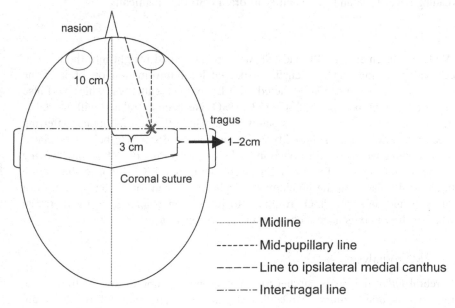

Figure 3   Ventriculostomy anatomy.

bony fragments are removed, the dura and pia are opened by abrading them gently with a to-and-fro twisting action of the drill. The hole must be drilled in the trajectory desired: if the skull is thick, it will influence the subsequent passage of the catheter. The catheter is directed toward the ipsilateral medial canthus in the medial-lateral plane and the ipsilateral tragus in the anterior-posterior plane. An alternative is to pass the catheter perfectly perpendicular to the skull surface. The catheter is then tunneled out through the skin through a separate stab incision to reduce the likelihood of infection. Even in the presence of a mass lesion or shift, the same landmarks and trajectory are used.

The catheter is never passed to a depth of more than 6 cm from the inner table. If the ventricle is not cannulated on the third attempt, the catheter is left in place and a CT scan is obtained to check the position. An overly lateral placement risks internal capsule injury, and an overly deep catheter placement risks injury to critical brain stem structures.

Other Monitoring Devices: Indications and Technique

When we are uncertain whether intracranial hypertension will be a problem, or when the ventricles are slit-like, an intraparenchymal monitor is placed. The scalp incision is made in the same location as for ventriculostomy, but a smaller drill bit is used. The dura is opened with a small stylet, and a fixation bolt is screwed in to hold the parenchymal fiberoptic catheter in place; the catheter itself is passed approximately 1 to 2 cm into the parenchyma. The hemorrhage and infection risks are lower than for ventriculostomy, but the disadvantages include drift of ICP readings over time and the inability to drain CSF therapeutically.

Licox

While measurement of CPP and ICP will provide broad insight into the level of cerebral perfusion and oxygenation, specific local information on brain tissue oxygenation ($PbtO_2$) can be gathered with Licox microcatheters, which will also provide brain temperature and ICP (73). $PbtO_2$ has been correlated with mortality outcomes, with prolonged values below 15 mmHg in the first 24 hours conferring greater than 50% risk of mortality and values above 35 mmHg being associated with good recovery (74,75). Importantly, Licox monitoring of $PbtO_2$ may provide predictive information for impending ischemic events (76). Licox catheters are traditionally placed in the nondominant right hemisphere or in the penumbra of the ischemic damage. $PbtO_2$ response to an oxygen challenge test will reveal whether the Licox is accurately measuring oxygenation in viable tissue.

Microdialysis

Cerebral microdialysis is another tool that allows for monitoring fluctuations in markers of brain injury. Molecules in the extracellular fluid of the brain passively diffuse across a semipermeable dialysis membrane at the tip of a double-lumen probe, providing a sampling of local neurochemical changes surrounding the probe. The commonly used parameters for the instrument are 10-mm catheter length, 20- or 100-kDa molecular weight cutoff, and a 0.3-μL/min flow rate (77). Among the most commonly used readouts, microdialysis provides information on the levels of glucose and glutamate. Microdialysate glucose concentrations of less than 0.2 mM are correlated with poor outcomes, despite the lack of this association with ischemia as measured by CPP or $SjvO_2$ (78). Increased glutamate, a proposed mediator of calcium-induced neuronal excitotoxicity, is also associated with cerebral ischemia and poor outcomes.

Near-Infrared Spectroscopy

Near-infrared spectroscopy relies on the differential absorption of light by deoxygenated and oxygenated hemoglobin to provide information on tissue oxygenation. However, this technique is not yet well supported, as studies have raised concerns as to whether it can provide consistent sensitive information when compared with the more invasive methods described above (79,80).

Management of Raised Intracranial Pressure

The goals in management of intracranial hypertension are the maintenance of satisfactory CPP and the avoidance of intracranial herniation. The clinical justification for ICP reduction is that elevated ICP is an independent predictor of poor neurologic outcome in patients with severe head injury (37,44,59,68). While this management principle is well supported, the particular threshold at which treatment is initiated varies. Incrementally worse outcomes were documented with increasing duration of ICP readings above 20 mmHg. In addition, worse outcomes were reported in patients with sustained ICP readings of greater than 25 mmHg (81). More recently, another group found that initial or sustained ICP readings of greater than 20 mmHg were effective predictors of poor neurologic outcome among patients with severe head injury (59,81). The Brain Trauma Foundation supports initiating treatment at ICP readings of between 20 and 25 mmHg while preserving adequate CBF (7). A caveat in the rigid adherence to these oft-quoted values is that herniation may occur at ICP readings below 20 mmHg, particularly with temporal lesions. On the other hand, a therapeutic CPP target may be reached with ICP readings as high as 25 mmHg. At our institution, we initiate treatment when ICP is greater than 25 mmHg, unless CPP is compromised at lower levels. We employ a stepwise approach, which begins with techniques to optimize venous outflow from the brain (head elevation) and is followed by pharmacotherapy and CSF drainage (Fig. 4).

Physical Positioning

We advocate elevating the head of the bed to 30° and maintaining a neutral head position to maximize venous return from the brain and thereby reduce CBV.

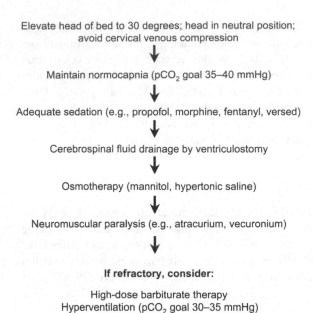

Elevate head of bed to 30 degrees; head in neutral position;
avoid cervical venous compression

Maintain normocapnia (pCO$_2$ goal 35–40 mmHg)

Adequate sedation (e.g., propofol, morphine, fentanyl, versed)

Cerebrospinal fluid drainage by ventriculostomy

Osmotherapy (mannitol, hypertonic saline)

Neuromuscular paralysis (e.g., atracurium, vecuronium)

If refractory, consider:

High-dose barbiturate therapy
Hyperventilation (pCO$_2$ goal 30–35 mmHg)
Decompressive hemicraniectomy

Figure 4 Stepwise protocol for management of intracranial pressure. *Abbreviation*: pCO$_2$, partial pressure of carbon dioxide.

CBV is to be differentiated from CBF. CBV represents the total amount of blood in the intracranial space and affects ICP, while CBF is the physiologic parameter that governs adequate brain tissue oxygenation. A reduction in CBV does not a priori suggest a reduction in CBF; it is possible to maintain adequate CBF and CPP while reducing CBV. While some advocate keeping the head of the bed flat to maximize CPP (82), other data have shown that CPP and CBF may be preserved and ICP reduced by elevating the head of the bed to 30° (83–85). In addition, raising the head of the bed over 30° significantly decreases the rate of pneumonia.

Avoidance of Hypoventilation: CO$_2$ Reactivity

CBF varies with CPP in pressure autoregulation and with CMRO$_2$ in metabolic autoregulation. Changes in arterial CO$_2$ also affect CBF and vascular caliber. For every millimeter-of-mercury change in PaCO$_2$, the CBF changes by 2% to 3%. These vascular effects are passively mediated through changes in pH in the perivascular space—not directly by PaCO$_2$ (86). Hypoventilation leads to an increase in PaCO$_2$, resulting in vasodilatation and an increase in CBF and ICP. Conversely, hyperventilation leads to a decrease in PaCO$_2$, arteriolar vasoconstriction, and a reduction in CBF and ICP.

Although pressure autoregulation may be deranged in severe head injury, CO$_2$ reactivity is preserved (24,87). The routine measurement of PaCO$_2$ in head-injured patients is strongly recommended. Hypoventilation raises $PaCO_2$ and ICP, while $PaCO_2$ levels below 35 mmHg may lower ICP but compromise CBF. The ideal $PaCO_2$ level in head-injured patients is normocapnia to avoid elevations in ICP from hypoventilation and decreased CBF and ischemia from hyperventilation.

Adequate Sedation, Analgesia, and Neuromuscular Paralysis

Sedation and analgesia may blunt the sympathetic stimulation provided by pain or agitation from traumatic injury, endotracheal irritation, or routine nursing care, all of which if untreated may increase ICP. An additional benefit of benzodiazepine sedation is the reduction of $CMRO_2$. The effects on MAP, CBF, and ICP of commonly used sedative and analgesic agents are shown in Table 4 (88–90). Narcotics (fentanyl, morphine) alone or in combination with short-acting benzodiazepines (i.e., midazolam) are commonly administered. The short-acting sedative-anesthetic propofol is being used with increasing frequency because its short half-life permits frequent neurologic examinations and because it appears to have superior effects on ICP reduction compared with narcotic-based regimens (91). Propofol is a potent vasodilator, and careful attention must be paid to MAP and CPP during its administration.

When intracranial hypertension becomes severe, patients may require pharmacologic paralysis by neuromuscular blockade for maximum muscle relaxation. Agents with short durations of effect (atracurium lasts for 30–45 minutes, and vecuronium lasts for 45–60 minutes) are preferred so that neurologic examinations may be conducted at frequent intervals (92,93). Their effects on cerebrovascular hemodynamics and ICP in normal conditions are shown in Table 4. Neuromuscular paralysis is reserved for use at the point at which all standard treatments have been exhausted (Fig. 4).

Occasionally observed in patients with severe head injury is the paradoxic "sympathetic storm," characterized by episodic hyperhidrosis, hypertension, hyperthermia, tachypnea, tachycardia, and posturing; this constellation is only

Table 4 Cerebrovascular Profiles of Commonly Used Sedatives and Analgesics

Agent	MAP	CBF	ICP
Morphine (1–5 mg/hr)	↓	↔	↑
Fentanyl (25–100 mcg/hr)	↓	↔	↑
Midazolam (0.05–5 mcg/kg/min)	↓	↓	↔/↓
Propofol (0–100 mcg/kg/min)	↓	↓	↓
Atracurium (20–50 mg/hr)	↔/↓	↔	↔
Vecuronium (4–10 mg/hr)	↔	↔	↔

↑ = Increase; ↓ = decrease; ↔ = No effect. *Abbreviations*: MAP, mean arterial pressure; CBF, cerebral blood flow; ICP, intracranial pressure.
Source: Refs. 88–90.

suggested after mass lesions, seizure, toxic/metabolic derangements, and infection have been excluded. The prevailing view is that these symptoms represent disruption of autonomic function in the diencephalon and brain stem. A combination of small doses of morphine for sedation and appropriate α 1- and β-receptor blockade with labetalol is particularly effective in addressing the clinical manifestations of these occasional sympathetic outbursts (94).

Drainage of Cerebrospinal Fluid by Ventriculostomy

CSF drainage via an external ventricular drain, or ventriculostomy, is a highly effective and physiologic method to reduce ICP in head-injured patients. The utility of the ventriculostomy catheter, however, may be compromised in the presence of considerable brain edema and subsequent ventricular collapse. When a ventriculostomy is in place, some of it drains CSF to its maximal capacity for increased ICP control before starting osmotherapy. However, when an intraparenchymal monitor is in place, osmotherapy may be instituted first. If large amounts of mannitol or hypertonic saline are required to control ICP, we replace the intraparenchymal device with a ventriculostomy, if possible.

Osmotherapy

The osmotic diuretic mannitol is a mainstay in the control of elevated ICP. We prefer to administer this drug in 0.25- to 1-g/kg boluses and expect maximal reduction of ICP within 15 minutes of administration, with effects lasting up to 4 hours. An osmotic diuretic, mannitol was commonly thought to reduce ICP by reducing intracranial water (95), but it is now recognized to also expand plasma volume and decrease viscosity. CBF increases and ICP is decreased by autoregulatory vasoconstriction (96–100). Furosemide (0.7 mg/kg), which can inhibit the production of CSF, may potentiate the effects of mannitol. When they are given together, a greater and more sustained decrease in ICP has been observed (101).

When using mannitol, intravascular volume status, serum osmolarity, sodium, and blood urea nitrogen and creatinine must be monitored for possible adverse effects. When the serum osmolarity is raised above 320 mOsm, mannitol (particularly in large doses) may precipitate acute tubular necrosis (102). With prolonged use, mannitol can also disrupt the blood-brain barrier and pass into the brain parenchyma, causing a rebound effect with subsequent increases in ICP (102–104).

Two studies have demonstrated effectiveness of mannitol in controlling ICP. A randomized controlled trial that compared mannitol with barbiturates in the management of high ICP in head-injured patients demonstrated superior ICP reduction, CPP preservation, and overall outcome in patients treated with mannitol (105). A smaller study showed the superior effects of mannitol in ICP reduction, CPP preservation, and $SjvO_2$ levels when compared with ventriculostomy drainage alone or hyperventilation (106).

Hypertonic Saline Solutions

Hypertonic saline solutions may be used as an adjunct or alternative to mannitol. One advantage of these agents compared with mannitol is a lower risk of rebound intracranial hypertension and renal failure. In hyperosmolar concentrations, sodium ions (which are less permeable to cross an intact blood-brain barrier than is mannitol) create a gradient that drives water from its interstitial and intracellular compartments into the intravascular space (107), reducing brain water and ICP. Hypertonic saline may also augment CBF and cardiac output, reducing secondary ischemia.

Data on the effectiveness of hypertonic saline solutions in the management of raised ICP in head-injured patients have been gathered only in small case series and controlled groups. One group has reported that 23.4% saline in doses of 30 to 60 mL over 20 minutes can markedly reduce ICP when standard treatments fail (108). In smaller studies, 7.5% hypertonic saline was particularly effective in ICP reduction and CPP elevation in patients with severe TBI whose intracranial pressures were refractory to standard therapy (109,110). Recently, a small prospective randomized study found that patients with TBI who were treated with 7.5% hypertonic saline boluses had fewer refractory ICP episodes than did patients who were treated with 20% mannitol boluses; however, the outcomes were the same (111).

Hypernatremia is commonly observed but usually resolves as renal free water clearance is reduced (112). Potential adverse consequences include central pontine myelinolysis and seizures, as well as hypernatremia, congestive heart failure from fluid shifts, and coagulopathy (108). At present, hypertonic saline use for the management of high ICP is primarily limited to patients in whom standard osmotherapy is ineffective. It is recognized, though, that more specific guidelines for the use of mannitol versus hypertonic saline for osmotherapy await findings from larger prospective studies (113).

Intracranial Hypertension Refractory to Standard Treatment:
Other Measures to Consider

The measures described above are routinely used to manage intracranial hypertension. When ICP begins to increase despite maximal treatment, other measures are considered, such as hyperventilation, decompressive craniectomy, or barbiturate-induced burst suppression. Prolonged hyperventilation can be harmful, and neither barbiturate-induced burst suppression nor decompressive hemicraniectomy have been proven to be beneficial. Therefore, these measures should be used in select situations only, after careful consideration and discussion with family members regarding the advantages and disadvantages of each. The practical consequences of these treatments must also be considered, including increased costs that result from prolonged ICU stays. (When a patient is placed into a barbiturate coma, withdrawal of ventilatory support cannot occur until the barbiturate level becomes low, which can take several days.)

Barbiturates

Barbiturates potentiate the effects of gamma-aminobutyric acid (GABA) at GABA receptors and thus reduce $CMRO_2$ by globally inhibiting neuronal transmission. With an intact metabolic autoregulatory mechanism, a reduction in $CMRO_2$ may be accompanied by a corresponding decrease in CBF and CBV and a concomitant reduction in ICP. Barbiturates may also decrease ICP by limiting free radical–mediated lipid peroxidation and limiting resultant cerebral edema (114,115).

The routine use of barbiturates as the prophylactic treatment of ICP is not indicated because two studies have shown no improvement in outcome (105,116). In one study, over half of the treated group developed clinically significant hypotension during pentobarbital administration. Conversely, barbiturates decreased ICP in two early studies (105,117). In a prospective randomized trial, it was shown that pentobarbital coma in patients with refractory intracranial hypertension had a 2:1 benefit in the control of ICP (118). In this trial, the recommended loading dose was 10 mg/kg over 30 minutes, followed by 5 mg/kg each hour for three doses and a maintenance dose of 1 mg/kg/hr. Because plasma and CSF pentobarbital levels correlate weakly with physiologic effects, pentobarbital dosing and effects are best monitored by electroencephalogram, with dose titration to achieve burst suppression (119). A recent Cochrane review of the literature found that barbiturate use did not result in a significant improvement in the outcome of patients with TBI (120).

The most frequently cited and clinically important side effects of barbiturate administration are hypotension and global oligemic hypoxia, followed by hypokalemia, respiratory depression, hepatic dysfunction, and renal dysfunction (121,122). For these reasons, this treatment should only be used in conjunction with a Swan–Ganz catheter.

Hyperventilation

In addition to pressure and metabolic autoregulation, CO_2 reactivity is a potent vasoactive agent. Vascular caliber and CBF are highly responsive to changes in arterial CO_2; CBF changes 2% to 3% for each millimeter of mercury of $PaCO_2$. Hypercarbia from hypoventilation leads to vasodilatation and increased CBF, whereas hypocarbia (hypoventilation) results in vasoconstriction, lower CBF, and lower ICP. Although pressure and metabolic autoregulation is sometimes impaired in patients with severe head injury, observers have noted a trend toward preservation of CO_2 reactivity (24,87). As such, hyperventilation was at one time routinely used as a prophylactic means of reducing intracranial hypertension. However, ICP reduction by hyperventilatory vasoconstriction poses the significant risk of inducing cerebral ischemia through inadequate CBF, particularly in the first 24 hours after injury, when CBF is already severely compromised. These physiologic effects have been tied to outcome, with one group reporting an improved outcome at three and six months, when prophylactic hyperventilation was avoided for five days after injury (123). While the routine use of hyperventilation should generally be avoided, it remains a rapid method of reducing ICP in emergency situations with acute neurologic deterioration and impending herniation. In such situations, hyperventilation should be maintained only as long as necessary to initiate other treatments.

Decompressive Hemicraniectomy

Delayed decompressive hemicraniectomy, where the bone is removed and the dura is opened to increase the size of the intracranial compartment, can lower ICP. The first large series of such intervention was the bifrontal decompressive craniotomy reported in 1971; outcomes, however, were generally poor (124). Prospective results on the use of bifrontal or hemicraniectomy were reported from a study that had more stringent inclusion criteria; patients over 40 years of age and those with GCS scores less than 5 were excluded. A 14% mortality rate and a 38% rate of "full restitution" were reported (125). Another group reported favorable outcomes in 60% of patients who present with GCS score between 3 and 8, intractable hypertension, ICP less than 40 mmHg, and underwent a modified Kjellberg procedure within 48 hours of injury (126). Other studies, without directly comparing patients who did not have the procedure, have noted favorable outcomes (127–131). A recent study assessed the outcome of patients who received decompressive craniectomy after the ICP was noted to be refractory to conventional management. The ICP decreased to below 20 mmHg as a result of the craniectomy, and the patients performed better (as gauged by the GOS) within the first three months when compared to published control cohorts (132). One small randomized controlled trial that involved pediatric patients found that early craniectomy (within 19.2 hours of the injury, on average) was associated with improved morbidity and mortality outcomes (133). The particular timing and indications for intervention are yet to be codified and await results of RESCUEicp (Randomised Evaluation of Surgery with Craniectomy for Uncontrollable Elevation of Intra-Cranial Pressure, Europe) and DECRAN (Australia), ongoing randomized controlled trials.

Steroid Use

Class I data do not support the use of steroids—dexamethasone, methylprednisolone, or tirilazad—to reduce ICP in head-injured patients. Side effects include gastrointestinal bleeding and hyperglycemia, with no benefit in ICP or outcome observed (134–137).

MANAGEMENT PARADIGMS

The principal goal of severe TBI management centers on limiting the extent of secondary brain injury from cerebral ischemia. Avoiding intracranial hypertension is essential to preventing both brain herniation and CPP reduction. This concept has led to what has been termed an ICP-based approach to patients with severe

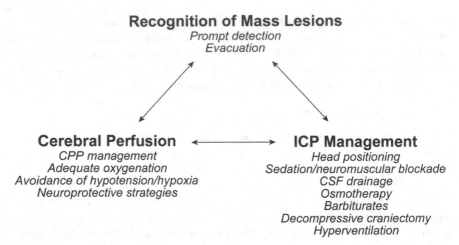

Figure 5 Cornerstones of management for severe TBI. *Abbreviations*: CPP, cerebral perfusion pressure; ICP, intracranial pressure; CSF, Cerebrospinal fluid.

TBI, wherein therapy focuses on maintaining a normal ICP, with the stepwise measures shown in Figure 4.

Others have stressed the importance of CPP-based management, in which maintaining a particular CPP is central rather than focusing on the ICP. This paradigm recognizes that a decrease in CPP—whether by an increase in ICP or a decrease in MAP—leads to compensatory vasodilatation and results in increased CBV, which further increases ICP and even further compromises CPP (Fig. 2). Initial favorable outcomes (28) have led to widespread adoption of CPP preservation in the management algorithms of severe TBI. While Rosner's original paper suggests maintaining a CPP greater than 70 mmHg, other reports have failed to document added benefit to maintaining a CPP greater than 60 mmHg. Studies have noted an increase in acute respiratory distress syndrome in their trial arm in which patients were maintained with CPPs greater than 70 mmHg (138,139).

Given these considerations, the three cornerstones of an integrated management paradigm that monitors and controls both ICP and CPP include (*i*) rapid identification and potential management of intra- or extra-axial mass lesions, (*ii*) ICP monitoring and treatment of intracranial hypertension, and (*iii*) CPP preservation and avoidance of cerebral ischemia (Fig. 5).

SYSTEMIC MEDICAL MANAGEMENT

Nutritional Support and Gastrointestinal Prophylaxis

The systemic response to multitrauma and severe TBI includes hypermetabolism, catabolism, and altered gastric voiding. Patients with severe head injury may need 140% of their normal caloric expenditures, while those in barbiturate coma may require between 100% and 120% of normal resting levels (140). Enteral alimentation should be established as soon as possible, with a goal of full caloric replacement by the end of the first week after injury. Full caloric replacement through seven days after injury, with at least 15% of calories representing protein, is correlated with improved outcome (141,142). Orogastric tubes are preferred to the nasogastric route in the presence of skull base fractures or sinus disease. Long-term feeding may require placement of a percutaneous endoscopic gastrostomy tube or jejunal tube if gastric emptying is compromised. While the enteral route diminishes the risk of bacterial translocation and sepsis, parenteral nutrition may serve as a temporary route for nutritional support until gastroparesis resolves.

An appropriate nutritional regimen also includes gastric ulcer prophylaxis. Ulcers are common complications in patients in the ICU, and the potential morbidity from hemorrhagic diathesis demands appropriate prophylaxis. Reduction of acid production by H2 antagonists or proton pump inhibitors is commonly performed, but neutralizing gastric acid pH carries the theoretical risk of increasing nosocomial pneumonias. Sucralfate, which strengthens gastric mucosa, may avoid this risk.

Sodium Derangements

Hypernatremia and hyponatremia are common disorders, and nearly 60% of patients experience electrolyte abnormalities following head injury (143). Careful distinction between the syndrome of inappropriate antidiuretic hormone secretion (SIADH) and cerebral salt wasting should be made in the head-injured patient; the former is euvolemic or hypervolemic, while the latter is likely to be hypovolemic. Fluid restriction in SIADH may be complemented by demeclocycline use. Cerebral salt wasting may require judicious use of hypertonic saline, should normal saline prove ineffective.

Diabetes insipidus from stalk dysfunction should also be considered in a hypernatremic patient. Great care should be taken when administering large, free water boluses, which may worsen cerebral edema. Desmopressin may be used to complement hypotonic therapy in such cases.

Intravenous Fluid Use

Isotonic saline (0.9% NaCl) remains the standard maintenance fluid in head-injured patients after initial resuscitation, with dextrose excluded from the solution if hyperglycemia becomes difficult to manage. Hypotonic fluids should be strictly avoided, as they may exacerbate cerebral edema. The presence of SIADH, salt wasting, or diabetes insipidus may prompt more specific alterations in fluid administration.

Hyperglycemia

Elevated glucose levels are common in all patients in the ICU, irrespective of the presence of diabetes. In head trauma patients this abnormality is thought to be related to a systemic surge in the sympathoadrenal axis. In fact, hyperglycemia has been correlated with the severity of injury and with poor outcome in patients with severe TBI (144,145). We aggressively correct serum glucose greater than 150 mg/dL with either sliding scale insulin or insulin infusions on the basis of recent data that demonstrate improved mortality and reduced infection rates in ICU patients with tight glucose control (146).

Seizure Prophylaxis

Between 4% and 53% of patients with TBI suffer at least one seizure (147), with onset described as either early or late, occurring either before or after the first seven days of injury, respectively. Risk factors for long-term seizures include the presence of cortical contusions; depressed skull fracture; subdural, epidural, or intracranial hematoma; penetrating injury; or seizure within 24 hours of injury (148,149). As seizures may dramatically increase $CMRO_2$ and ICP, a large number of prevention studies in patients with head trauma have been conducted. The current literature supports the use of phenytoin or carbamazepine for preventing seizures only within the first seven days after injury (150,151). Otherwise, seizures are managed as any first-time seizure in another patient population.

Hyperpyrexia

Fever increases cerebral metabolism. In cases in which metabolic autoregulation is uncoupled and CBF does not match $CMRO_2$, significant secondary ischemia may result. Fever is a negative predictor of outcome in head-injured patients (152) and must be aggressively controlled with antipyretics and cooling blankets. Infectious sources should be aggressively investigated as in any other type of patient.

Prophylaxis for Deep Venous Thrombosis

Patients with severe head injury are at high risk for deep venous thrombosis (DVT) and pulmonary embolism. Prophylaxis by low-dose heparin or venous compression devices was shown to decrease the incidence of DVT in trauma patients (153). More recent data demonstrate the safety of using subcutaneous heparin for DVT prophylaxis in patients with severe head injury (154). Because of the high frequency of this complication in severe TBI, we have recently begun to routinely place temporary inferior vena cava filters in these patients. These devices have demonstrated efficacy and safety (155) and, when combined with compression devices and low-dose heparin, may significantly prevent morbidity and mortality associated with pulmonary emboli in this high-risk patient population. No definitive class I data support any particular preventative measure.

CONCLUSIONS AND FUTURE DIRECTIONS

Current clinical management of severe TBI has been appropriately guided by evidence-based algorithms to preserve normal physiology in the face of nervous system derangement. Future directions in brain injury management include the formulation of strategies to "protect" the head-injured brain from further secondary injury and to repair injured neural tissue. An early attempt at neuroprotection was cooling, or hypothermia, which produces proportionate reductions in energy production and use, $CMRO_2$, and CBF. Although early pilot studies demonstrated favorable outcomes in head-injured patients (156,157), a multicentered, prospective randomized controlled trial failed to show improvement in outcome (158). However, a follow-up study in a subgroup of patients who may have benefited is currently in progress.

Therapeutic strategies have also been developed to antagonize the glutamate excitotoxic pathway by inhibiting calcium entry through N-methyl-D-aspartate (NMDA) receptors into neurons, but no convincing effect on outcome has been demonstrated to date (159,160). However, current studies are under way to examine the efficacy of antagonists that target specific subclasses of NMDA receptors (such as those containing NR2B subunits) (161). Tirilazad, a 21-aminosteroid that inhibits lipid peroxidation, and the free radical scavenger PEGSOD were both studied in large clinical trials, with no benefit on outcome reported (137,162). Large clinical trials of compounds that inhibit calpains— calcium-activated proteolytic enzymes—and pro-apoptotic enzymes of the caspase family may be conducted in the future (163,164). Animal models suggest that the therapeutic window for calpain inhibitors is within three to six hours of the initial insult (165).

Another exciting possibility is the stimulation of endogenous neurogenesis or engraftment of exogenous neural stem cells to repair damaged brain by cell replacement or growth factor release (166–168). In the coming years, current TBI management paradigms will surely be complemented by highly selective neuroprotective and neurorestorative strategies to enhance the likelihood of meaningful functional recovery.

REFERENCES

1. Sosin DM, Sniezek JE, Waxweiler RJ. Trends in death associated with traumatic brain injury, 1979 through 1992. Success and failure. JAMA 1995; 273(22): 1778–1780.
2. Consensus conference. Rehabilitation of persons with traumatic brain injury. NIH Consensus Development Panel on Rehabilitation of Persons With Traumatic Brain Injury. JAMA 1999; 282(10):974–983 (review).
3. Adekoya N, Thurman DJ, White DD, et al. Surveillance for traumatic brain injury deaths–United States, 1989-1998. MMWR Surveill Summ 2002; 51(10):1–14.
4. Jennett B, Teasdale G, Galbraith S, et al. Severe head injuries in three countries. J Neurol Neurosurg Psychiatry 1977; 40(3):291–298.

5. Marshall LF, Becker DP, Bowers SA, et al. The National Traumatic Coma Data Bank. Part 1: design, purpose, goals, and results. J Neurosurg 1983; 59(2):276–284.

6. Brain Trauma Foundation, American Association of Neurological Surgeons, Joint Section on Neurotrauma and Critical Care. Guidelines for the management of severe head injury. J Neurotrauma 1996; 13(11):641–734.

7. The Brain Trauma Foundation. The American Association of Neurological Surgeons. The Joint Section on Neurotrauma and Critical Care. Trauma systems. J Neurotrauma 2000; 17(6–7):457–627.

8. Teasdale G, Jennett B. Assessment of coma and impaired consciousness. A practical scale. Lancet 1974; 2(7872):81–84.

9. Choi SC, Narayan RK, Anderson RL, et al. Enhanced specificity of prognosis in severe head injury. J Neurosurg 1988; 69(3):381–385.

10. Fearnside MR, Cook RJ, McDougall P, et al. The Westmead Head Injury Project outcome in severe head injury. A comparative analysis of pre-hospital, clinical and CT variables. Br J Neurosurg 1993; 7(3):267–279.

11. Narayan RK, Greenberg RP, Miller JD, et al. Improved confidence of outcome prediction in severe head injury. A comparative analysis of the clinical examination, multimodality evoked potentials, CT scanning, and intracranial pressure. J Neurosurg 1981; 54(6):751–762.

12. Servadei F, Nasi MT, Cremonini AM, et al. Importance of a reliable admission Glasgow Coma Scale score for determining the need for evacuation of post-traumatic subdural hematomas: a prospective study of 65 patients. J Trauma 1998; 44(5):868–873.

13. Foreman BP, Caesar RR, Parks J, et al. Usefulness of the abbreviated injury score and the injury severity score in comparison to the Glasgow Coma Scale in predicting outcome after traumatic brain injury. J Trauma 2007; 62(4):946–950.

14. The Brain Trauma Foundation. The American Association of Neurological Surgeons. The Joint Section on Neurotrauma and Critical Care. Pupillary diameter and light reflex. J Neurotrauma 2000; 17(6–7):583–590.

15. Chesnut RM, Marshall LF, Klauber MR, et al. The role of secondary brain injury in determining outcome from severe head injury. J Trauma 1993; 34(2):216–222.

16. Hovda DA, Becker DP, Katayama Y. Secondary injury and acidosis. J Neurotrauma 1992; 9(suppl 1):S47–S60.

17. Foulkes MA, Eisenberg HM, Jane JA, et al. The Traumatic Coma Data Bank: design, methods, and baseline characteristics. J Neurosurg 1991; 75(suppl):S8–S13.

18. Wardlaw JM, Easton VJ, Statham P. Which CT features help predict outcome after head injury? J Neurol Neurosurg Psychiatry 2002; 72(2):188–192.

19. Andrews PJ, Piper IR, Dearden NM, et al. Secondary insults during intrahospital transport of head-injured patients. Lancet 1990; 335(8685):327–30.

20. Adams J. Graham DI. The pathology of blunt head injury. In: Critchley M, ed. Scientific Foundation of Neurology. London: Heinemann Medical, 1972.

21. Robertson C. Nitrous oxide saturation technique for CBF measurement. In: Narayan RK, Wilbert JE, Povlishcok JT, eds. Neurotrauma. New York: McGraw-Hill, 1996.

22. Gopinath SP, Robertson CS, Contant CF, et al. Jugular venous desaturation and outcome after head injury. J Neurol Neurosurg Psychiatry 1994; 57(6):717–723.

23. Cormio M, Valadka AB, Robertson CS. Elevated jugular venous oxygen saturation after severe head injury. J Neurosurg 1999; 90(1):9–15.

24. Fieschi C, Battistini N, Beduschi A, et al. Regional cerebral blood flow and intraventricular pressure in acute head injuries. J Neurol Neurosurg Psychiatry 1974; 37(12):1378–1388.

25. Wintermark M, Chiolero R, Van Melle G, et al. Cerebral vascular autoregulation assessed by perfusion-CT in severe head trauma patients. J Neuroradiol 2006; 33(1): 27–37.

26. Bouma GJ, Muizelaar JP. Cerebral blood flow, cerebral blood volume, and cerebrovascular reactivity after severe head injury. J Neurotrauma 1992; 9(suppl 1): S333–S348.

27. Gray WJ, Rosner MJ. Pressure-volume index as a function of cerebral perfusion pressure. Part 2: the effects of low cerebral perfusion pressure and autoregulation. J Neurosurg 1987; 67(3):377–380.

28. Rosner MJ. Introduction to cerebral perfusion pressure management. Neurosurg Clin N Am 1995; 6(4):761–773.

29. Obrist WD, Langfitt TW, Jaggi JL, et al. Cerebral blood flow and metabolism in comatose patients with acute head injury. Relationship to intracranial hypertension. J Neurosurg 1984; 61(2):241–253.

30. Weber M, Grolimund P, Seiler RW. Evaluation of posttraumatic cerebral blood flow velocities by transcranial Doppler ultrasonography. Neurosurgery 1990; 27(1): 106–112.

31. Bouma GJ, Muizelaar JP, Choi SC, et al. Cerebral circulation and metabolism after severe traumatic brain injury: the elusive role of ischemia. J Neurosurg 1991; 75(5): 685–693.

32. Jones TH, Morawetz RB, Crowell RM, et al. Thresholds of focal cerebral ischemia in awake monkeys. J Neurosurg 1981; 54(6):773–782.

33. Schroder ML, Muizelaar JP, Kuta AJ, et al. Thresholds for cerebral ischemia after severe head injury: relationship with late CT findings and outcome. J Neurotrauma 1996; 13(1):17–23.

34. Bouma GJ, Muizelaar JP, Bandoh K, et al. Blood pressure and intracranial pressure-volume dynamics in severe head injury: Relationship with cerebral blood flow. J Neurosurg 1992; 77(1):15–19.

35. Salvant JB Jr., Muizelaar JP. Changes in cerebral blood flow and metabolism related to the presence of subdural hematoma. Neurosurgery 1993; 33(3):387–393.

36. Bouma GJ, Muizelaar JP, Stringer WA, et al. Ultra-early evaluation of regional cerebral blood flow in severely head-injured patients using xenon-enhanced computerized tomography. J Neurosurg 1992; 77(3):360–368.

37. Jaggi JL, Obrist WD, Gennarelli TA, et al. Relationship of early cerebral blood flow and metabolism to outcome in acute head injury. J Neurosurg 1990; 72(2):176–82.

38. Kelly DF, Martin NA, Kordestani R, et al. Cerebral blood flow as a predictor of outcome following traumatic brain injury. J Neurosurg 1997; 86(4):633–641.

39. Robertson CS, Contant CF, Gokaslan ZL, et al. Cerebral blood flow, arteriovenous oxygen difference, and outcome in head injured patients. J Neurol Neurosurg Psychiatry 1992; 55(7):594–603.

40. Chan KH, Miller JD, Dearden NM, et al. The effect of changes in cerebral perfusion pressure upon middle cerebral artery blood flow velocity and jugular bulb venous oxygen saturation after severe brain injury. J Neurosurg 1992; 77(1):55–61.

41. Juul N, Morris GF, Marshall SB, et al. Intracranial hypertension and cerebral perfusion pressure: Influence on neurological deterioration and outcome in severe head

injury. The Executive Committee of the International Selfotel Trial. J Neurosurg 2000; 92(1):1–6.

42. McGraw CP. A cerebral perfusion pressure greater than 80 mmHg is more beneficial. In: Hoff JT, Betz AL, eds. Intracranial Pressure VII. Berlin: McGraw-Hill, 1989.

43. Henzler D, Cooper DJ, Tremayne AB, et al. Early modifiable factors associated with fatal outcome in patients with severe traumatic brain injury: a case control study. Crit Care Med 2007; 35(4):1027–1031.

44. Marmarou A, Anderson RL, Ward JD, et al. Impact of ICP instability and hypotension outcome in patients with severe head trauma. J Neurosurg 1991; S59–S66.

45. Miller JD, Sweet RC, Narayan R, et al. Early insults to the injured brain. JAMA 1978; 240(5):439–442.

46. Butcher I, Maas AI, Lu J, et al. Prognostic value of admission blood pressure in traumatic brain injury: Results from the IMPACT study. J Neurotrauma 2007; 24(2):294–302.

47. Stocchetti N, Furlan A, Volta F. Hypoxemia and arterial hypotension at the accident scene in head injury. J Trauma 1996; 40(5):764–767.

48. Winchell RJ, Hoyt DB. Endotracheal intubation in the field improves survival in patients with severe head injury. Trauma Research and Education Foundation of San Diego. Arch Surg 1997; 132(6):592–597.

49. Alvarez del Castillo M. Monitoring neurologic patients in intensive care. Curr Opin Crit Care 2001; 7(2):49–60.

50. Matz PG, Pitts L. Monitoring in traumatic brain injury. Clin Neurosurg 1997; 44:267–294.

51. Berre J, De Backer D, Moraine JJ, et al. Effects of dobutamine and prostacyclin on cerebral blood flow velocity in septic patients. J Crit Care 1994; 9(1):1–6.

52. Myburgh JA, Upton RN, Grant C, et al. A comparison of the effects of norepinephrine, epinephrine, and dopamine on cerebral blood flow and oxygen utilisation. Acta Neurochir Suppl 1998; 71:19–21.

53. Robertson C. Critical care management of traumatic brain injury. In: Winn HR, ed. Youmans Neurological Surgery. 5th ed. Philadelphia: Saunders, 2004.

54. von Essen C, Zervas NT, Brown DR, et al. Local cerebral blood flow in the dog during intravenous infusion of dopamine. Surg Neurol 1980; 13(3):181–188.

55. Kroppenstedt SN, Kern M, Thomale UW, et al. Effect of cerebral perfusion pressure on contusion volume following impact injury. J Neurosurg 1999; 90(3):520–526.

56. Kee DB Jr., Wood JH. Rheology of the cerebral circulation. Neurosurgery 1984; 15(1):125–131.

57. Becker DP, Miller JD, Ward JD, et al. The outcome from severe head injury with early diagnosis and intensive management. J Neurosurg 1977; 47(4):491–502.

58. Miller JD, Becker DP, Ward JD, et al. Significance of intracranial hypertension in severe head injury. J Neurosurg 1977; 47(4):503–516.

59. Saul TG, Ducker TB. Effect of intracranial pressure monitoring and aggressive treatment on mortality in severe head injury. J Neurosurg 1982; 56(4):498–503.

60. Kellie G. On death from cold, and on congestions of the brain: an account of the appearances observed in the dissection of two of three individuals presumed to have perished in the storm of 3rd November 1821; with some reflections on the pathology of the brain. Trans Med Chir Soc Edinb 1824; 84–169.

61. Monro A. Observations on the structure and function of the nervous system. Edinburgh: Creech and Johnson, 1823.
62. Marmarou A. Increased intracranial pressure in head injury and influence of blood volume. J Neurotrauma 1992; 9(suppl 1):S327–S332.
63. Marmarou A, Shulman K, Rosende RM. A nonlinear analysis of the cerebrospinal fluid system and intracranial pressure dynamics. J Neurosurg 1978; 48(3):332–344.
64. Marmarou A. Pathophysiology of intracranial pressure. In: Narayan RK, Wilberger JE, Povlishock JT, eds. Neurotrauma. New York: McGraw-Hill, 1996.
65. Marmarou A, Maset AL, Ward JD, et al. Contribution of CSF and vascular factors to elevation of ICP in severely head-injured patients. J Neurosurg 1987; 66(6): 883–890.
66. Lundberg N, Troupp H, Lorin H. Continuous recording of the ventricular-fluid pressure in patients with severe acute traumatic brain injury. A preliminary report. J Neurosurg 1965; 22(6):581–590.
67. Rosner MJ, Rosner SD, Johnson AH. Cerebral perfusion pressure: management protocol and clinical results. J Neurosurg 1995; 83(6):949–962.
68. Narayan RK, Kishore PR, Becker DP, et al. Intracranial pressure: to monitor or not to monitor? A review of our experience with severe head injury. J Neurosurg 1982; 56(5):650–659.
69. Eisenberg HM, Gary HE Jr., Aldrich EF, et al. Initial CT findings in 753 patients with severe head injury. A report from the NIH Traumatic Coma Data Bank. J Neurosurg 1990; 73(5):688–698.
70. Wiesmann M, Mayer TE. Intracranial bleeding rates associated with two methods of external ventricular drainage. J Clin Neurosci 2001; 8(2):126–128.
71. Zabramski JM, Whiting D, Darouiche RO, et al. Efficacy of antimicrobial-impregnated external ventricular drain catheters: a prospective, randomized, controlled trial. J Neurosurg 2003; 98(4):725–730.
72. Lozier AP, Sciacca RR, Romagnoli MF, et al. Ventriculostomy-related infections: a critical review of the literature. Neurosurgery 2002; 51(1):170–181.
73. Stevens WJ. Multimodal monitoring: head injury management using SjvO$_2$ and LICOX. J Neurosci Nurs 2004; 36(6):332–339.
74. Valadka AB, Gopinath SP, Contant CF, et al. Relationship of brain tissue PO$_2$ to outcome after severe head injury. Crit Care Med 1998; 26(9):1576–1581.
75. van den Brink WA, van Santbrink H, Avezaat CJ, et al. Monitoring brain oxygen tension in severe head injury: The Rotterdam experience. Acta Neurochir Suppl 1998; 71:190–194.
76. Meixensberger J, Dings J, Kuhnigk H, et al. Studies of tissue PO$_2$ in normal and pathological human brain cortex. Acta Neurochir Suppl (Wien) 1993; 59:58–63.
77. Tisdall MM, Smith M. Cerebral microdialysis: research technique or clinical tool. Br J Anaesth 2006; 97(1):18–25.
78. Vespa PM, McArthur D, O'Phelan K, et al. Persistently low extracellular glucose correlates with poor outcome 6 months after human traumatic brain injury despite a lack of increased lactate: a microdialysis study. J Cereb Blood Flow Metab 2003; 23(7):865–877.
79. Buchner K, Meixensberger J, Dings J, et al. Near-infrared spectroscopy—not useful to monitor cerebral oxygenation after severe brain injury. Zentralbl Neurochir 2000; 61(2):69–73.

80. Rothoerl RD, Faltermeier R, Burger R, et al. Dynamic correlation between tissue PO_2 and near infrared spectroscopy. Acta Neurochir Suppl 2002; 81:311–313.

81. Contant CF, Robertson CS, Gopinath SP, et al. Determination of clinically important thresholds in continuously monitored patients with head injury [abstract]. J Neurotrauma 1993; 10(suppl 1):S57.

82. Rosner MJ, Coley IB. Cerebral perfusion pressure, intracranial pressure, and head elevation. J Neurosurg 1986; 65(5):636–641.

83. Durward QJ, Amacher AL, Del Maestro RF, et al. Cerebral and cardiovascular responses to changes in head elevation in patients with intracranial hypertension. J Neurosurg 1983; 59(6):938–944.

84. Feldman Z, Kanter MJ, Robertson CS, et al. Effect of head elevation on intracranial pressure, cerebral perfusion pressure, and cerebral blood flow in head-injured patients. J Neurosurg 1992; 76(2):207–211.

85. Meixensberger J, Baunach S, Amschler J, et al. Influence of body position on tissue-pO_2, cerebral perfusion pressure and intracranial pressure in patients with acute brain injury. Neurol Res 1997; 19(3):249–253.

86. Muizelaar JP, van der Poel HG, Li ZC, et al. Pial arteriolar vessel diameter and CO_2 reactivity during prolonged hyperventilation in the rabbit. J Neurosurg 1988; 69(6): 923–927.

87. Enevoldsen EM, Jensen FT. Autoregulation and CO_2 responses of cerebral blood flow in patients with acute severe head injury. J Neurosurg 1978; 48(5):689–703.

88. Griffin JP, Cottrell JE, Hartung J, et al. Intracranial pressure during nifedipine-induced hypotension. Anesth Analg 1983; 62(12):1078–1080.

89. Moyer JH, Pontius R, Morris G, et al. Effect of morphine and n-allylnormorphine on cerebral hemodynamics and oxygen metabolism. Circulation 1957; 15(3):379–384.

90. Sperry RJ, Bailey PL, Reichman MV, et al. Fentanyl and sufentanil increase intracranial pressure in head trauma patients. Anesthesiology 1992; 77(3):416–420.

91. Kelly DF, Goodale DB, Williams J, et al. Propofol in the treatment of moderate and severe head injury: a randomized, prospective double-blinded pilot trial. J Neurosurg 1999; 90(6):1042–1052.

92. Rosa G, Orfei P, Sanfilippo M, et al. The effects of atracurium besylate (Tracrium) on intracranial pressure and cerebral perfusion pressure. Anesth Analg 1986; 65(4): 381–384.

93. Rosa G, Sanfilippo M, Vilardi V, et al. Effects of vecuronium bromide on intra-cranial pressure and cerebral perfusion pressure. A preliminary report. Br J Anaesth 1986; 58(4):437–440.

94. Do D, Sheen VL, Bromfield E. Treatment of paroxysmal sympathetic storm with labetalol. J Neurol Neurosurg Psychiatry 2000; 69(6):832–833.

95. Hartwell RC, Sutton LN. Mannitol, intracranial pressure, and vasogenic edema. Neurosurgery 1993; 32(3):444–450.

96. Barry KG, Berman AR. Mannitol infusion. III. The acute effect of the intravenous infusion of mannitol on blood and plasma volumes. N Engl J Med 1961; 264: 1085–1088.

97. Brown FD, Johns L, Jafar JJ, et al. Detailed monitoring of the effects of mannitol following experimental head injury. J Neurosurg 1979; 50(4):423–432.

98. Israel RS, Marx JA, Moore EE, et al. Hemodynamic effect of mannitol in a canine model of concomitant increased intracranial pressure and hemorrhagic shock. Ann Emerg Med 1988; 17(6):560–566.

99. Kassell NF, Baumann KW, Hitchon PW, et al. The effects of high dose mannitol on cerebral blood flow in dogs with normal intracranial pressure. Stroke 1982; 13(1): 59–61.

100. Muizelaar JP, Lutz HA III, Becker DP. Effect of mannitol on ICP and CBF and correlation with pressure autoregulation in severely head-injured patients. J Neurosurg 1984; 61(4):700–706.

101. Pollay M, Fullenwider C, Roberts PA, et al. Effect of mannitol and furosemide on blood-brain osmotic gradient and intracranial pressure. J Neurosurg 1983; 59(6): 945–950.

102. Feig PU, McCurdy DK. The hypertonic state. N Engl J Med 1977; 297(26): 1444–1454.

103. Kaufmann AM, Cardoso ER. Aggravation of vasogenic cerebral edema by multiple-dose mannitol. J Neurosurg 1992; 77(4):584–589.

104. Shackford SR, Norton CH, Todd MM. Renal, cerebral, and pulmonary effects of hypertonic resuscitation in a porcine model of hemorrhagic shock. Surgery 1988; 104(3):553–560.

105. Schwartz ML, Tator CH, Rowed DW, et al. The University of Toronto head injury treatment study: A prospective, randomized comparison of pentobarbital and mannitol. Can J Neurol Sci 1984; 11(4):434–440.

106. Smith HP, Kelly DL Jr., McWhorter JM, et al. Comparison of mannitol regimens in patients with severe head injury undergoing intracranial monitoring. J Neurosurg 1986; 65(6):820–824.

107. Zornow MH. Hypertonic saline as a safe and efficacious treatment of intracranial hypertension. J Neurosurg Anesthesiol 1996; 8(2):175–177.

108. Qureshi AI, Suarez JI. Use of hypertonic saline solutions in treatment of cerebral edema and intracranial hypertension. Crit Care Med 2000; 28(9):3301–3313.

109. Hartl R, Medary MB, Ruge M, et al. Hypertonic/hyperoncotic saline attenuates microcirculatory disturbances after traumatic brain injury. J Trauma 1997; 42 (5 suppl):S41–S47.

110. Horn P, Munch E, Vajkoczy P, et al. Hypertonic saline solution for control of elevated intracranial pressure in patients with exhausted response to mannitol and barbiturates. Neurol Res 1999; 21(8):758–764.

111. Vialet R, Albanese J, Thomachot L, et al. Isovolume hypertonic solutes (sodium chloride or mannitol) in the treatment of refractory posttraumatic intracranial hypertension: 2 mL/kg 7.5% saline is more effective than 2 mL/kg 20% mannitol. Crit Care Med 2003; 31(6):1683–1687.

112. Shackford SR, Fortlage DA, Peters RM, et al. Serum osmolar and electrolyte changes associated with large infusions of hypertonic sodium lactate for intravascular volume expansion of patients undergoing aortic reconstruction. Surg Gynecol Obstet 1987; 164(2):127–136.

113. Ogden AT, Mayer SA, Connolly ES Jr. Hyperosmolar agents in neurosurgical practice: the evolving role of hypertonic saline. Neurosurgery 2005; 57(2):207–15.

114. Demopoulos HB, Flamm ES, Pietronigro DD, et al. The free radical pathology and the microcirculation in the major central nervous system disorders. Acta Physiol Scand Suppl 1980; 492:91–119.

115. Kassell NF, Hitchon PW, Gerk MK, et al. Alterations in cerebral blood flow, oxygen metabolism, and electrical activity produced by high dose sodium thiopental. Neurosurgery 1980; 7(6):598–603.

116. Ward JD, Becker DP, Miller JD, et al. Failure of prophylactic barbiturate coma in the treatment of severe head injury. J Neurosurg 1985; 62(3):383–388.
117. Marshall LF, Smith RW, Shapiro HM. The outcome with aggressive treatment in severe head injuries. Part II: acute and chronic barbiturate administration in the management of head injury. J Neurosurg 1979; 50(1):26–30.
118. Eisenberg HM, Frankowski RF, Contant CF, et al. High-dose barbiturate control of elevated intracranial pressure in patients with severe head injury. J Neurosurg 1988; 69(1):15–23.
119. Winer JW, Rosenwasser RH, Jimenez F. Electroencephalographic activity and serum and cerebrospinal fluid pentobarbital levels in determining the therapeutic end point during barbiturate coma. Neurosurgery 1991; 29(5):739–741.
120. Roberts I. Barbiturates for acute traumatic brain injury. In: Cochrane Library. Chicester: Wiley & Sons, 2005.
121. Cruz J. Adverse effects of pentobarbital on cerebral venous oxygenation of comatose patients with acute traumatic brain swelling: relationship to outcome. J Neurosurg 1996; 85(5):758–761.
122. Schalen W, Messeter K, Nordstrom CH. Complications and side effects during thiopentone therapy in patients with severe head injuries. Acta Anaesthesiol Scand 1992; 36(4):369–377.
123. Muizelaar JP, Marmarou A, Ward JD, et al. Adverse effects of prolonged hyperventilation in patients with severe head injury: a randomized clinical trial. J Neurosurg 1991; 75(5):731–739.
124. Kjellberg RN, Prieto A Jr. Bifrontal decompressive craniotomy for massive cerebral edema. J Neurosurg 1971; 34(4):488–493.
125. Gaab MR, Rittierodt M, Lorenz M, et al. Traumatic brain swelling and operative decompression: a prospective investigation. Acta Neurochir Suppl (Wien) 1990; 51:326–328.
126. Polin RS, Shaffrey ME, Bogaev CA, et al. Decompressive bifrontal craniectomy in the treatment of severe refractory posttraumatic cerebral edema. Neurosurgery 1997; 41(1):84–92.
127. Albanese J, Leone M, Alliez JR, et al. Decompressive craniectomy for severe traumatic brain injury: evaluation of the effects at one year. Crit Care Med 2003; 31 (10):2535–2538.
128. Coplin WM, Cullen NK, Policherla PN, et al. Safety and feasibility of craniectomy with duraplasty as the initial surgical intervention for severe traumatic brain injury. J Trauma 2001; 50(6):1050–1059.
129. De Luca GP, Volpin L, Fornezza U, et al. The role of decompressive craniectomy in the treatment of uncontrollable post-traumatic intracranial hypertension. Acta Neurochir Suppl 2000; 76:401–404.
130. Guerra WK, Gaab MR, Dietz H, et al. Surgical decompression for traumatic brain swelling: indications and results. J Neurosurg 1999; 90(2):187–196.
131. Meier U, Zeilinger FS, Henzka O. The use of decompressive craniectomy for the management of severe head injuries. Acta Neurochir Suppl 2000; 76:475–478.
132. Aarabi B, Hesdorffer DC, Ahn ES, et al. Outcome following decompressive craniectomy for malignant swelling due to severe head injury. J Neurosurg 2006; 104(4):469–479.

133. Taylor A, Butt W, Rosenfeld J, et al. A randomized trial of very early decompressive craniectomy in children with traumatic brain injury and sustained intracranial hypertension. Childs Nerv Syst 2001; 17(3):154–162.
134. Cooper PR, Moody S, Clark WK, et al. Dexamethasone and severe head injury. A prospective double-blind study. J Neurosurg 1979; 51(3):307–316.
135. Dearden NM, Gibson JS, McDowall DG, et al. Effect of high-dose dexamethasone on outcome from severe head injury. J Neurosurg 1986; 64(1):81–88.
136. Gudeman SK, Miller JD, Becker DP. Failure of high-dose steroid therapy to influence intracranial pressure in patients with severe head injury. J Neurosurg 1979; 51(3):301–306.
137. Marshall LF, Maas AI, Marshall SB, et al. A multicenter trial on the efficacy of using tirilazad mesylate in cases of head injury. J Neurosurg 1998; 89(4):519–525.
138. Robertson CS, Valadka AB, Hannay HJ, et al. Prevention of secondary ischemic insults after severe head injury. Crit Care Med 1999; 27(10):2086–2095.
139. Huang SJ, Hong WC, Han YY, et al. Clinical outcome of severe head injury in different protocol-driven therapies. J Clin Neurosci 2007; 14(5):449–454.
140. Clifton GL, Robertson CS, Choi SC. Assessment of nutritional requirements of head-injured patients. J Neurosurg 1986; 64(6):895–901.
141. Deutschman CS, Konstantinides FN, Raup S, et al. Physiological and metabolic response to isolated closed-head injury. Part 1: Basal metabolic state: correlations of metabolic and physiological parameters with fasting and stressed controls. J Neurosurg 1986; 64(1):89–98.
142. Rapp RP, Young B, Twyman D, et al. The favorable effect of early parenteral feeding on survival in head-injured patients. J Neurosurg 1983; 58(6):906–912.
143. Piek J, Chesnut RM, Marshall LF, et al. Extracranial complications of severe head injury. J Neurosurg 1992; 77(6):901–907.
144. Lam AM, Winn HR, Cullen BF, et al. Hyperglycemia and neurological outcome in patients with head injury. J Neurosurg 1991; 75(4):545–551.
145. Young B, Ott L, Dempsey R, et al. Relationship between admission hyperglycemia and neurologic outcome of severely brain-injured patients. Ann Surg 1989; 210(4):466–472.
146. van den Berghe G, Wouters P, Weekers F, et al. Intensive insulin therapy in the critically ill patients. N Engl J Med 2001; 345(19):1359–1367.
147. Frey LC. Epidemiology of posttraumatic epilepsy: a critical review. Epilepsia 2003; 44(suppl 10):11–17.
148. Temkin NR, Dikmen SS, Winn HR. Management of head injury. Posttraumatic seizures. Neurosurg Clin N Am 1991; 2(2):425–435.
149. Yablon SA. Posttraumatic seizures. Arch Phys Med Rehabil 1993; 74(9):983–1001.
150. Glotzner FL, Haubitz I, Miltner F, et al. [Seizure prevention using carbamazepine following severe brain injuries]. Neurochirurgia (Stuttg) 1983; 26(3):66–79.
151. Temkin NR, Dikmen SS, Wilensky AJ, et al. A randomized, double-blind study of phenytoin for the prevention of post-traumatic seizures. N Engl J Med 1990; 323(8):497–502.
152. Jones PA, Andrews PJ, Midgley S, et al. Measuring the burden of secondary insults in head-injured patients during intensive care. J Neurosurg Anesthesiol 1994; 6(1):4–14.

153. Dennis JW, Menawat S. Von Thron J, et al. Efficacy of deep venous thrombosis prophylaxis in trauma patients and identification of high-risk groups. J Trauma 1993; 35(1):132–138.

154. Kim J, Gearhart MM, Zurick A, et al. Preliminary report on the safety of heparin for deep venous thrombosis prophylaxis after severe head injury. J Trauma 2002; 53(1): 38–42.

155. Langan EM III, Miller RS, Casey WJ III, et al. Prophylactic inferior vena cava filters in trauma patients at high risk: follow-up examination and risk/benefit assessment. J Vasc Surg 1999; 30(3):484–488.

156. Clifton GL, Allen S, Barrodale P, et al. A phase II study of moderate hypothermia in severe brain injury. J Neurotrauma 1993; 10(3):263–271.

157. Marion DW, Obrist WD, Carlier PM, et al. The use of moderate therapeutic hypothermia for patients with severe head injuries: a preliminary report. J Neurosurg 1993; 79(3):354–362.

158. Clifton GL, Miller ER, Choi SC, et al. Lack of effect of induction of hypothermia after acute brain injury. N Engl J Med 2001; 344(8):556–563.

159. Maas AI, Steyerberg EW, Murray GD, et al. Why have recent trials of neuroprotective agents in head injury failed to show convincing efficacy? A pragmatic analysis and theoretical considerations. Neurosurgery 1999; 44(6):1286–1298.

160. Morris GF, Bullock R, Marshall SB, et al. Failure of the competitive N-methyl-D-aspartate antagonist Selfotel (CGS 19755) in the treatment of severe head injury: results of two phase III clinical trials. The Selfotel Investigators. J Neurosurg 1999; 91(5):737–743.

161. Yurkewicz L, Weaver J, Bullock MR, et al. The effect of the selective NMDA receptor antagonist traxoprodil in the treatment of traumatic brain injury. J Neurotrauma 2005; 22(12):1428–1443.

162. Young B, Runge JW, Waxman KS, et al. Effects of pegorgotein on neurologic outcome of patients with severe head injury. A multicenter, randomized controlled trial. JAMA 1996; 276(7):538–543.

163. Raghupathi R, Graham DI, McIntosh TK. Apoptosis after traumatic brain injury. J Neurotrauma 2000; 17(10):927–938.

164. Ray SK, Banik NL. Calpain and its involvement in the pathophysiology of CNS injuries and diseases: therapeutic potential of calpain inhibitors for prevention of neurodegeneration. Curr Drug Targets CNS Neurol Disord 2003; 2(3):173–189.

165. Wang KK, Larner SF, Robinson G, et al. Neuroprotection targets after traumatic brain injury. Curr Opin Neurol 2006; 19(6):514–519.

166. Dash PK, Mach SA, Moore AN. Enhanced neurogenesis in the rodent hippocampus following traumatic brain injury. J Neurosci Res 2001; 63(4):313–319.

167. Hagan M, Wennersten A, Meijer X, et al. Neuroprotection by human neural progenitor cells after experimental contusion in rats. Neurosci Lett 2003; 351(3): 149–152.

168. Riess P, Zhang C, Saatman KE, et al. Transplanted neural stem cells survive, differentiate, and improve neurological motor function after experimental traumatic brain injury. Neurosurgery 2002; 51(4):1043–1052.

3

Diffuse Axonal Injury and Dysautonomia

Richard H. Singleton, MD, PhD, Senior Resident
David O. Okonkwo, MD, PhD, Assistant Professor
Department of Neurosurgery, University of Pittsburgh School of Medicine,
Pittsburgh, Pennsylvania, U.S.A.

P. David Adelson, MD, FACS, FAAP, Professor[a] and Vice Chairman[b]
A. Leland Albright Professor of [a]Neurological Surgery and
[b]Pediatric Neurosurgery, Children's Hospital of Pittsburgh,
University of Pittsburgh School of Medicine, Pittsburgh,
Pennsylvania, U.S.A.

DIFFUSE AXONAL INJURY

Background

Significant progress has been made over the last few decades toward our understanding the pathobiological mechanisms that underlie traumatic brain injury (TBI). The progress into our understanding of diffuse axonal injury (DAI) parallels that of TBI, given that significant experimental advances have been made in various animal and in vitro models. However, the application of these findings into the clinical arena has proven challenging.

The initial clinical definition of DAI was posttraumatic loss of consciousness lasting longer than six hours. DAI was presumed in cases in which no mass lesion was present to explain the comatose state of the patient. In the computed tomography (CT) era, DAI was at times detected as scattered petechial hemorrhages, most commonly at the cortical gray-white junction, the corpus callosum, and in the brain stem. At present, DAI may be detected with high sensitivity by magnetic resonance imaging (MRI) or by neurophysiological testing such as somatosensory-evoked potentials or brain stem auditory-evoked responses (1).

Perhaps the most important recent discovery in the field of axonal injury that challenges longstanding dogma has been that axonal disconnection is primarily a delayed phenomenon and does not occur primarily at the time of initial injury. The identification of this delayed injury has permitted researchers to identify several different experimental therapies that can reduce axonal injury if given within the therapeutic window. Clinical exploration of these therapies is still relatively immature, and, to date, no clinical evidence of efficacy exists for any studied therapies.

The first histopathological description of DAI was provided in 1956 by Strich, who identified five severely disabled individuals surviving for between five and 15 months after TBI (2). Postmortem gross examination revealed only minor pathological changes that were inconsistent with the level of neurological disability. Using various histological techniques, Strich was able to microscopically identify "diffuse degeneration" of axons within various white matter tracts of these brain-injured patients. In a follow-up study five years later, Strich identified 15 additional patients with the same pathological findings at both the microscopic and macroscopic levels (3). She posited that the pathology, in which large spheroidal and torpedo shaped-axonal varicosities were observed in various white matter tracts, including the corpus callosum, the internal capsule, and the pyramidal and medial lemniscal tracts of the brain stem, occurred as a result of immediate axonal tearing at the moment of injury, with extrusion of the axoplasm into the cytoplasmic space. With little evidence on which to base her suppositions, she correctly posited that the axonal damage was a consequence of shear forces generated by angular acceleration of the brain as a result of rapid head rotation (2,3).

Significant further progress into the understanding of DAI did not occur until the early 1980s when Gennarelli et al. created a model of primate brain injury involving rapid rotation of the head in the sagittal, coronal, and oblique planes (4). It was found that rapid rotation in the sagittal plane caused the least degree of injury, while coronal injury caused the worst degree of neurological impairment, DAI, and duration of coma, with oblique movements resulting in an intermediate degree of impairment. It was also described in the study that the length of posttraumatic coma was directly associated with neurological disability and burden of DAI. It was in this publication as well as another human neuropathological study identifying axonal injury in fatal nonpenetrating TBI appearing in the same journal (5) that the term "diffuse axonal injury" was coined.

Since that time, other in vivo models of (TBI) have been developed, all of which are based on rapid, dynamic deformation of the brain and its associated structures. Some of these models, such as optic nerve stretch (6), have been developed with the intent of creating pure axonal injury. Others, such as fluid percussion injury (7–10), cortical contusion (11,12), and impact acceleration (13,14) have been created to mimic more generalized forms of TBI, with DAI noted to occur in concert with other forms of traumatic intracranial pathology. The development of these numerous models has permitted further understanding into the pathobiology that underlies the development of DAI and permits testing of various neuroprotective strategies.

Epidemiology, Finanacial and Societal Impact

Approximately 1.5 to 2 million individuals are estimated to sustain TBI yearly. Of these, 70,000 to 90,000 suffer significant long-term loss of function and 300,000 require admission for mild and moderate TBI, and there are 52,000 deaths (15). The proportion of individuals sustaining DAI after severe TBI is between 12.9% and 42.5% based on pathological examination (16–22). Non-invasive radiographic examination of individuals with less severe forms of TBI also reveals white matter changes consistent with DAI in some patients (23,24).

To date, no study has evaluated the financial impact of (DAI) as it relates to the overall costs of TBI to the United States. We do know, however, that TBI affects approximately 1.5 to 2 million individuals yearly. A significant subset of these individuals sustains severe TBI. DAI is most prevalent in this population (18,19,25–28). The population most at risk for sustaining severe TBI is more likely to be young and of the male gender (29). DAI most commonly occurs secondary to high-velocity events, such as motor vehicle accidents, although it has also been reported in the presence of other inciting factors.

Given, then, that DAI is more likely to impact young individuals and that it is more commonly associated with severe disability and persistent vegetative state, DAI is an underlying pathophysiology in TBI survivors with severe life-long disabilities and limited functional independence.

Pathobiology

Previous thought held that the forces associated with diffuse injury caused immediate renting and disruption of the axonal membrane, resulting in "primary axotomy," which is analogous to the focal axonal injury caused by direct mechanical axonal transection, as would be seen in penetrating brain injury. The current concept, referred to as "secondary axotomy," involves the initial generation of diffuse shear and tensile forces within the brain as a result of angular acceleration caused by the traumatic insult. These shear and tensile forces result in focal perturbation but not overt disruption of axonal membranes. Membrane disruption then initiates multiple pathological processes that result in cessation of axonal transport, degradation of the axonal cytoskeleton, and ultimate axonal disconnection in the hours and days after injury. While it is certainly possible that immediate disconnection can occur with extraordinary shear forces, the majority of axons are now thought to remain physically intact after the initial trauma (30–32).

The initiating step in the process of axonal injury and disconnection involves traumatic perturbation of the axonal membrane (33). As a result of axolemmal perturbation, the electrochemical homeostasis generated by various axonal transport systems is disrupted because of uncontrolled passage of multiple ionic species down their respective concentration gradients (30,33–37). The most important of these ions in the generation of axonal injury is calcium. In the uninjured axon, intracellular calcium levels are tightly controlled by multiple axolemmal and organelle-based transporters, all of which operate in a coordinated fashion to keep axoplasmic calcium low with respect to the extracellular environment (38). The uncontrolled inward flux of calcium that occurs because of axolemmal perturbation is thought to overwhelm the capacity of these endogenous buffering systems, resulting in a rapid rise in cytosolic calcium levels (35,36,39,40).

Increased cytoplasmic levels of calcium can initiate multiple pathological processes via activation of several different pathways. Calpains are a group of calcium-dependent proteases that are activated by elevated levels of intracellular calcium. These proteases have numerous intracellular targets and can result in degradation of both the neuronal and axonal cytoskeleton. Detailed studies of animal models of DAI have demonstrated the activity of calpains in regions of focal axonal swellings. In the setting of human TBI, calpain activity has been identified in the spinal fluid of traumatically brain-injured individuals.

Mitochondria are also essential to the maintenance of intracellular calcium levels, in addition to their primary role in intracellular energy metabolism and oxidative phosphorylation. In the presence of an overwhelming cytosolic load of calcium, rapid and overwhelming mitochondrial uptake of calcium results in mitochondrial swelling and loss of electrochemical potential across the mitochondrial membrane. This results in loss of oxidative phosphorylation and cessation of adenosine triphosphate production. Another important consequence of mitochondrial swelling is opening of the mitochondrial permeability transition pore. It has been shown that opening of this pore results in release of cytochrome c from the mitochondrial intermembrane space into the cytosol.

Caspases, a family of cysteine proteases activated by various intra- and extracellular signals, are essential to the process of apoptotic cell death. In the setting of trauma, the orderly activation of these effectors, which can be initiated by cytochrome c in concert with other proteins, is disrupted, causing degradation of numerous intracellular proteins (41). Caspase-3, one of the major terminal effectors of the caspase pathway, is responsible for degradation of the subaxolemmal cytoskeleton in the setting of axonal injury (42). Putative therapeutic agents targeting each of these pathophysiological mechanisms of traumatic axonal injury (calpain activation, caspase activation, mitochondrial damage) are at various stages of preclinical testing.

Although neuronal and axonal membranes are perturbed by traumatic injury, resulting in loss of ionic homeostasis, they typically do not remain disrupted. Like most other cell types in the body, neurons and axons are capable of resealing after membrane disruption (43–50). The difference between axons and other cell types is that whereas cellular resealing typically occurs within seconds (51), axonal resealing in the central nervous system can require a significantly longer period of time (44). The implications of this observation as it relates to DAI are unclear at this time, but it appears reasonable to assume that a persistent loss of membrane integrity is not desirable.

Research into the pathological cascades responsible for the evolution of DAI has done little to shed light on the response of the linked neuronal cell body. In contrast to the long-held idea that traumatic axonal injury results in the ultimate death of the associated neuronal cell body, current experimental data indicate that neurons may sustain proximal axonal injury and disconnection without evidence of cell death (52). Although these neuronal somata show initial morphological signs of injury, they also demonstrate evidence of attempted regeneration of synaptic contacts. The implications of this finding as it relates to outcome after severe TBI with DAI are unknown at this time. It is hoped that the survival of neurons sustaining axonal injury would allow them to be recruited by future therapies as a component of neuronrehabilitation.

Diagnosis

Prior to the introduction of CT, the diagnosis of DAI could be made only via microscopic examination at the time of autopsy. Following the development of CT technology, it was recognized that DAI was associated with scattered petechial hemorrhages in the centrum semiovale, corpus callosum, basal ganglia, and/or brain stem (53). The most sensitive modality to date for the detection of DAI has been MRI, which has only become more effective as newer sequences have been developed to identify specific characteristics of DAI.

The initial experience with MRI found that while it is equally effective in detecting hemorrhagic areas of injury when compared with CT scanning, it is much more effective than CT in detecting areas of nonhemorrhagic injury and brain stem injury (54,55). The identification of T2 hyperintensity in the splenium of the corpus callosum and the dorsolateral brain stem in severe DAI represents the best example of this improved detection of nonhemorrhagic injury (Fig. 1). With the development of T2*-weighted gradient-echo sequencing, micro-hemorrhages not evident with CT scanning were resolved (56) (Fig. 2). Even newer imaging modalities based on fractional anisotropy, which detect limits on the movement of intracerebral water, have further increased the sensitivity of MRI with respect to the detection of DAI.

Anisotropy-based techniques rely on the detection of either restricted diffusion of water [increased anisotropy, diffusion-weighted imaging (DWI)], or decreased restrictions on water movement [decreased anisotropy, diffusion tensor imaging (DTI)]. DWI has been demonstrated to identify lesions associated with DAI that are not detected by any other MRI sequences (57,58). DTI has

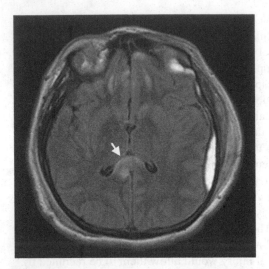

Figure 1 T2 hyperintensity in the splenium after severe traumatic brain injury. Axial T2 FLAIR MRI of a 21-year-old female sustaining severe traumatic brain injury. Note the hyperintense T2 signal in the splenium of the corpus callosum (*arrow*), consistent with diffuse axonal injury. The patient also has a resolving left subdural hematoma. *Abbreviation*: MRI, magnetic resonance imaging.

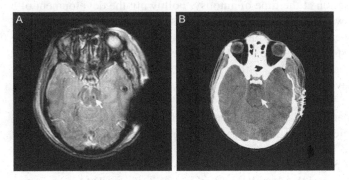

Figure 2 MRI is superior to CT in the detection of intracerebral microhemorrhage. Axial T2*-weighted gradient-echo MRI (**A**) and noncontrasted CT (**B**) images at the level of the midbrain from an individual sustaining severe traumatic brain injury with diffuse axonal injury show the presence of a left mesencephalic microhemorrhage (*arrow*). The lesion, which is apparent on MRI, is not detected via CT imaging. *Abbreviations*: MRI, magnetic resonance imaging; CT, computed tomography.

been found to be especially sensitive to disruptions in the normal orderly arrangement of parallel axonal fibers in the white matter pathways (59–61). Other techniques such as magnetization transfer imaging may also prove useful in the future detection of axonal injury (62).

Treatment

As of writing this chapter, there have been no effective treatments reported for DAI. Current clinical efforts are primarily focused on limiting secondary injury, which is known to worsen outcome after TBI (63). In the broader context of severe TBI, a recently completed phase II clinical trial of the immunophilin ligand cyclosporin A (CsA) has shown preliminary evidence of improvement of brain metabolic parameters (64). CsA is a medication primarily known for its role in the prevention of transplant rejection. However, under experimental conditions it has been shown to mitigate a variety of posttraumatic neuronal and axonal pathologies, including DAI (65–70). The targets through which CsA is thought to mediate its neuroprotective activity are (1) prevention of mitochondrial permeability transition in response to elevated intra-axonal calcium and (2) inhibition of calcineurin, a protein phosphatase that has been shown to reduce DAI independent of mitochondrial effects (71–73). It is hoped that a phase III clinical trial will be initiated shortly to ascertain the potential for CsA to ameliorate both DAI as well as other sequelae of TBI.

DYSAUTONOMIA

Background

Although DAI occurs exclusively in patients sustaining TBI, dysautonomia can occur in the setting of both traumatic and, to a lesser extent, nontraumatic brain injury. The constellation of symptoms associated with dysautonomia has been reported for some time (2). It was not recognized until recent times that these symptoms, taken together, constituted a single syndrome that was based on autonomic dysfunction. Part of the reason for the delay in the widespread recognition of dysautonomia may have been the lack of a common terminology to describe the syndrome. The multiple descriptors coined by various clinicians (Table 1) likely prevented other practitioners in the fields of neural injury and rehabilitation from recognizing that they were dealing with a common entity. In addition, there are several other neurological conditions, including malignant hyperthermia, neuroleptic malignant syndrome, autonomic dysreflexia, and narcotic withdrawal, which mimic many of the symptoms associated with dysautonomia (74,75). Some debate among practitioners still exists with respect to an appropriate single name for this syndrome, but for the purpose of this review, dysautonomia will be used.

Epidemiology

To date, the collective literature on dysautonomia is restricted mainly to small case-control series, observational studies, and case series/reports. As such, the incidence of dysautonomia after TBI is not firmly established. The limited data available at this time suggest that dysautonomia occurs in an estimated 10% to 30% of cases of severe TBI (76–78). Dysautonomia is reported to occur more

Table 1   Dysautonomia Syndrome Synonyms

Sympathetic storming
Paroxysmal sympathetic storming
Neurostorming
Paroxysmal autonomic instability with dystonia (PAID)
Autonomic dysfunction syndrome (ADS)
Acute midbrain syndrome
Midbrain dysregulatory syndrome
Brain stem attack
Hypothalamic-midbrain dysregulation syndrome
Acute hypothalmic instability
Diencephalic seizures
Central dysregulation
Tonic decerebrate spasms
Sympathoadrenal response
Tonic cerebellar fits
Hyperpyrexia associated with muscle contraction
Fever of central origin

commonly after severe TBI, and is associated with DAI, brain stem injury, younger age, and preadmission hypoxia (74–76,79). The reported association between dysautonomia and severe TBI is most likely a reflection of the fact that DAI, brain stem injury, and hypoxia are most common with severe injuries.

Pathophysiology

The pathological basis for dysautonomia has not yet been defined. A significant reason for this lack of scientific exploration lies in the fact that no model of injury exists that reproducibly generates posttraumatic autonomic dysfunction. Thus, the search for a pathological basis for dysautonomia is limited primarily to autopsy specimens from individuals clinically diagnosed with the condition.

While dysautonomia occurs primarily as a consequence of TBI, some of the earliest descriptions of the syndrome were in the setting of brain tumors. Specifically, tumors involving the diencephalon and hypothalamus were noted to be associated with paroxysmal autonomic dysregulation (80,81). Over the years, dysautonomia has also been noted in association with hydrocephalus, hypoxic-ischemic injury, and subarachnoid/intracerebral hemorrhages (74,75).

While many theories have been advanced as to pathological mechanism underlying the development of dysautonomia, the current evidence supports two potentially interrelated mechanisms. First, given the association between hypothalamic injury and autonomic dysregulation (82), it is reasonable to posit that TBI can result in direct injury to the hypothalamus, resulting in the development of dysautonomia. Second, dysautonomia may also manifest as a result of a functional disconnection of the hypothalamus and diencephalon from the rest of the central nervous system, possibly because of axonal injury of the afferent and efferent pathways. This would also stand to reason, given the reported association between DAI and dysautonomia.

Diagnosis

The diagnosis of dysautonomia is based on patient history in combination with specific physical examination findings. The seven main findings associated with the dysautonomia syndrome are presented in Table 2. It has been suggested that the diagnosis of dysautonomic syndrome is the presence of at least five of the seven findings. It should also be noted that pupillary dilation is also common in patients with dysautonomia (75,83,84), although this is not one of the criteria.

Many of the signs noted above are relatively nonspecific when taken individually, and even when occurring in combination may represent a problem other than dysautonomia. Infection is a common problem in intensive care unit (ICU) patients that typically results in fever, tachycardia, tachypnea, and diaphoresis. Fever in patients with neurological injuries is known to worsen the mental status examination, which may result in posturing. As such, it is imperative that patients with suspected dysautonomia undergo adequate fever work up, including blood, urine, cerebrospinal fluid (CSF), and sputum cultures. Dysautonomia may be diagnosed only after infection has been treated adequately or ruled out via negative cultures.

Dysautonomia typically presents with delayed onset. The signs of dysautonomia are usually not detected until patients have been weaned from sedation and paralytics in the ICU (74). The symptoms may be relatively minor at first, but can become florid if left untreated. Not uncommonly, the initial signs of dysautonomia are mistaken for agitation and result in increased sedation, prolonging an individual's ICU stay and time of intubation/ventilation. It is not until the syndrome is appropriately recognized and treated that progress can be made toward successfully discontinuing sedation and transferring the patient out of the ICU.

It has been suggested that the natural history of dysautonomia be divided into three phases. Phase I is the time in which the patient remains intubated and sedated with or without chemical paralysis. During this time dysautonomia is usually unrecognized. Phase II occurs after the stoppage of sedation and is the time when the above-mentioned symptoms of dysautonomia present. Phase III begins with the stoppage of diaphoresis, at which point the paroxysmal episodes of autonomic dysfunction subside. Transition to phase III is proposed to represent "burnt out" dysautonomia, leaving behind an individual with variable dystonia and/or spasticity (74). The average duration of phase I is reported to be approximately one week, while phase II averages 74 days, but can be quite variable (74).

Treatment

The treatment of dysautonomia seldom starts with diagnosis. More typically, individuals who have sustained severe TBI begin to develop fever, tachycardia,

Table 2   Findings in Dysautonomia Syndrome

Tachycardia
Tachypnea
Hypertension
Fever
Diaphoresis
Rigidity
Posturing

hypertension, and agitation as their initial sedation is weaned. This prompts a fever work up as well as increased sedation to control the episodes of "agitation." Only after multiple days of additional sedation, prolonged treatment with empiric antibiotics, and multiple blood, urine, CSF, and sputum cultures remain negative is the diagnosis of dysautonomia made. Early recognition and treatment of dysautonomia can mitigate the need for additional testing and an extended stay in the ICU.

The goals of dysautonomia treatment are to prevent secondary injury caused by the paroxysmal autonomic episodes. There are three main mechanisms by which dysautonomia can worsen secondary brain injury after TBI. First, hyperthermia in brain-injured patients is associated with worsened outcomes (85–87). Given that dysautonomic episodes can be associated with high fever, this represents an especially important component of the syndrome to control. Second, the rigidity and posturing associated with dysautonomia result in markedly increased energy expenditures, up to 150% to 200% over baseline at one week and 200% to 250% at two weeks (88,89). The increased expenditure may not be accounted for in the individual's feeding regimen and may result in an insufficient number of calories being delivered. This relative malnutrition has been demonstrated to worsen outcomes for all types of traumatic injury (88–91). Finally, the paroxysms associated with dysautonomia are associated with elevations in circulating catecholamine levels, which are independent predictors of poor outcome after TBI (88). However, no studies have been conducted to show that treatment of dysautonomia improves functional outcome.

Numerous pharmacological interventions have been employed in attempts to treat dysautonomia (Table 3). Narcotics and benzodiazepines, when used either alone or in combination, successfully reduce the number and frequency of autonomic paroxysms (76). This reduction likely occurs via a generalized suppression of brain activity (i.e., sedation). While sedation is a viable treatment for dysautonomia in the acute setting, it is not desirable as a long-term solution, given that sedation treats the symptoms of dysautonomia rather than the underlying pathophysiology. Many other medications have been used to attempt to control autonomic paroxysms without success. These medications include antiepileptics [phenytoin, phenobarbital, and carbamazepine (79,84,92–94), dopamine antagonists (haloperidol and chlorpromazine (93,95), antipyretics (acetaminophen) (96), and gamma-aminobutyric acid agonists (oral baclofen) (96)].

Other medications have shown evidence of successful control of various components of the autonomic paroxysms associated with dysautonomia.

Table 3 Medical Therapy for Dysautonomia

Medication	Dose	Symptoms treated	Typical adverse effects
Clonidine	Adults: 0.1 mg PO BID to start, max 1.2 mg PO BID Peds: 5–10 mcg/kg/day in divided doses, max 25 mcg/kg/day	Hypertension Tachycardia Agitation	Hypotension Sedation Rebound hypertension
Hydralazine	Adults: 10 mg Q10 min PRN Peds: 0.1–0.5 mg/kg IM/IV Q4-6hr	Hypertension	↑ ICP Hypotension Tachycardia
Labetalol	Adults: 10 mg Q10 min PRN Peds: 0.4–1 mg/kg/hr IV infusion max: 3 mg/kg/hr	Hypertension Tachycardia	Bradycardia Hypotension Bronchospasm
Bromocriptine	1.25 mg PO BID to start, max 40 mg/day	Rigidity Posturing Diaphoresis	Hypotension Hallucinations
IT Baclofen	Adults: start 50–400 mcg/day to start, titrate final dose based on symptoms/side effects (77,100) Peds: start 10 200 mcg/day to start, titrate final dose based on symptoms/side effects	Hypertension Tachycardia Rigidity Diaphoresis Hyperthermia	
Propranolol	Adults: 20–40 mg PO BID initially, max 640mg/day Peds: 0.5–1 mg/kg/day PO div BID, max: 8 mg/kg/day	Hypertension Tachycardia ↑ Energy expenditure Hyperthermia Rigidity	Bradycardia Hypotension Bronchospasm
Dantrolene	Adult: 25 mg PO QD to start, titrated up to goal dose of 100 mg PO BID-TID. 400 mg/day max Peds: 0.5 mg/kg/day PO to start, titrated up to goal dose of 2 mg/kg BID-TID. 12 mg/kg/day max	Rigidity Posturing	Somnolence Hepatotoxicity Fatigue

References are shown in parenthesis.

Clonidine, an α2-adrenergic agonist, causes decreased central sympathetic out-flow, resulting in decreased blood pressure and reduced levels of circulating catecholamines (74,79,96,97). Dantrolene is a medication used primarily for the treatment of malignant hyperthermia via inhibition of intracellular release of calcium, causing decreased muscle contraction. It has shown limited success in reducing rigidity and posturing in dysautonomia (84). The hypertensive and tachycardic component of dysautonomia can be effectively controlled via the use of β blockers like labetalol (98).

Yet other groups of medications potentially show the most promise with respect to the control of dysautonomia. These medications include bromocriptine, a dopamine D2 agonist that has been shown to be effective in the control of the fever and diaphoresis that occurs with autonomic dysfunction (79,83,84,99). Although oral baclofen has not proven successful in the treatment of dysautonomia, intrathecal baclofen appears to be quite effective at controlling autonomic dysfunction in the limited number of patients in whom it has been tried (77,100). Finally, the nonselective β blocker propranolol also appears quite useful at controlling multiple components of autonomic dysfunction. Namely, it has been shown to reduce blood pressure, heart rate, temperature, muscle tone, circulating catecholamines, cardiac work, and resting energy expenditure (92,96,97,101–103).

CONCLUSION

In the setting of severe TBI, both DAI and dysautonomia can exert a profound negative influence on the ultimate outcome of affected individuals. Although the staggering monetary and psychosocial impact of TBI has been previously described, the contribution of DAI and dysautonomia to this overall cost has not been defined. Given that the incidence of both these sequelae increases with worsening injury, it stands to reason that the most severely injured individuals are disproportionately impacted by these pathologies from both a medical and a financial perspective.

REFERENCES

1. Rumpl E, Prugger M, Gerstenbrand F, et al. Central somatosensory conduction time and short latency somatosensory evoked potentials in post-traumatic coma. Electroencephalogr Clin Neurophysiol 1983; 56(6):583–596.
2. Strich SJ. Diffuse degeneration of the cerebral white matter in severe dementia following head injury. J Neurol Neurosurg Psychiatry 1956; 19:163–185.
3. Strich SJ. Shearing of nerve fibers as a cause of brain damage due to head injury: a pathological study of twenty cases. Lancet 1961; 2:443–448.
4. Gennarelli TA, Thibault LE, Adams JH, et al. Diffuse axonal injury and traumatic coma in the primate. Ann Neurol 1982; 12(6):564–574.
5. Adams JH, Graham DI, Murray LS, et al. Diffuse axonal injury due to nonmissile head injury in humans: an analysis of 45 cases. Ann Neurol 1982; 12(6):557–563.
6. Tomei G, Spagnoli D, Ducati A, et al. Morphology and neurophysiology of focal axonal injury experimentally induced in the guinea pig optic nerve. Acta Neuropathol (Berl) 1990; 80(5):506–13.
7. Sullivan HG, Martinez J, Becker DP, et al. Fluid-percussion model of mechanical brain injury in the cat. J Neurosurg 1976; 45(5):521–534.
8. Dixon CE, Lyeth BG, Povlishock JT, et al. A fluid percussion model of experimental brain injury in the rat. J Neurosurg 1987; 67(1):110–119.

9. McIntosh TK, Noble L, Andrews B, et al. Traumatic brain injury in the rat: characterization of a midline fluid-percussion model. Cent Nerv Syst Trauma 1987; 4(2):119–134.

10. Dixon CE, Lighthall JW, Anderson TE. Physiologic, histopathologic, and cineradiographic characterization of a new fluid-percussion model of experimental brain injury in the rat. J Neurotrauma 1988; 5(2):91–104.

11. Lighthall JW. Controlled cortical impact: a new experimental brain injury model. J Neurotrauma 1988; 5(1):1–15.

12. Dixon CE, Clifton GL, Lighthall JW, et al. A controlled cortical impact model of traumatic brain injury in the rat. J Neurosci Methods 1991; 39(3):253–262.

13. Foda MA, Marmarou A. A new model of diffuse brain injury in rats. Part II: Morphological characterization. J Neurosurg 1994; 80(2):301–313.

14. Marmarou A, Foda MA, van den Brink W, et al. A new model of diffuse brain injury in rats. Part I: Pathophysiology and biomechanics. J Neurosurg 1994; 80(2): 291–300.

15. NIH Consensus Development Panel on Rehabilitation of Persons with Traumatic Brain Injury. Rehabilitation of persons with traumatic brain injury. JAMA 1999; 282(10):974–983.

16. Adams JH, Doyle D, Ford I, et al. Diffuse axonal injury in head injury: definition, diagnosis and grading. Histopathology 1989; 15(1):49–59.

17. Adams JH, Doyle D, Graham DI, et al. Diffuse axonal injury in head injuries caused by a fall. Lancet 1984; 2(8417-18):1420–1422.

18. Lobato RD, Cordobes F, Rivas JJ, et al. Outcome from severe head injury related to the type of intracranial lesion. A computerized tomography study. J Neurosurg 1983; 59(5):762–774.

19. Cordobes F, Lobato RD, Rivas JJ, et al. Post-traumatic diffuse axonal brain injury. Analysis of 78 patients studied with computed tomography. Acta Neurochir (Wien) 1986; 81(1-2):27–35.

20. Blumbergs PC, Jones NR, North JB Diffuse axonal injury in head trauma. J Neurol Neurosurg Psychiatry 1989; 52(7):838–841.

21. Wang H, Duan G, Zhang J, et al. Clinical studies on diffuse axonal injury in patients with severe closed head injury. Chin Med J (Engl) 1998; 111(1):59–62.

22. Pilz P. Axonal injury in head injury. Acta Neurochir Suppl (Wien) 1983; 32:119–123.

23. Arfanakis K, Haughton VM, Carew JD, et al. Diffusion tensor MR imaging in diffuse axonal injury. AJNR Am J Neuroradiol 2002; 23(5):794–802.

24. Mittl RL, Grossman RI, Hiehle JF, et al. Prevalence of MR evidence of diffuse axonal injury in patients with mild head injury and normal head CT findings. AJNR Am J Neuroradiol 1994; 15(8):1583–1589.

25. Gennarelli TA. Head injury in man and experimental animals: clinical aspects. Acta Neurochir Suppl (Wien) 1983; 32:1–13.

26. McLellan DR, Adams JH, Graham DI, et al. The structural basis of the vegetative state and prolonged coma after non-missile head injury. In: Le Coma Traumatique. Liviana Editrice: Padova, 1986:165–185.

27. Sahuquillo J, Vilalta J, Lamarca J, et al. Diffuse axonal injury after severe head trauma. A clinico-pathological study. Acta Neurochir(Wien) 1989; 101(3–4):149–158.

28. Shigemori M, Kikuchi N, Tokutomi T, et al. Coexisting diffuse axonal injury (DAI) and outcome of severe head injury. Acta Neurochir. Suppl (Wien) 1992; 55:37–39.

29. Traumatic Brain Injury In the United States: A Report to Congress. 1999, Division of Acute Care, Rehabilitation Research, and Disability Prevention, National Center for Injury Prevention and Control, Centers for Disease Control and Prevention, U.S. Department of Health and Human Services.

30. Maxwell WL, Povlishock JT, Graham DL. A mechanistic analysis of nondisruptive axonal injury: a review [published erratum appears in J Neurotrauma 1997 Oct;14 (10):755]. J.Neurotrauma 1997; 14(7):419–440.

31. Povlishock JT, Becker DP, Cheng CL, et al. Axonal change in minor head injury. J Neuropathol Exp Neurol 1983; 42(3):225–242.

32. Povlishock JT and Christman CW. The pathobiology of traumatically induced axonal injury in animals and humans: a review of current thoughts. J. Neurotrauma 1995; 12(4):555–564.

33. Pettus EH, Christman CW, Giebel ML, et al. Traumatically induced altered membrane permeability: its relationship to traumatically induced reactive axonal change. J Neurotrauma 1994; 11(5):507–522.

34. Agrawal SK, Nashmi R, Fehlings MG. Role of L- and N-type calcium channels in the pathophysiology of traumatic spinal cord white matter injury. Neuroscience 2000; 99(1):179–188.

35. Wolf JA, Stys PK, Lusardi T, et al. Traumatic axonal injury induces calcium influx modulated by tetrodotoxin-sensitive sodium channels. J Neurosci 2001; 21(6): 1923–1930.

36. He X, Yi S, Zhang X, et al. Intra-axonal overloading of calcium ion in rat diffuse axonal injury and therapeutic effect of calcium antagonist. Chin J Traumatol 1999; 2(1):25–29.

37. Pettus EH, Povlishock JT. Characterization of a distinct set of intra-axonal ultra-structural changes associated with traumatically induced alteration in axolemmal permeability. Brain Res 1996; 722(1-2):1–11.

38. Kandel ES, Schwartz JH, Jessell TM. Principles of Neural Science. New York: McGraw-Hill, 2000.

39. Tymianski M, Tator CH. Normal and abnormal calcium homeostasis in neurons: a basis for the pathophysiology of traumatic and ischemic central nervous system injury. Neurosurgery 1996; 38(6):1176–1195.

40. Maxwell WL, McCreath BJ, Graham DI, et al. Cytochemical evidence for redis-tribution of membrane pump calcium- ATPase and ecto-Ca-ATPase activity, and calcium influx in myelinated nerve fibres of the optic nerve after stretch injury. J Neurocytol 1995; 24(12):925–942.

41. Springer JE, Nottingham SA, McEwen ML, et al. Caspase-3 apoptotic signaling following injury to the central nervous system. Clin Chem Lab Med 2001; 39 (4):299–307.

42. Buki A, Okonkwo DO, Wang KK, et al. Cytochrome c release and caspase acti-vation in traumatic axonal injury. J Neurosci 2000; 20(8):2825–2834.

43. Singleton RH, Povlishock JT, Identification and characterization of heterogeneous neuronal injury and death in regions of diffuse brain injury: evidence for multiple independent injury phenotypes. J Neurosci 2004; 24(14):3543–3553.

44. Ahmed FA, Ingoglia NA, Sharma SC. Axon resealing following transection takes longer in central axons than in peripheral axons: implications for axonal regener-ation. Exp Neurol 2001; 167(2):451–455.

45. Detrait E, Eddleman CS, Yoo S, et al. Axolemmal repair requires proteins that mediate synaptic vesicle fusion. J Neurobiol 2000; 44(4):382–391.

46. Eddleman CS, Ballinger ML, Smyers ME, et al. Endocytotic formation of vesicles and other membranous structures induced by Ca2+ and axolemmal injury. J Neurosci 1998; 18(11):4029–4041.
47. Godell CM, Smyers ME, Eddleman CS, et al. Calpain activity promotes the sealing of severed giant axons. Proc Natl Acad Sci U S A 1997; 94(9):4751–4756.
48. Shi R, Pryor JD. Temperature dependence of membrane sealing following transection in mammalian spinal cord axons. Neuroscience 2000; 98(1):157–166.
49. Xie XY, Barrett JN. Membrane resealing in cultured rat septal neurons after neurite transection: evidence for enhancement by Ca(2+)-triggered protease activity and cytoskeletal disassembly. J Neurosci 1991; 11(10):3257–3267.
50. Howard MJ, David G, Barrett JN. Resealing of transected myelinated mammalian axons in vivo: evidence for involvement of calpain. Neuroscience 1999; 93(2): 807–15.
51. McNeil PL, Terasaki M. Coping with the inevitable: how cells repair a torn surface membrane. Nat Cell Biol 2001; 3(5):E124–E129.
52. Singleton RH, Zhu J, Stone JR, et al. Traumatically induced axotomy adjacent to the soma does not result in acute neuronal death. J Neurosci 2002; 22(3):791–802.
53. Parizel PM, Ozsarlak, Van Goethem JW, et al. Imaging findings in diffuse axonal injury after closed head trauma. Eur Radiol 1998; 8(6):960–965.
54. Gentry LR, Godersky JC, Thompson B. MR imaging of head trauma: review of the distribution and radiopathologic features of traumatic lesions. AJR Am J Roentgenol 1988; 150(3):663–672.
55. Gentry LR, Godersky JC, Thompson B, et al. Prospective comparative study of intermediate-field MR and CT in the evaluation of closed head trauma. AJR Am J Roentgenol 1988; 150(3):673–682.
56. Mittl RL, Grossman RI, Hiehle JF, et al. Prevalence of MR evidence of diffuse axonal injury in patients with mild head injury and normal head CT findings. AJNR Am J Neuroradiol 1994; 15(8):1583–1589.
57. Ezaki Y, Tsutsumi K, Morikawa M, et al. Role of diffusion-weighted magnetic resonance imaging in diffuse axonal injury. Acta Radiol 2006; 47(7):733–740.
58. Huisman TA, Sorensen AG, Hergan K, et al. Diffusion-weighted imaging for the evaluation of diffuse axonal injury in closed head injury. J Comput Assist Tomogr 2003; 27(1):5–11.
59. Arfanakis K, Haughton VM, Carew JD, et al. Diffusion tensor MR imaging in diffuse axonal injury. AJNR Am J Neuroradiol 2002; 23(5):794–802.
60. Inglese M, Makani S, Johnson G, et al. Diffuse axonal injury in mild traumatic brain injury: a diffusion tensor imaging study. J Neurosurg 2005; 103(2):298–303.
61. Le TH, Mukherjee P, Henry RG, et al. Diffusion tensor imaging with three-dimensional fiber tractography of traumatic axonal shearing injury: an imaging correlate for the posterior callosal "disconnection" syndrome: case report. Neurosurgery 2005; 56(1):189.
62. Sinson G, Bagley LJ, Cecil KM, et al. Magnetization transfer imaging and proton MR spectroscopy in the evaluation of axonal injury: correlation with clinical outcome after traumatic brain injury. AJNR Am J Neuroradiol 2001; 22(1):143–151.
63. Brain Trauma Foundation I, American Association of Neurological Surgeons, Part 1: guidelines for the management of severe traumatic brain injury. New York: Brain Trauma Foundation, 2000.
64. Merenda A, Bullock R. Clinical treatments for mitochondrial dysfunctions after brain injury. Curr Opin Crit Care 2006; 12(2):90–96.

65. Okonkwo DO, Buki A, Siman R, et al. Cyclosporin A limits calcium-induced axonal damage following traumatic brain injury. Neuroreport 1999; 10(2):353–358.
66. Buki A, Okonkwo DO, Povlishock JT. Postinjury cyclosporin A administration limits axonal damage and disconnection in traumatic brain injury. J Neurotrauma 1999; 16(6):511–521.
67. Scheff SW, Sullivan PG. Cyclosporin A significantly ameliorates cortical damage following experimental traumatic brain injury in rodents. J Neurotrauma 1999; 16 (9):783–792.
68. Sullivan PG, Thompson MB, Scheff SW. Cyclosporin A attenuates acute mitochondrial dysfunction following traumatic brain injury. Exp Neurol 1999; 160(1): 226–234.
69. Sullivan PG, Thompson M, Scheff SW. Continuous infusion of cyclosporin A postinjury significantly ameliorates cortical damage following traumatic brain injury. Exp Neurol 2000; 161(2):631–637.
70. Suehiro E, Povlishock JT. Exacerbation of traumatically induced axonal injury by rapid posthypothermic rewarming and attenuation of axonal change by cyclosporin A. J Neurosurg 2001; 94(3):493–498.
71. Singleton RH, Stone JR, Okonkwo DO, et al. The immunophilin ligand FK506 attenuates axonal injury in an impact-acceleration model of traumatic brain injury. J Neurotrauma 2001; 18(6):607–614.
72. Bavetta S, Hamlyn PJ, Burnstock G, et al. The effects of FK506 on dorsal column axons following spinal cord injury in adult rats: neuroprotection and local regeneration. Exp Neurol 1999; 158(2):382–393.
73. Suehiro E, Singleton RH, Stone JR, et al. The immunophilin ligand FK506 attenuates the axonal damage associated with rapid rewarming following posttraumatic hypothermia. Exp Neurol 2001; 172(1):199–210.
74. Baguley IJ, Nicholls JL, Felmingham KL, et al. Dysautonomia after traumatic brain injury: a forgotten syndrome? J Neurol Neurosurg Psychiatry 1999; 67(1):39–43.
75. Blackman JA, Patrick PD, Buck ML, et al. Paroxysmal autonomic instability with dystonia after brain injury. Arch Neurol 2004; 61(3):321–328.
76. Baguley IJ, Cameron ID, Green AM, et al. Pharmacological management of Dysautonomia following traumatic brain injury. Brain Inj 2004; 18(5):409–417.
77. Cuny E, Richer E, and Castel JP. Dysautonomia syndrome in the acute recovery phase after traumatic brain injury: relief with intrathecal Baclofen therapy. Brain Inj 2001; 15(10):917–25.
78. Fernandez-Ortega JF, Prieto-Palomino MA, Munoz-Lopez A, et al. Prognostic influence and computed tomography findings in dysautonomic crises after traumatic brain injury. J Trauma 2006; 61(5):1129–1133.
79. Boeve BF, Wijdicks EF, Benarroch EE, et al. Paroxysmal sympathetic storms ("diencephalic seizures") after severe diffuse axonal head injury. Mayo Clin Proc 1998; 73(2):148–152.
80. Penfield W. Diencephalic autonomic epilepsy. Arch Neurol Psychiatry 1929; 22:358–374.
81. Solomon GE. Diencephalic autonomic epilepsy caused by a neoplasm. J Pediatr 1973; 83(2):277–280.
82. Benarroch EE. The central autonomic network: functional organization, dysfunction, and perspective. Mayo Clin Proc 1993; 68(10):988–1001.

83. Bullard DE. Diencephalic seizures: responsiveness to bromocriptine and morphine. Ann Neurol 1987; 21(6):609–611.

84. Rossitch E Jr., Bullard DE. The autonomic dysfunction syndrome: aetiology and treatment. Br J Neurosurg 1988; 2(4):471–478.

85. Jiang JY, Gao GY, Li WP, et al. Early indicators of prognosis in 846 cases of severe traumatic brain injury. J Neurotrauma 2002; 19(7):869–874.

86. Natale JE, Joseph JG, Helfaer MA, et al. Early hyperthermia after traumatic brain injury in children: risk factors, influence on length of stay, and effect on short-term neurologic status. Crit Care Med 2000; 28(7):2608–2615.

87. Suz P, Vavilala MS, Souter M, et al. Clinical features of fever associated with poor outcome in severe pediatric traumatic brain injury. J Neurosurg Anesthesiol 2006; 18(1):5–10.

88. Clifton GL, Ziegler MG, Grossman RG. Circulating catecholamines and sympathetic activity after head injury. Neurosurgery 1981; 8(1):10–14.

89. Moore R, Najarian MP, Konvolinka CW. Measured energy expenditure in severe head trauma. J Trauma 1989; 29(12):1633–1636.

90. Biffl WL, Moore EE, Haenel JB. Nutrition support of the trauma patient. Nutrition 2002; 18(11-12):960–965.

91. Wilson RF, Tyburski JG. Metabolic responses and nutritional therapy in patients with severe head injuries. J Head Trauma Rehabil 1998; 13(1):11–27.

92. Sandel ME, Abrams PL, Horn LJ. Hypertension after brain injury: case report. Arch Phys Med Rehabil 1986; 67(7):469–472.

93. Sneed RC. Hyperpyrexia associated with sustained muscle contractions: an alternative diagnosis to central fever. Arch Phys Med Rehabil 1995; 76(1):101–103.

94. Talman WT, Florek G, Bullard DE. A hyperthermic syndrome in two subjects with acute hydrocephalus. Arch Neurol 1988; 45(9):1037–1040.

95. Scott JS, Ockey RR, Holmes GE, et al. Autonomic dysfunction associated with locked-in syndrome in a child. Am J Phys Med Rehabil 1997; 76(3):200–203.

96. Pranzatelli MR, Pavlakis SG, Gould RJ, et al. Hypothalamic-midbrain dysregulation syndrome: hypertension, hyperthermia, hyperventilation, and decerebration. J Child Neurol 1991; 6(2):115–122.

97. Silver JK, Lux WE. Early onset dystonia following traumatic brain injury. Arch Phys Med Rehabil 1994; 75(8):885–888.

98. Do D, Sheen VL, and Bromfield E. Treatment of paroxysmal sympathetic storm with labetalol. J Neurol Neurosurg Psychiatry 2000; 69(6):832–833.

99. Russo RN, O'Flaherty S. Bromocriptine for the management of autonomic dysfunction after severe traumatic brain injury. J Paediatr Child Health 2000; 36 (3):283–285.

100. Francois B, Vacher P, Roustan J, et al. Intrathecal baclofen after traumatic brain injury: early treatment using a new technique to prevent spasticity. J Trauma 2001; 50(1):158–161.

101. Chiolero RL, Breitenstein E, Thorin D, et al. Effects of propranolol on resting metabolic rate after severe head injury. Crit Care Med 1989; 17(4):328–334.

102. Meythaler JM, Stinson AM III. Fever of central origin in traumatic brain injury controlled with propranolol. Arch Phys Med Rehabil 1994; 75(7):816–818.

103. Robertson CS, Clifton GL, Taylor AA, et al. Treatment of hypertension associated with head injury. J Neurosurg 1983; 59(3):455–460.

4

Neuromonitoring in Traumatic Brain Injury

Rene Celis, MD, Research Assistant
Claudia S. Robertson, MD, Professor
Department of Neurosurgery, Baylor College of Medicine,
Houston, Texas, U.S.A.

Although the incidence of traumatic brain injury (TBI) has steadily decreased over the past decade, each year an estimated 1.5 million people in the United States sustain a TBI. Approximately 5% of the population (5.3 million Americans) lives with a disability as a result of TBI, and one in four adults with TBI are unable to return to work one year after injury (1).

Prevention is the only way to reduce the incidence of TBI. Once the primary insult has occurred, the main goal of the neurointensivist is to prevent additional brain damage through prompt detection and individualized treatment of secondary insults such as intracranial hypertension and cerebral ischemia. To achieve this goal, multimodality neuromonitoring is employed. Neuromonitoring constitutes any technique that can provide information about a patient's neurologic status, from the simple and inexpensive serial neurologic assessments to the most complex and invasive forms of neuromonitoring. Invasive neuromonitoring technologies fall into three general categories: pressure, flow, and metabolism (Table 1).

CLINICAL ASSESSMENTS

A thorough and systematic neurologic examination must include evaluation of mental status, cranial and pupillary reflexes, and motor responses. The Glasgow

Table 1 Neuromonitoring Techniques

Monitors of Pressure
    Intracranial pressure
    Cerebral perfusion pressure
Monitors of Flow
    Direct
        Stable xenon CT imaging
        Perfusion CT imaging
        Transcranial Doppler
    Indirect
        Jugular venous oxygen saturation
        Brain tissue pO_2
Monitors of Metabolism
    Electroencephalogram
    Microdialysis

Coma Scale (GCS), measured at the field or site of accident and in the emergency center as first-line assessment and for triage purposes (2) or as a routine assessment at the neonatal intensive care unit provides the physician with valuable data on the patient's neurologic status. A GCS score of 13 to 15 is considered a mild head injury, scores between 9 and 12 are considered moderate, whereas a patient with a GCS score less than or equal to 8 is considered to have a severe TBI (3).

Although widely used, the GCS has well-known limitations. GCS measurements vary, depending on the skills and expertise of the examiner (4). It is unrealistic for a neurointensivist to assess GCS at the bedside on an hourly basis, and as more than one physician and nurse usually perform the assessment, even the most standardized examination presents significant variations between examiners. How the examination is conducted, the level of stimulus applied to the patient, and the perception of pupillary reactivity performed with different light intensities can result in variable results. Drug and/or alcohol intoxication can confound early neurologic assessment. Sedation and neuromuscular-blocking agents used to intubate and to control ventilation can also obscure the neurologic examination (5). The infrared pupillometer is a new technology that may allow more objective assessment of pupillary reactivity (6). Several pupil characteristics, including maximum and minimum apertures, constriction and dilation velocities, and latency period, can be measured accurately (7). Subtle changes in the velocity of the pupils correlate with changes in intracranial pressure (ICP) (8).

MEASURES OF PRESSURE

ICP

Intracranial hypertension cannot be accurately predicted from clinical signs and symptoms after trauma. Classic presentation of headache, nausea, projectile vomiting, and papilledema are not consistent, and intracranial hypertension can

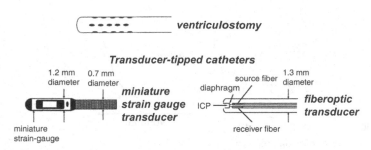

Figure 1 Common technologies for monitoring ICP include the ventriculostomy (*top*) and parenchymal catheters that incorporate a miniature pressure transducer at the tip of the catheter (*bottom*). *Abbreviation*: ICP, intracranial pressure.

occur in the absence of these signs and symptoms. Furthermore, symptoms cannot be evaluated in an obtunded, sedated, or comatose patient. CT signs of brain swelling, such as midline shift and compressed basal cisterns, are predictive of raised ICP, but intracranial hypertension can occur without these observations (9). As no clinical assessment accurately quantifies ICP, it must actually be measured when the information is critical.

Since 1960, a ventricular catheter has been the gold standard for measuring ICP (10). Ventriculostomy placement can be performed at the bedside under local anesthesia and is a quick and effective method to reduce raised ICP by draining cerebrospinal fluid (CSF) (11). Through a burr hole, the ventricular catheter is positioned in the frontal horn of the lateral ventricle and coupled by a fluid-filled pressurized tubing to an external strain gauge transducer that can be easily zeroed and recalibrated.

Although measurement of ICP has traditionally been performed through a ventriculostomy catheter, new technologic advances that allow the pressure transducer to be incorporated into the tip of the catheter offer alternative approaches (Fig. 1). Although several noninvasive technologies for estimating ICP, including tympanic membrane displacement (12), venous ophthalmodynamometry (13), tissue resonance analysis (14), ultrasound measurement of cranial diameter pulsations (15), and latency of visual evoked potentials (16), have been developed, none are sufficiently reliable at present to monitor ICP in the critically ill patient. While invasive ICP monitoring lacks randomized trial data, it remains the gold standard for monitoring ICP and the physiologic measure that distinguishes the neurointensivist.

According to the Monro (1783)–Kellie (1824) doctrine, ICP is determined by the volume of brain, CSF, and intravascular blood contained within the rigid skull vault. An increase in any of these three components or the development of an intracranial mass lesion must be met by a corresponding decrease in the volume of another component, or ICP increases, providing a small amount of compensation as intracranial volume expands. Once this compensation is exhausted, ICP rapidly increases with further expansion of intracranial volume

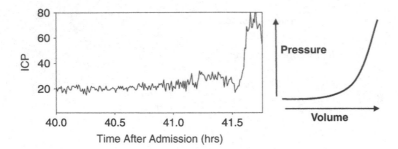

Figure 2 (*Right*) Exponential relationship between volume of intracranial contents and ICP. (*Left*) The change in ICP over time in a patient with an expanding mass lesion. Initially, the rise in ICP is very gradual, but when compensatory mechanisms are exhausted, ICP increases rapidly. *Abbreviation*: ICP, intracranial pressure.

(Fig. 2). Raised ICP is an important secondary insult in patients who are brain injured and a predictor of poor outcome after TBI.

ICP of a healthy individual in a supine position is maintained between 3 and 10 mmHg, with an upper limit of 15 mmHg. ICP can sometimes reach levels of 25 mmHg in morbidly obese individuals. Valsalva maneuver, straining, sneezing, or coughing can result in transient pressure elevations up to 60 mmHg. For a patient with a brain injury, ICP values of 20 to 30 mmHg represent intracranial hypertension that is mild but requires treatment. ICP values of 30 to 40 mmHg represent moderately severe intracranial hypertension, and ICP values greater than 40 mmHg represent severe, potentially life-threatening intracranial hypertension.

The most common reason for not monitoring ICP is the risk of serious complication, including ventriculitis and hemorrhage. The risk of infection is directly related to the duration of catheterization. A number of practices include periodic replacement of catheters (17–20), daily monitoring of CSF cell counts and chemistries (21), and the use of prophylactic antibiotics (17,19,20,22). The use of prophylactic antibiotics has not shown a reduction in the incidence of ventriculitis associated with ventriculostomy catheters. However, recent use of a ventricular catheter impregnated with minocycline and rifampin was shown to significantly decrease the infection rate from 9.4% to 1.3% (23).

The risk of hemorrhage following placement of a ventriculostomy catheter is increased when a coagulopathy is present, and severe coagulopathy is a relative contraindication to placement of an ICP monitor. When the international normalized ratio is less than or equal to 1.6, the risk of hemorrhage is not significantly increased and correction of the coagulopathy is not necessary prior to insertion of an ICP monitor (24).

ICP monitors are usually placed by neurosurgeons. However, when properly trained and supervised, midlevel practitioners or nonneurosurgeon physicians can safely place ICP monitors (25,26).

Cerebral Perfusion Pressure

ICP is also used to calculate cerebral perfusion pressure (CPP) (27), the difference between mean arterial pressure (MAP) and ICP (CPP = MAP − ICP). CPP describes the pressure gradient across the cerebral vascular bed and constitutes the driving pressure for blood flow to the brain. Under normal conditions, the brain is capable of maintaining a constant blood flow over a wide range of CPP values (50–150 mmHg) through the process of pressure autoregulation. Following TBI, however, pressure autoregulation can be impaired or absent, and blood flow may be more dependent on an adequate CPP. Current TBI guidelines recommend maintaining CPP at at least 60 mmHg (28,29).

DIRECT MEASUREMENT OF CEREBRAL BLOOD FLOW

Perfusion CT and Stable Xenon CT

Cerebral blood flow (CBF) can be measured directly using a diffusible or a nondiffusible indicator. Global CBF and cerebral metabolic rate of oxygen (CMRO$_2$) were first quantified by Kety and Schmidt, who used a diffusible indicator method based on the Fick principle. CBF was quantified by having the subject inhale nitrous oxide, while arterial and internal jugular blood was simultaneously sampled during the saturation phase. Another method by which to quantify CBF is the injection of contrast agents such as 133 Xenon (^{133}Xe) into the carotid artery and intravenously. The major disadvantages of this method are the invasive nature and the radioactivity of the indicator. Stable xenon has also been used to quantify CBF, with the enhancement of the CT scan image induced by xenon diffusion into the brain being used as the measurement of the tissue concentration of xenon in the Kety–Schmidt equation.

A perfusion CT study is performed by acquiring sequential images of stationary brain CT slices during intravenous administration of an iodinated contrast bolus. Analysis of the resulting contrast enhancement curves, using the central volume principle, allows calculation of three cerebral hemodynamic parameters in each pixel of the CT slice: the regional cerebral blood volume, the blood mean transit time through cerebral capillaries, and the regional CBF.

For the patient with TBI in whom CT is routinely used for anatomic imaging, stable xenon CT and CT perfusion are convenient methods for imaging regional CBF. Stable xenon CT is the more accurate quantitative measure of regional CBF, but perfusion CT is faster and easier. Incorporation of either of these methodologies with a mobile CT scanner transforms regional CBF imaging into a technology that can be used at the bedside of a critically ill patient.

A characteristic pattern of changes in CBF following TBI has been described. In the first few hours after injury, CBF is usually low (30). During this time, the CBF level correlates with outcome, with every 10 mL/100 g/min increase in global CBF being associated with a threefold increase in the probability of survival (31). CBF gradually increases following this initial period of hypoperfusion, peaking on day 2 or 3 after injury (32). CBF can also be low in and surrounding areas of contusion (33). In one recent study, the response of CBF in contused brain to treatment with induced hypertension was quite variable, with some increasing and others decreasing with treatment (34). Such a variable response has not been observed by others (35), but it illustrates the potential usefulness of measurement of regional CBF in assessing the effectiveness of treatment in individuals.

Transcranial Doppler

In 1959, Satomura and Kaneko were interested in measuring CBF; however, they were unable to bypass the bony barrier of the skull. Therefore, they concentrated their efforts on the extracranial carotid arteries. In 1982, Aaslid and colleagues, with the use of an optimized Doppler ultrasound with a lower frequency (2 MHz) and pulsed Doppler range technology, reported the first successful recordings of cerebral blood vessels (36). This technology employs ultrasound and Doppler principles and can be used to distinguish the presence or absence of flow, flow velocity (FV), and the direction of the flow. The transcranial Doppler (TCD) study is performed using a 2-MHz ultrasonic sound wave produced from one crystal of the continuous wave transducer, which is then reflected from the erythrocytes flowing in the intravascular space and received by a second crystal that generated a graphic waveform. The display indicates the depth, angle of insonation, mean FV, and pulsatility index. Flow volume is directly proportional to the FV and may be obtained by multiplying the velocity by the cross-sectional area of the vessel insonated.

Several studies have assessed the relationship between peak FV and changes in CBF, suggesting that changes in middle cerebral artery FV (mcaFV) may be used as an indicator of relative changes in blood flow. A study investigated the relationship between mcaFV and CBF as assessed by stable xenon–CT during balloon test occlusion of the carotid artery in 31 patients and found a significant correlation in the alteration of flow detected by the two methods (37). More recently, correlation has been shown between changes in mcaFV and changes in stable xenon–CT CBF in patients with various intracranial pathologies, including eight with closed-head injury, (38).

With vasospasm, FV increases through the narrowed segment proportional to the reduction in the vessel's diameter. Severe vasospasm, with a greater than 50% reduction in vessel diameter, is associated with FV greater than 200 cm/sec (39). An increase in FV may also indicate hyperemia, especially in the posttrauma setting. To differentiate between the two hemodynamic phenomena in the absence of direct CBF measurements, FV ratio of the middle cerebral artery to the extracranial internal carotid artery, also known as the Lindegaard or hemispheric index, has been used. With hyperemia, raised FV in both extracranial and intracranial vessels does not alter the ratio; however, with vasospasm, FV is high only in the intracranial vessels, resulting in a high hemispheric index. The mean hemispheric index in normal individuals is 1.76 ± 0.1, and pathologic values suggestive of vasospasm are generally above 3 (40).

Doppler devices capable of accurately measuring the diameter of the vessel that is being insonated may provide a better method by which to differentiate between these two hemodynamic causes of increased FV by calculating flow volume. Flow volume of the internal carotid artery has a close correlation to hemispheric CBF measured by the ^{133}Xe clearance technique (41) and may be useful as a bedside estimation of hemispheric CBF.

Doppler techniques may also be useful in assessing dynamic pressure autoregulation. Sudden deflation of blood pressure cuffs that have been inflated around both thighs results in a small, transient drop in blood pressure. FV in the middle cerebral artery measured immediately following the cuff deflation provides an assessment of the ability of the cerebral vasculature to compensate for this blood pressure drop. FV normally recovers more rapidly than blood pressure. If pressure autoregulation is impaired, FV recovery will parallel blood pressure recovery. Using this methodology, pressure autoregulation has been assessed serially after severe TBI. At the nadir of the impairment of pressure autoregulation at 36 to 48 hours postinjury, 87% of the patients had impaired autoregulation (42).

INDIRECT MEASURES OF CBF

Jugular Venous Oxygen Saturation

One tool for continuously monitoring global CBF adequacy is jugular venous oxygen saturation ($SjvO_2$). A fiberoptic oxygen saturation catheter is placed in the internal jugular vein so that the oxygen-sensing tip of the catheter is positioned in the jugular bulb. If cerebral oxygen delivery decreases or cerebral oxygen consumption increases, a greater amount of the total arterial oxygen content will be extracted during the transport of blood through the brain, and the outflow venous oxygen saturation will be lower. A low $SjvO_2$ value is not an indicator of a specific problem but should initiate a search for causes of reduced oxygen delivery (hypotension, intracranial hypertension, hypoxia, hypocapnia, or anemia) and/or causes of increased oxygen consumption (seizures, fever).

Two important limitations of $SjvO_2$ monitoring are that jugular venous blood may not be completely mixed with cerebral venous blood (43) and that extracerebral tissues can contribute to the blood in the jugular bulb, falsely elevating the oxygen saturation. Extracerebral contamination can be minimized but not completely eliminated by proper positioning of the catheter and slow drawing of blood through the catheter (44). Studies that compare bilateral measurements of $SjvO_2$ or that compare $SjvO_2$ with oxygen saturation in the confluence of the cerebral sinuses clearly indicate that when focal lesions are present after TBI, significant differences may be seen in the oxygen saturation between the left and right jugular bulbs (45,46). If the monitoring strategy is to use SjvO$_2$ as a monitor of global oxygenation, then cannulating the dominant jugular vein is the best choice because it will be the most representative of the whole brain. If the monitoring strategy is to identify the most abnormal oxygen saturation, then the recommendations of Metz et al. should be followed (46). Even if jugular venous blood were perfectly mixed and saturation values in the left and right jugular bulbs were always identical, it would still be unreasonable to expect that a global measure such as SjvO$_2$ could reliably detect an area of regional ischemia. Therefore, the former monitoring strategy is probably the most logical.

Normal values for SjvO$_2$ have been assessed in several studies. In a study of 50 normal young males, it was observed that their SjvO$_2$ ranged from 55% to 71% (mean of 61.8%) (47). More recent studies in which catheter placement was confirmed radiographically suggest that SjvO$_2$ in normal subjects may be even lower (52–62%; mean value 57%, with 95% confidence intervals). In patients with head injury, the average SjvO$_2$ is higher than normal and the range for SjvO$_2$ is wider than in normal subjects. In a series of 116 patients with continuous measurement of SjvO$_2$ for the first 5 to 10 days after a severe head injury (48), SjvO$_2$ averaged 68.1 ± 9.7% (range 32–96%) in 1329 measurements. Jugular venous oxygen partial pressure (PjvO$_2$) averaged 37 ± 7 mmHg (range 22–85 mmHg).

Experimental studies have extensively examined the ischemic thresholds for blood flow. In contrast, only a few studies have examined the SjvO$_2$ threshold associated with the depletion of energy stores, alterations in brain metabolism, and suppression of brain function (49–51). From the available studies, it appears that normal brain metabolism and function can be altered at SjvO$_2$ values less than 45% to 50%, but values less than 20% are required for irreversible ischemic injury to occur.

Carotid puncture is reported as the most common complication of jugular bulb catheterization, usually without any sequelae (52–54). Other adjacent structures that are susceptible to puncture are stellate ganglion, the cervical sympathetic trunk, phrenic nerve, and pleural dome. As with any intravascular catheter, the risk of bacterial colonization is directly related to catheterization duration. Thrombosis of the internal jugular vein occurs commonly with cannulation of the jugular bulb, but is usually not symptomatic (55).

Brain Tissue Oxygen Tension

Another method by which to continuously monitor CBF adequacy is placement of a partial pressure oxygen (PO$_2$) catheter directly into brain tissue. Unlike the global information obtained from a jugular bulb catheter, a PO$_2$ probe gives information about oxygenation in the brain immediately surrounding the probe. For this reason, the precise position of the PO$_2$ probe determines the nature of the data, and knowledge of the probe position is critical to accurate interpretation of the PO$_2$.

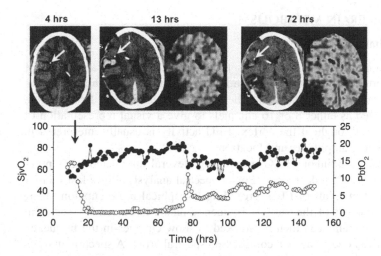

Figure 3 SjvO$_2$ (*closed circles*) and PbtO$_2$ (*open circles*) tracings from a patient who developed evolving contusions following evacuation of subdural hematoma (*surgery indicated by the black arrow*). Initially normal, PbtO$_2$ rapidly decreases postoperatively, but SjvO$_2$ remains normal. A stable xenon-CT image shows normal average cortical CBF but large areas of hypoperfusion in the right hemisphere. *Abbreviations*: SjvO$_2$, jugular venous oxygen saturation; PbtO$_2$, brain tissue oxygen tension; CBF, cerebral blood flow.

The major limitation of SjvO$_2$ as a monitor of CBF adequacy is that regional ischemia will not be identified. In circumstances such as brain trauma, in which regional differences in CBF commonly occur, the local nature of the values obtained from a PO$_2$ catheter implanted in the brain may provide an important advantage (56,57). When a PO$_2$ catheter is placed in a relatively normal area of the brain, the information obtained generally correlates with global oxygenation. However, when a PO$_2$ catheter is strategically placed in an area of interest, the values provide unique information about the surrounding tissue. The changes in brain tissue oxygen tension (PbtO$_2$) in a focal area of evolving contusions are illustrated in Figure 3. Global CBF was normal and SjvO$_2$ remained well preserved despite marked hypoperfusion in contused areas of the brain.

Because the PO$_2$ probe is an invasive monitor, limited data are available regarding brain PO$_2$ values in normal awake subjects. In anesthetized subjects, brain tissue PO$_2$ values of 20 to 40 mmHg have been recorded. Several sources suggest that PbtO$_2$ values less than 8 to 10 mmHg are abnormally low. PbtO$_2$ in patients with ischemia was found by single photoemission CT to average 10 ± 5 mmHg compared with 37 ± 12 mmHg in normal brain (58). Another group found that the likelihood of death following a severe head injury increased with increasing duration of time with PbtO$_2$ less than 15 mmHg and with any occurrence of a PbtO$_2$ less than 6 mmHg (59). Others correlated serial measurements of both SjvO$_2$ and PbtO$_2$ and found that an SjvO$_2$ of 50% in general correlates with a PbtO$_2$ of 8.5 mmHg (60).

MEASURES OF BRAIN METABOLISM

Electroencephalogram

Electroencephalogram (EEG) represents the spontaneous electrical activity of the cerebral cortex, generated by summation of excitatory and inhibitory post-synaptic potentials of cortical neurons. The electrical signal is amplified, filtered, and then displayed as either 8 or 16 channels to give a visual representation of electrical activity throughout the cortex. EEG activity is usually interpreted in terms of frequency, amplitude, and location.

To facilitate continuous EEG monitoring, several automated EEG processing systems have been developed. Power spectral analysis allows fast Fourier transformation of intervals of EEG, providing a graphical representation of the relative power content of the various frequency bands in each EEG segment. These spectral diagrams can then be stacked to show changes in the frequency content of the EEG over time as a compressed spectral array. A spectral analysis can also give a summary number, such as the mean frequency or the frequency below which 95% of the signal lies, which can be plotted over time.

Continuous EEG monitoring in patients with TBI during the first week postinjury identified the occurrence of seizure activity in more than 20% of those monitored (61). These seizures occurred despite prophylactic administration of phenytoin at therapeutic levels and were often subclinical, so that the EEG findings would have been the only clinical sign. Electrocorticography with the electrodes placed on contused brain has revealed the occurrence of waves of spreading depression in 50% of patients monitored (62). Studies are currently underway to better understand the clinical importance of these observations, but it is likely that they contribute to the secondary injury of the brain following trauma.

Microdialysis

Microdialysis is a technique widely used in animal physiology and pharmacology research. In the human brain, microdialysis monitoring has been progressively adopted as a neuromonitoring technique that can provide insight into neurophysiologic and neuropathologic events. However, as recently reviewed, application of microdialysis in the ICU remains primarily a research tool (63).

The technique consists of placing a small catheter, simulating a capillary in the brain parenchyma via a burr hole or at the time of craniectomy. The tip of the catheter is constructed of a dialysis membrane. When artificial CSF solution is slowly pumped through the catheter at a rate of 0.3 ml/min, small molecules present in the brain tissue can pass through the dialysis membrane and equilibrate with dialysate fluid in the catheter. The fluid that exits the catheter is collected and analyzed at the bedside for substrates (glucose, pyruvate), metabolites (lactate), neurotransmitters (glutamate), or other substances of interest. The use of microdialysis has enabled a better understanding of the neurochemical changes that follow TBI, such as those that occur during secondary ischemic insults.

The concentration of substances in the dialysate depends on the flow rate and chemical composition of the perfusate, the length of the dialysis membrane, the type of dialysis membrane, and the diffusion coefficient or "tortuosity" of the tissue. The recovery of a particular substance is defined as the concentration in the dialysate divided by the concentration in the interstitial fluid. If the membrane is long enough and the flow is slow enough, the concentration in the perfusate will be the same as in the interstitial fluid, i.e., the recovery rate is 100%. The parameters that are commonly used in clinical studies (10-mm membrane, perfusion with Ringer solution, and flow rate of 0.3 μL/min) provide an in vivo recovery rate (extrapolation to zero-flow method) of approximately 70% (64).

SUMMARY

Several brain-specific monitoring techniques are readily available for assessing the injured brain's physiology. Some of these techniques, such as ICP, have established roles in the management of critically ill patients with TBI. For others, such as microdialysis, it is not clear what the eventual role, if any, will be. Imaging of CBF in the ICU has just recently become possible, but it is likely to become an important tool for assessing regional CBF. The use of these neurologic monitoring techniques should be based on an understanding of the nature of the patient's brain injury, knowledge of the type of secondary injury processes that are likely to complicate the patient's course, and the characteristics of the monitoring technique.

REFERENCES

1. CDC. Traumatic Brain Injury in America. CDC 2001.
2. Menegazzi JJ, Davis EA, Sucov AN, et al. Reliability of the Glasgow Coma Scale when used by emergency physicians and paramedics. J Trauma 1993; 34(1):46–48.
3. Valadka AB, Mattox KL. Injury to the cranium. In: Mattox KL, Moore EE, eds. Trauma, 4th ed. New York: McGraw-Hill, 2000:377–399.
4. Rowley G, Fielding K. Reliability and accuracy of the Glasgow Coma Scale with experienced and inexperienced users. Lancet 1991; 337(8740):535–538.
5. Stocchetti N, Pagan F, Calappi E, et al. Inaccurate early assessment of neurological severity in head injury. J Neurotrauma 2004; 21(9):1131–1140.
6. Fountas KN, Kapsalaki EZ, Machinis TG, et al. Clinical implications of quantitative infrared pupillometry in neurosurgical patients. Neurocrit Care 2006; 5(1):55–60.
7. Meeker M, Du R, Bacchetti P, et al. Pupil examination: Validity and clinical utility of an automated pupillometer. J Neurosci Nurs 2005; 37(1):34–40.
8. Taylor WR, Chen JW, Meltzer H, et al. Quantitative pupillometry, a new technology: Normative data and preliminary observations in patients with acute head injury. Technical note. J Neurosurg 2003; 98(1):205–213.
9. Kishore PR, Lipper MH, Becker DP, et al. Significance of CT in head injury: correlation with intracranial pressure. AJR Am J Roentgenol 1981; 137(4):829–833.

10. Lundberg N. Continuous recording and control of ventricular fluid pressure in neurosurgical practice. Acta Psychiatr Neurol Scand 1960; 149(suppl 36):1–193.
11. Fortune JB, Feustel PJ, Graca L, et al. Effect of hyperventilation, mannitol, and ventriculostomy drainage on cerebral blood flow after head injury. J Trauma 1995; 39(6):1091–1097.
12. Shimbles S, Dodd C, Banister K, et al. Clinical comparison of tympanic membrane displacement with invasive intracranial pressure measurements. Physiol Meas 2005; 26(6):1085–1092.
13. Firsching R, Schutze M, Motschmann M, et al. Venous opthalmodynamometry: a noninvasive method for assessment of intracranial pressure. J Neurosurg 2000; 93(1): 33–36.
14. Michaeli D, Rappaport ZH. Tissue resonance analysis; a novel method for non-invasive monitoring of intracranial pressure. Technical note. J Neurosurg 2002; 96(6):1132–1137.
15. Ueno T, Ballard RE, Macias BR, et al. Cranial diameter pulsations measured by non-invasive ultrasound decrease with tilt. Aviat Space Environ Med 2003; 74(8):882–885.
16. Zhao YL, Zhou JY, Zhu GH. Clinical experience with the noninvasive ICP monitoring system. Acta Neurochir Suppl 2005; 95:351–355.
17. Mayhall CG, Archer NH, Lamb VA, et al. Ventriculostomy-related infections. A prospective epidemiologic study. N Engl J Med 1984; 310(9):553–559.
18. Paramore CG, Turner DA. Relative risks of ventriculostomy infection and morbidity. Acta Neurochir (Wien) 1994; 127(1–2):79–84.
19. Holloway KL, Barnes T, Choi S, et al. Ventriculostomy infections: the effect of monitoring duration and catheter exchange in 584 patients. J Neurosurg 1996; 85(3): 419–424.
20. Lozier AP, Sciacca RR, Romagnoli MF, et al. Ventriculostomy-related infections: a critical review of the literature. Neurosurgery 2002; 51(1):170–181.
21. Schade RP, Schinkel J, Roelandse FW, et al. Lack of value of routine analysis of cerebrospinal fluid for prediction and diagnosis of external drainage-related bacterial meningitis. J Neurosurg 2006; 104(1):101–108.
22. Schade RP, Schinkel J, Visser LG, et al. Bacterial meningitis caused by the use of ventricular or lumbar cerebrospinal fluid catheters. J Neurosurg 2005; 102(2): 229–234.
23. Zabramski JM, Whiting D, Darouiche RO, et al. Efficacy of antimicrobial-impregnated external ventricular drain catheters: a prospective, randomized, controlled trial. J Neurosurg 2003; 98(4):725–730.
24. Davis JW, Davis IC, Bennink LD, et al. Placement of intracranial pressure monitors: Are "normal" coagulation parameters necessary? J Trauma 2004; 57(6):1173–1177.
25. Bochicchio M, Latronico N, Zappa S, et al. Bedside burr hole for intracranial pressure monitoring performed by intensive care physicians. A 5-year experience. Intensive Care Med 1996; 22(10):1070–1074.
26. Ko K, Conforti A. Training protocol for intracranial pressure monitor placement by nonneurosurgeons: 5-year experience. J Trauma 2003; 55(3):480–483.
27. Steiner LA, Andrews PJ. Monitoring the injured brain: ICP and CBF. Br J Anaesth 2006; 97(1):26–38.
28. Bullock RM, Chesnut R, Clifton GL, et al. Management and prognosis of severe yraumatic brain injury. Part 1: guidelines for the management of severe traumatic brain injury. J Neurotrauma 2000; 17(6/7):451–553.

29. Maas AIR, Dearden M, Teasdale GM, et al. EBIC-guidelines for management of severe head injury in adults. Acta Neurochir (Wien) 1997; 139:286–294.
30. Bouma GJ, Muizelaar JP, Stringer WA, et al. Ultra-early evaluation of regional cerebral blood flow in severely head-injured patients using xenon-enhanced computerized tomography. J Neurosurg 1992; 77(3):360–368.
31. Hlatky R, Contant CF, Diaz-Marchan P, et al. Significance of a reduced CBF during the first 12 hours following traumatic brain injury. Neurocritical Care 2004; 1(1):69–84.
32. Martin NA, Patwardhan RV, Alexander MJ, et al. Characterization of cerebral hemodynamic phases following severe head he trauma: Hypoperfusion, hyperemia, and vasospasm. J Neurosurg 1997; 87(1):9–19.
33. McLaughlin MR, Marion DW. Cerebral blood flow and vasoresponsivity within and around cerebral contusions. J Neurosurg 1996; 85(5):871–876.
34. Chieregato A, Tanfani A, Compagnone C, et al. Cerebral blood flow in traumatic contusions is predominantly reduced after an induced acute elevation of cerebral perfusion pressure. Neurosurgery 2007; 60(1):115–122.
35. Johnston AJ, Steiner LA, Coles JP, et al. Effect of cerebral perfusion pressure augmentation on regional oxygenation and metabolism after head injury. Crit Care Med 2005; 33(1):189–195.
36. Aaslid R, Markwalder TM, and Nornes H. Noninvasive transcranial Doppler ultrasound recording of flow velocity in basal cerebral arteries. J Neurosurg 1982; 57(6):769–774.
37. Kofke WA, Brauer P, Policare R, et al. Middle cerebral artery blood flow velocity and stable xenon-enhanced computed tomographic blood flow during balloon test occlusion of the internal carotid artery. Stroke 1995; 26(9):1603–1606.
38. Brauer P, Kochs E, Werner C, et al. Correlation of transcranial Doppler sonography mean flow velocity with cerebral blood flow in patients with intracranial pathology. J Neurosurg Anesth 1998; 10(2):80–85.
39. Newell DW, Winn HR. Transcranial Doppler in cerebral vasospasm. Neursurg Clin N Am 1990; 1(2):316–328.
40. Lindegaard KF, Nornes H, Bakke SJ, et al. Cerebral vasospasm diagnosis by means of angiography and blood velocity measurements. Acta Neurochir (Wien) 1989; 100: 12–24.
41. Soustiel JF, Glenn TC, Vespa P, et al. Assessment of cerebral blood flow by means of blood-flow-volume measurement in the internal carotid artery: comparative study with a 133xenon clearance technique. Stroke 2003; 34(8):1876–1880.
42. Hlatky R, Furuya Y, Valadka AB, et al. Dynamic autoregulatory response after severe head injury. J Neurosurg 2002; 97(5):1054–1061.
43. Beards SC, Yule S, Kassner A, et al. Anatomical variation of cerebral venous drainage: the theoretical effect on jugular bulb blood samples. Anaesthesia 1998; 53(7):627–633.
44. Matta BF, Lam AM. The rate of blood withdrawal affects the accuracy of jugular venous bulb. Oxygen saturation measurements. Anesthesiology 1997; 86(4): 806–808.
45. Stocchetti N, Paparella A, Bridelli F, et al. Cerebral venous oxygen saturation studied using bilateral samples in the jugular veins. Neurosurgery 1994; 34(1):38–44.
46. Metz C, Holzschuh M, Bein T, et al. Monitoring of cerebral oxygen metabolism in the jugular bulb: reliability of unilateral measurements in severe head injury. J Cereb Blood Flow Metab 1998; 18(3):332–343.

47. Gibbs EL, Lennox WG, Nims LF, et al. Arterial and cerebral venous blood. Arterial-venous differences in man. J Biol Chem 1942; 144:325–332.
48. Gopinath SP, Robertson CS, Contant CF, et al. Jugular venous desaturation and outcome after head injury. J Neurol Neurosurg Psych 1994; 57(6):717–723.
49. Sutton LN, McLaughlin AC, Dante S, et al. Cerebral venous oxygen content as a measure of brain energy metabolism with increased intracranial pressure and hyperventilation. J Neurosurg 1990; 73(6):927–932.
50. Sapire KJ, Gopinath SP, Farhat G, et al. Cerebral oxygenation during warming after cardiopulmonary bypass. Crit Care Med 1997; 25(10):1655–1662.
51. Cruz J. On-line monitoring of global cerebral hypoxia in acute brain injury: relationship to intracranial hypertension. J Neurosurg 1993; 79(2):228–233.
52. Goetting MG, Preston G. Jugular bulb catheterization: experience with 123 patients. Crit Care Med 1990; 18(11):1220–1223.
53. Stocchetti N, Barbagallo M, Gordon CR, et al. Arterio-jugular difference of oxygen and intracranial pressure in comatose, head injured patients. I. Technical aspects and complications. Minerva Anestesiol 1991; 57(6):319–326.
54. Gemma M, Beretta L, De VA, et al. Complications of internal jugular vein retrograde catheterization. Acta Neurochir Suppl 1998; 71:320–323.
55. Coplin WM, O'Keefe GE, Grady MS, et al. Thrombotic, infectious, and procedural complications of the jugular bulb catheter in the intensive care unit. Neurosurgery 1997; 41(1):101–107.
56. Dings J, Meixensberger J, Roosen K. Brain tissue pO_2-monitoring: catheter stability and complications. Neurol Res 1997; 19(3):241–245.
57. Zauner A, Doppenberg E, Woodward JJ, et al. Multiparametric continuous monitoring of brain metabolism and substrate delivery in neurosurgical patients. Neurol Res 1997; 19(3):265–273.
58. Hoffman WE, Charbel FT, Edelman G. Brain tissue oxygen, carbon dioxide, and pH in neurosurgical patients at risk for ischemia. Anesth Analg 1996; 82(3):582–586.
59. Valadka A, Gopinath SP, Contant CF, et al. Relationship of brain tissue PO_2 to outcome after severe head injury. Crit Care Med 1998; 26(9):1576–1581.
60. Kiening KL, Unterberg AW, Bardt TF, et al. Monitoring of cerebral oxygenation in patients with severe head injuries: brain tissue PO_2 versus jugular vein oxygen saturation. J Neurosurg 1996; 85(5):751–757.
61. Vespa PM, Nuwer MR, Nenov V, et al. Increased incidence and impact of nonconvulsive and convulsive seizures after traumatic brain injury as detected by continuous electroencephalographic monitoring. J Neurosurg 1999; 91(5):750–760.
62. Fabricius M, Fuhr S, Bhatia R, et al. Cortical spreading depression and peri-infarct depolarization in acutely injured human cerebral cortex. Brain 2006; 129(pt 3): 778–790.
63. Hillered L, Vespa PM, and Hovda DA. Translational neurochemical research in acute human brain injury: The current status and potential future for cerebral microdialysis. J Neurotrauma 2005; 22(1):3–41.
64. Hutchinson PJ, O'Connell MT, Al-Rawi PG, et al. Clinical cerebral microdialysis—determining the true extracellular concentration. Acta Neurochir Suppl 2002; 81: 359–362.

5

Hypothermia and Pharmacologic Coma in the Treatment of Traumatic Brain Injury

Gordon Li, MD, Resident
Shivanand P. Lad, MD, PhD, Resident
Roland A. Torres, MD, Clinical Professor
Department of Neurosurgery, Stanford University School of Medicine, Palo Alto, California, U.S.A.

Gary K. Steinberg, MD, PhD, Professor[a] and Chairman[b]

[a]Bernard and Ronni Lacroute-William Randolph Hearst Professor of Neurosurgery and the Neurosciences, [b]Department of Neurosurgery, Stanford University School of Medicine, Palo Alto, California, U.S.A.

Traumatic brain injury (TBI) is a leading cause of trauma morbidity and mortality with an estimated 10 million people experiencing head injuries worldwide each year (1). In the United States, TBI accounts for approximately 1% of all injuries and annual visits to the emergency department, with an estimated 1.9 million cases per year. Of this number,

- approximately 800,000 receive only outpatient care
- approximately 270,000 require hospital admission
- mortality is greater than 60,000
- approximately 80,000 adults and children are permanently disabled each year

Most patients with TBI are young, healthy males; therefore, TBI constitutes the leading cause of morbidity and mortality in this patient population. In addition, TBIs account for as much as 50% of all deaths from acute injuries. In the United States direct costs are estimated at $4 billion annually, with indirect costs approximately 10 times that amount (2). Preventative measures have reduced the overall death rate from TBI; however, no equivalent effective therapy has been shown to reduce mortality and improve neurologic outcome once the injury has occurred. Current treatment modals include hyperventilation, osmotherapy (mannitol and/or hypertonic saline), drainage of cerebrospinal fluid, pharmacologic coma, decompressive craniectomy, and therapeutic hypothermia (3). The roles of hypothermia and pharmacologic coma in the treatment of TBI will be evaluated in this chapter.

HYPOTHERMIA FOR TREATMENT OF TBI

The therapeutic potential of hypothermia to treat TBI was first noted by Hippocrates (460–377 BCE), who advocated that wounded patients be packed in snow and ice to prevent hemorrhage. He stated that ''a man will survive longer in winter than in summer, whatever be the part of the head in which the wound is situated'' (3). Napoleon's surgeon general, Baron Dominique Larrey, during the retreat from Russia in the winter of 1812, used refrigeration by ice and snow to alleviate wounded soldiers' pain during amputations. He also observed that injured patients who were hypothermic and put close to a fire died more rapidly than those who remained hypothermic. The first clinical application was reported in 1938 by Fay, who cooled metastatic cancer patients to 27°C and noted tumor shrinkage and pain relief (4). This report was followed in the 1940s by the research of Wilfred Bigelow, who initiated cardiac surgery and hypothermia (predating the bypass machine). Induced hypothermia (IH) was first used in clinical practice as an adjunct to TBI therapy by Fay over 50 years ago (5,6). Between 1950 and 1960, several (uncontrolled) series were reported in which IH was included in the management of patients with TBI (6–9). Ultimately, this research led to the widespread use of hypothermia in cardiothoracic and neurosurgical patients for neuroprotection. Unfortunately, patients were cooled to 15°C to 22°C (deep hypothermia), which led to systemic complications. Although IH is still commonly used for neurologic protection during cardiac surgery (9), deep hypothermia for neuroprotection during neurosurgical procedures was abandoned in the 1960s because of perceived problems of sepsis, cardiac dysrhythmias, and coagulopathy. While deep hypothermia with total circulatory arrest is still occasionally used for select giant intracranial aneurysm cases, mild-to-moderate hypothermia is more frequently utilized in patients who undergo cerebrovascular surgery rather than in those with severe TBI.

BENEFITS OF HYPOTHERMIA

Animal studies and early single-centered randomized trials showed encouraging results; however, hypothermia as a treatment for TBI remains controversial (3). A recent, large, multicentered randomized trial and meta-analysis of the multiple hypothermia trials have not supported earlier smaller trials or animal data (10).

Nevertheless, a recent survey of the Neuroanaesthesia Society of Great Britain and Ireland showed that 41% of respondents induced mild or moderate hypothermia in patients with head injury (11).

MECHANISM

The mechanism(s) of hypothermic protection is debatable and likely multifactorial. Primarily, it had been thought to be a result of reduced cerebral metabolic rate: for each 1°C decrease in temperature, the cerebral metabolic rate decreases by 6% to 7% (12). A decrease in metabolic rate leads to decreased oxygen and glucose demand and decreased hypoxemia and ischemia. However, TBI animal model data suggest other possible mechanisms, including reduced blood-brain barrier dysfunction with decreased extravasation of hemoglobin following TBI (13), reduction in cerebral edema (14), reduction in levels of excitatory neurotransmitters and free radical production (15), reduced inflammatory response (16), and decreased intracranial pressure (ICP) (3).

INDICATIONS AND TECHNIQUE

Precisely, how hypothermia should be used to treat TBI is an issue of debate. In randomized trials, patients with severe TBI defined as a Glasgow Coma Scale (GCS) score of less than or equal to 8 were chosen (1,2). Trials to date have excluded those younger than 16 years or those older than 65 years. Patients with severe cardiac instability of other severe multisystem trauma are also excluded. All patients had ICP monitoring, and ICP was kept less than or equal to 25 mmHg in most trials. Cerebral perfusion was greater than 70 mmHg, and appropriate paralytics and pain medications were administered. The trials had heterogeneity regarding the temperature to which patients were cooled, the onset of cooling, the duration of cooling, and the speed at which they were rewarmed. Some studies cooled patients to 32°C–33°C, while other studies cooled patients to 33°C–34°C (1,2). In some studies, patients were cooled as early as six hours postinjury and reached a target temperature at approximately eight hours postinjury, but the ranges of these data varied widely between studies and even between centers within the same study. While some studies cooled patients for 24 hours, others cooled patients for 48 hours, and some cooled patients for 48 hours and kept them cool until the ICP normalized (1,2).

COMPLICATIONS

Risks of hypothermia include hypotension, sepsis, pneumonia, renal failure, potassium fluxes, coagulation abnormalities, and possible myocardial infarction and atrial fibrillation (2,3). However, experimental data show less chance of complications with temperatures greater than or equal to 32°C (17); therefore, most of the recent clinical trials have cooled patients to no lower than 32°C (1,2).

Controversies Regarding Efficacy

After animal studies and early observations from several small randomized clinical trials demonstrated improved survival and neurologic outcome results with mild-to-moderate hypothermia (18–21), a large, multicentered randomized controlled trial was undertaken [National Acute Brain Injury Study: Hypothermia (NABIS:H)] (10). However, the NABIS:H study was terminated after enrollment of 392 of the planned 500 patients, when the study showed no difference in neurologic outcomes after six months. Patients were treated with either moderate hypothermia (33°C) within eight hours of injury or kept at normal temperature (37°C). Thirty-eight percent of the patients were randomized with waiver of consent. Although ICP was lower in patients who were treated with hypothermia, these patients stayed in the hospital longer because of complications such as pneumonia. No difference in overall mortality or neurologic outcome was noted. Since the NABIS:H study, three meta-analysis studies have evaluated the role of hypothermia in TBI. One meta-analysis study suggests an overall beneficial effect from moderate hypothermia in the treatment of severe TBI (22), while two other meta-analyses (2,23) and a Cochrane database review (1) concluded that no benefit results.

In 2002, Polderman suggested that variability in the management of complications such as hypotension, fluids, electrolytes, and medications among the 11 centers involved in the NABIS:H trial may have contributed to poor results. Polderman, in his own randomized prospective clinical trial of 136 patients who suffered severe head injuries, was able to conclude that "artificial cooling can significantly improve survival and neurologic outcome in patients with severe head injury when used in a protocol with great attention to the prevention of side effects" (24).

In some experimental brain injury models, hypothermia must be initiated within 90 minutes of injury to have any effect (14). The most likely explanation for the negative effect of hypothermia in the NABIS:H study was that the intervention was initiated too late following the initial injury, with hypothermia achieved after the window of therapeutic effectiveness. Post hoc analysis revealed a sensitive subgroup of patients who benefited from hypothermia: those who were aged 16 to 45, had an admission GCS of three to eight and were hypothermic on admission with temperatures less than or equal to_35°C. In this subgroup, those subjects randomized to hypothermia showed a 24% decrease in the absolute percentage of poor outcome ($n = 81$; normothermia, 76% poor outcome; hypothermia, 52%; $p = 0.02$). The outcome measure was based on the dichotomized Glasgow Outcome Scale. Improvement was due to a shift of patients from a severe disability category (poor outcome) to a moderate disability category (good outcome), with no change in the percentages of vegetative or dead categories. Based on these findings, NABIS:H II was approved and funded by the National Institutes of Neurologic Disorders and Stroke in 2001. Enrollment in NABIS:H II was suspended, and a feasibility trial of early cooling was initiated at the Houston and Calgary study centers in October 2004 and January 2005, respectively, and successfully completed by August 2005 (personal communication).

NABIS:H IIR was developed as a result of the data obtained in 2005. It is a National Institutes of Health randomized clinical trial of 240 patients with severe TBI (GCS, 3–8), aged 16 to 45. In the summer of 2006, patients who were accessed within two hours of injury were randomized to hypothermia or normothermia. The objective of the protocol was to test the effect of very early mild hypothermia followed by more prolonged moderate hypothermia on patients with severe brain injury (personal communication).

DISCUSSION

Despite numerous studies much debate remains over the role of hypothermia in treating TBI (1–3,22,23). Significant heterogeneity between the studies and institutions performing the trials may explain the contradictions. For instance, larger institutions/hospitals more adept at handling hypothermia had better outcomes. Some hospitals were better at randomizing patients with timely protocols. Moreover, specific subsets of patients fared better than others. For example, certain studies revealed that patients who arrived cool (<35°C) did better than those who did not. Patients initially presenting with GCS of three to four did not improve with hypothermia, while patients with an initial GCS of five to seven experienced improved neurologic outcome (10). Different studies cooled patients to different temperatures. For example, the Clifton study in 2001 cooled patients down to 33°C, while the Shiozaki study cooled patients to between 34°C and 35°C (2). Animal studies revealed that the cooler the temperature, the more protective the treatment. For example, sheep studies have shown that cooling down to 34°C is more protective than 36°C (normothermia for sheep is 39°C) (25). However, the possibility of greater protection must be balanced with the higher chance of complications as the patient is cooled to a lower temperature. The time at which the target temperature was reached also varied. Animal studies in gerbils, sheep, and rats showed that adverse outcome was prevented by hypothermia only if cooling was achieved within two to six hours of the injury (26–28). Cooling (normothermia of 39–34°C) of sheep for 72 hours was protective if achieved within 90 minutes, partially effective if achieved within 5.5 hours, and ineffective if achieved within 8.5 hours. The large multicentered trial did not reach the target temperature until an average of 8.4 hours postinjury (10). Achieving early hypothermia in brain-injured patients has been problematic in the past because of the risk of early hypothermia induction causing increased bleeding complications in patients with unrecognized multisystem trauma. Another problem has been the requirement to delay randomization while attempts were made to obtain family consent for research. One other variable not well controlled was the duration of cooling. As mentioned earlier, some trials cooled for 24 hours, some for 48 hours, and others for a minimum of 48 hours without rewarming until the ICP was normalized. As part of the protective effect of hypothermia for TBI may be secondary to decreased ICP, cooling until the ICP normalizes seems rational.

Currently, hypothermia is not recommended for treatment of TBI, as the large, multicentered randomized trial and meta-analyses data do not support it. In fact, hypothermia is shown to increase hospitalization length and increase chance of pneumonia, hypotension, and other complications. However, hypothermia for TBI is still controversial, as many early studies and experimental trials were very encouraging, and further trials are needed to determine if different cooling parameters or different TBI subgroups will respond better to hypothermia. Outcomes in some of these studies were influenced by depth and duration of hypothermia and rate of rewarming ($\leq$24 hours) after discontinuation of hypothermia.

Future trials should target larger centers that are more adept at reaching cooler temperatures more quickly. Results from various population subsets, including initial GCS of patient, age, and initial temperature should be evaluated. Patients should also be cooled for 48 hours, and then rewarmed only when the ICP normalizes. Further improvements in outcome may be possible if IH could be used for longer periods, but the effects of prolonged IH have not been well described in the literature. Significant improvement in survival and neurologic outcome for patients with severe head injury may also derive from a protocol with a strict focus on the prevention of side effects (24).

PHARMACOLOGIC COMA FOR TREATMENT OF TRAUMATIC BRAIN INJURY

Approximately 10% to 15% of all patients with TBIs will develop intractable intracranial hypertension i.e., elevated ICP resistant to standard forms of treatment (sedation, paralysis, hyperventilation, hypothermia, cerebrospinal fluid drainage, osmotic diuretics, and surgery). The use of pharmacologic coma to treat refractory elevations in ICP began in the 1970s with Shapiro and colleagues examining the use of pentobarbital and hypothermia to control high ICP (29). This early work laid the foundation for a number of subsequent randomized research studies. In general, no differences in outcome or mortality between barbiturate coma and control groups were noted, although hypotension occurred more frequently in the pentobarbital-treated group (30–32). The use of barbiturate-induced coma for the management of intractable intracranial hypertension remains controversial. The assessment of the therapeutic value of barbiturates in patients with intractable intracranial hypertension is difficult. Many of the trials in the literature are nonblinded and nonrandomized, and it is difficult to make comparisons between these trials because of differences in conventional treatments used, measurements of outcomes, and types and doses of barbiturates.

The Guidelines for the Management of Severe Head Injury (33) suggest that the use of high-dose barbiturate therapy should be considered in the hemodynamically stable patient with elevated ICP that is refractory to all other medical and surgical treatment. A randomized study in 1988 examined the use of pento-barbital in patients with refractory ICP who had exhausted all first-tier treatment, including hyperventilation, mannitol, decompressive hemicraniectomies, and cerebrospinal fluid diversion (34). The pentobarbital treatment group was com-pared to a control group that received standard therapies. Refractory ICP was defined as (*i*) an ICP greater than 25 mmHg for 30 minutes, greater than 30 mmHg for 15 minutes, or greater than 40 mmHg for 1 minute in closed skulls, and (*ii*) an ICP greater than 15 mmHg for 15 minutes, greater than 20 mmHg for 10 minutes, or greater than 30 mmHg for 1 minute in decompressed skulls. The dosing for the study included a vigorous regimen: 10 mg/kg IV over 30 minutes, 5 mg/kg IV over 60 minutes × 3, then 1 mg/kg/hr. Of the 925 patients eligible for the study, only 12% met the ICP inclusion thresholds. Results of the study showed that patients who were treated with barbiturates had a twofold increase in successful control of ICP when compared to the standard treatment group. Cardiac complications (e.g., presence of hypotension or hypertension prerandomization) negatively impacted outcomes in the groups. In the absence of cardiac complications, the pento-barbital group showed a fourfold increase in successful control compared with the group of patients with cardiac complications.

Another study retrospectively examined 21 head-injured patients who had failed conventional ICP management and required barbiturate coma; 67% of the patients regained control of ICP (35). Patients with ICP control in a barbiturate coma had a 71% survival rate compared with 14% survival in the group of patients who did not maintain ICP control. A number of studies have demon-strated the ability of barbiturate coma to lower refractory ICP, and therefore resulted in this therapy becoming an adjunctive therapy in the overall treatment of the TBI patient. However, in a prospective-controlled study, investigators concluded that no improvement in survivability was achieved with the use of barbiturate-induced coma (32). To effectively use this modal, a good under-standing of mechanisms of action, dosing protocol, potential adverse effects, and monitoring strategies is needed.

Mechanism

Since the 1930s it has been known that high-dose barbiturates are effective in reducing ICP. The two most commonly used barbiturates for the production of barbiturate-induced coma are thiopental and pentobarbital. Barbiturates reduce ICP by decreasing cerebral blood flow (CBF), cerebral metabolic usage of oxygen ($CMRO_2$), and cerebral glucose by up to 50%, and by acting as a free oxygen radical scavenger (29,35,36). As the barbiturate load increases, the conductance of GABA-regulating chloride channels is increased, and the wave and frequency distribution in the electroencephalogram (EEG) is altered, effectively decreasing neuronal activity. The decrease in EEG activity produces burst suppression, where the EEG has bursts of activity followed by periods of isoelectric activity. The goal in barbiturate-induced coma is to achieve periods of absent EEG activity from 6 to 10 seconds, with three to five bursts of EEG activity per minute. Barbiturates can also alter cerebrovascular tone and inhibit free radical-mediated lipid peroxidation. However, high-dose barbiturate therapy is associated with a number of potential adverse effects, including hypotension, myocardial depression, direct vasodilatation, decrease in immune response, and reduction in jugular venous oxygen saturation. The most common adverse side effect is hypotension, with approximately 25% of patients under barbiturate-induced coma becoming markedly hypotensive.

Pentobarbital is one of the more frequently used drugs to induce barbiturate coma. Pentobarbital has a rapid onset of action, prolonged effect on CBF, metabolic rate, and ICP, and is seen by some to be safer than thiopental because of a more gradual impact on the cardiovascular system. Injection of pentobarbital produces an effect in the central nervous system within 10 to 60 seconds, with a half-life of 20 hours (37). Monitoring the effects of the barbiturate-induced coma includes regularly assessing physiologic parameters and following serum drug levels. Pentobarbital doses are to be adjusted to maintain serum levels of 3 mg/dL.

Through induction of the hepatic microsomal cytochrome P450 system, pentobarbital increases the metabolism of multiple compounds. Among these are other anticonvulsant medications such as warfarin, steroids, metoprolol, and vitamin K. Concurrent administration of other central nervous system depressants will potentiate the sedative, respiratory, and hemodynamic effects of pentobarbital (38,39).

Indications, Techniques, and Complications

A number of regimens are used for dosing pentobarbital to produce barbiturate-induced coma. One commonly used regimen includes the following: a loading dose of 10 mg/kg IV over 30 minutes, followed by 5 mg/kg IV over 60 min × 3 doses, a maintenance dose of 1 to 3 mg/kg/hr adjusted for optimal ICP control, a titration dose to maintain EEG-burst suppression at 3 to 5 bursts/min, and measurement of serum pentobarbital level in the 3%–4 mg% range (40).

Patients require continuous ICP monitoring because of the loss of neurologic examination as a result of the barbiturate effect and EEG monitoring. Barbiturate infusion is titrated to maintain a burst-suppression pattern on EEG. Patients often require invasive cardiovascular monitoring, including central venous and pulmonary artery catheters to monitor intravascular volume and cardiac function because of myocardial suppression. Although brain tissue oxygen requirements are lowered with barbiturate coma, a brain oxygenation monitor (LICOX) should also be placed to ensure adequate oxygenation. The escalation of critical care and complications associated with the use of barbiturates can mean costly therapy. For every four patients treated, one may become hypotensive, requiring aggressive cardiovascular support (38).

DISCUSSION

Barbiturate therapy is utilized as a treatment for those patients in whom ICP remains refractory to other treatments. Many of the randomized trials that examined barbiturate therapy were conducted in the 1980s and 1990s when standard intensive care management differed significantly from today's practice (39). Variations in dosing regimens and outcome measurements also contributed to the wide variability in results. At that time, for example, the profound adverse effect of even a single episode of systemic hypotension on neurologic outcome was not well recognized, and this may have contributed to increased mortality in barbiturate-treated patients. The contemporary relevance of these studies is therefore unclear (39). In summary, no evidence supports prophylactic high-dose barbiturate therapy. Barbiturates are often used to control refractory intracranial hypertension, but side effects are significant, and there is no definitive evidence to support improved neurologic outcomes.

CONCLUSION AND FUTURE DIRECTIONS

While experimental studies and early single-centered randomized trials have demonstrated encouraging results hypothermia as a treatment for TBI remains controversial at this juncture. At present, hypothermia is not recommended for treatment of TBI, as the large, multicentered randomized trial and meta-analyses data do not demonstrate efficacy. Future trials should take into account important variables such as methods to reach cooler temperatures more rapidly and optimal duration of IH. Barbiturate therapy continues to be utilized as a therapeutic modality in patients with refractory intracranial hypertension.

REFERENCES

1. Alderson P, Gadkary C, Signorini DF. Therapeutic hypothermia for head injury. Cochrane Database Syst Rev. 2004; (4):CD001048 (review).
2. Harris OA, Colford JM Jr., Good MC, et al. The role of hypothermia in the management of severe brain injury: a meta-analysis. Arch Neurol 2002; 59(7):1077–1083.
3. Adamides AA, Winter CD, Lewis PM, et al. Current controversies in the management of patients with severe traumatic brain injury. ANZ J Surg 2006; 76(3):163–174.
4. Fay T. Early experiences with local and generalized refrigeration of the human brain. J Neurosurg 1959; 16(3):239–259 (discussion 259–260).
5. Fay T. Observations on prolonged human refrigeration. N Y St J Med 1940; 40: 1351–1354.
6. Fay T. Observations on generalized refrigeration in cases of severe cerebral trauma. Res Publ Assoc Nerv Dis 1945; 4:611–619.
7. Lazorthes G, Campan L. Hypothermia in the treatment of craniocerebral traumatism. J Neurosurg 1958; 15:162–168.
8. Sedzimir CB. Therapeutic hypothermia in cases of head injury. J Neurosurg 1959; 16:407–414.

9. Hendrick EB. The use of hypothermia in severe head injuries in childhood. Ann Surg 1959; 79:362–364.

10. Clifton GL, Miller ER, Choi SC, et al. Lack of effect of induction of hypothermia after acute brain injury. N Engl J Med 2001; 344(8):556–563.

11. Pemberton PL, Dinsmore J. The use of hypothermia as a method of neuroprotection during neurosurgical procedures and after traumatic brain injury: a survey of clinical practice in Great Britain and Ireland. Anaesthesia 2003; 58(4):370–373.

12. Rosomoff HL, Holaday DA. Cerebral blood flow and cerebral oxygen consumption during hypothermia. Am J Physiol 1954; 179(1):85–88.

13. Smith SL, Hall ED. Mild pre- and posttraumatic hypothermia attenuates blood-brain barrier damage following controlled cortical impact injury in the rat. J Neurotrauma 1996; 13(1):1–9.

14. Markgraf CG, Clifton GL, Moody MR. Treatment window for hypothermia in brain injury. J Neurosurg 2001; 95(6):979–983.

15. Globus MY, Alonso O, Dietrich WD, et al. Glutamate release and free radical production following brain injury: effects of posttraumatic hypothermia. J Neurochem 1995; 65(4):1704–1711.

16. Chatzipanteli K, Alonso OF, Kraydieh S, et al. Importance of posttraumatic hypothermia and hyperthermia on the inflammatory response after fluid percussion brain injury: Biochemical and immunocytochemical studies. J Cereb Blood Flow Metab 2000; 20(3):531–542.

17. Michenfelder JD, Terry HR, Daw EF, et al. Induced hypothermia: Physiological effects, indications and techniques. Surg Clin North Am 1965; 45:889–898.

18. Jiang J, Yu M, Zhu C. Effect of long-term mild hypothermia therapy in patients with severe traumatic brain injury: 1-year follow-up review of 87 cases. J Neurosurg 2000; 93(4):546–549.

19. Marion DW, Penrod LE, Kelsey SF, et al. Treatment of traumatic brain injury with moderate hypothermia. N Engl J Med 1997; 336(8):540–546.

20. Clifton GL, Allen S, Barrodale P, et al. A phase II study of moderate hypothermia in severe brain injury. J Neurotrauma 1993; 10(3):263–271 (discussion 273).

21. Shiozaki T, Sugimoto H, Taneda M, et al. Effect of mild hypothermia on uncontrollable intracranial hypertension after severe head injury. J Neurosurg 1993; 79(3):363–368.

22. McIntyre LA, Fergusson DA, Hebert PC, et al. Prolonged therapeutic hypothermia after traumatic brain injury in adults: a systematic review. JAMA 2003; 289(22):2992–2999.

23. Henderson WR, Dhingra VK, Chittock DR, et al. Hypothermia in the management of traumatic brain injury. A systematic review and meta-analysis. Intensive Care Med 2003; 29(10):1637–1644.

24. Polderman KH, Tjong Tjin Joe R, Peerdeman SM, et al. Effects of therapeutic hypothermia on intracranial pressure and outcome in patients with severe head injury. Intensive Care Med 2002; 28(11):1563–73.

25. Shann F. Hypothermia for traumatic brain injury: how soon, how cold, and how long? Lancet 2003; 362(9400):1950–1951.

26. Colbourne F, Li H, Buchan AM. Indefatigable CA1 sector neuroprotection with mild hypothermia induced 6 hours after severe forebrain ischemia in rats. J Cereb Blood Flow Metab 1999; 19(7):742–749.

27. Colbourne F, Auer RN, Sutherland GR. Behavioral testing does not exacerbate ischemic CA1 damage in gerbils. Stroke 1998; 29(9):1967–1970 (discussion 1971).

28. Gunn AJ. Cerebral hypothermia for prevention of brain injury following perinatal asphyxia. Curr Opin Pediatr 2000; 12(2):111–115.
29. Shapiro HM, Wyte SR, Loeser J. Barbiturate-augmented hypothermia for reduction of persistent intracranial hypertension. J Neurosurg 1974; 40(1):90–100.
30. Saul TG, Ducker TB. Effect of intracranial pressure monitoring and aggressive treatment on mortality in severe head injury. J Neurosurg 1982; 56(4):498–503.
31. Schwartz ML, Tator CH, Rowed DW, et al. The University of Toronto head injury treatment study: a prospective, randomized comparison of pentobarbital and mannitol. Can J Neurol Sci 1984; 11(4):434–440.
32. Ward JD, Becker DP, Miller JD, et al. Failure of prophylactic barbiturate coma in the treatment of severe head injury. J Neurosurg 1985; 62(3):383–388.
33. Brain Trauma Foundation. Prognosis of Severe Traumatic Brain Injury: Part 1 Guidelines for the Management of Severe Brain Trauma and Part 2 Early Indicators of Prognosis in Severe Traumatic Brain Injury, 2000.
34. Eisenberg HM, Frankowski RF, Contant CF, et al. High-dose barbiturate control of elevated intracranial pressure in patients with severe head injury. J Neurosurg 1988; 69(1):15–23.
35. Lee MW, Deppe SA, Sipperly ME, et al. The efficacy of barbiturate coma in the management of uncontrolled intracranial hypertension following neurosurgical trauma. J Neurotrauma 1994; 11(3):325–331.
36. Nordstrom CH, Messeter K, Nordström CH, et al. Cerebral blood flow, vasoreactivity, and oxygen consumption during barbiturate therapy in severe traumatic brain lesions. J Neurosurg 1988; 68(3):424–431.
37. Winer JW, Rosenwasser RH, Jimenez F. Electroencephalographic activity and serum and cerebrospinal fluid pentobarbital levels in determining the therapeutic end point during barbiturate coma. Neurosurgery 1991; 29(5):739–741 (discussion 741–742).
38. Feen ES, Suarez JI. Raised intracranial pressure. Curr Treat Options Neurol 2005; 7(2):109–117.
39. Roberts I. Barbiturates for acute traumatic brain injury. Cochrane Database Syst Rev, 2000(2):CD000033.
40. Bader MK, Arbour R, Palmer S. Refractory increased intracranial pressure in severe traumatic brain injury: barbiturate coma and bispectral index monitoring. AACN Clin Issues 2005; 16(4):526–541.

6

Pediatric Traumatic Brain Injury

Zachary N. Litvack, MD, Senior Resident

*Department of Neurological Surgery,
Oregon Health & Science University, Portland, Oregon, U.S.A.*

Nathan R. Selden, MD, PhD, FACS, FAAP, Associate Professor[a], Vice-Chairman[b], and Head[c]

[a]*Mario and Edith Campagna Associate Professor,* [b]*Education and Program Director,* [c]*Division of Pediatric Neurosurgery, and Department of Neurological Surgery, Oregon Health & Science University, Portland, Oregon, U.S.A.*

INTRODUCTION

Traumatic brain injury (TBI) represents one of the leading causes of injury, hospitalization, and death among pediatric patients. The U.S. Centers for Disease Control and Prevention estimates 475,000 children (younger than 14 years) sustain TBI each year, resulting in 37,000 hospital admissions and over 2600 deaths (1). Young male children (younger than 4 years) have the highest combined prevalence of TBI (1353/100,000) that results in emergency department visits, hospitalization, or death of any subgroup in the U.S. population. However, within the pediatric population, adolescents have the highest incidence of death (24.3/100,000) because of TBI (1).

The average length of stay for a TBI admission is 4.5 days, with an average cost of approximately $20,000 (2). In a single year, pediatric hospitalizations for TBI consumed over 1 billion health care dollars. However, the true cost of childhood TBI is largely unknown. When factoring in long-term effects on learning, cognition, and behavior, which consume further health care, rehabilitation, and education resources, the true economic burden of pediatric TBI is estimated at $20 billion/yr (3). Despite the economic and social burden of pediatric TBI, public funding for research is extremely limited, representing less than 1% of the economic burden of the disease (4,5).

In 2003, after multidisciplinary review of the existing literature, the evidence-based "Guidelines for the acute medical management of severe traumatic brain injury in infants, children, and adolescents" (The Guidelines) were published (6). Despite inclusion of over 350 class I–III studies and reviews and exclusion of thousands more, only six treatment guidelines (Class II) and no treatment standards (Class I) were formulated, suggesting that pediatric neurotrauma research remains an emerging field. In this chapter, recent research into TBI treatment paradigms will be reviewed, particularly that which has changed our understanding of traumatic injury to the developing brain.

PLASTICITY AND RESPONSE TO INJURY

It is a common but inaccurate belief that children with TBI have a better chance for recovery than do adults with the same injury. In contrast to the correlation between young age and positive outcome from TBI in the adult population, a discontinuity exists between age and outcome in children. Subgroups within the pediatric population have varying mechanisms for injury, response to injury, and potential for recovery. A review of the Trauma Coma Databank demonstrates a nonlinear relationship between age and outcome in children: infants and toddlers (aged 0–4 years) have the worst outcomes for a given injury, while children (aged 5–10 years) have the best outcomes (5,7).

Some of this discontinuity may be attributed to the unique mechanism of and response to nonaccidental trauma seen in patients younger than 4 years. For example, children exposed to nonaccidental TBI may suffer from sudden, secondary, and often catastrophic edema of one or both hemispheres ("black brain" syndrome) (8) (Fig. 1). Anecdotally, this event may occur in the presence of acute subdural blood over the cerebral hemispheric surface, even in the case of very thin subdural collections with relatively limited mass effect (9). However, the efficacy of subdural hematoma evacuation and other surgical or medical interventions to prevent black brain syndrome are unknown.

Most existing models of TBI and cognitive measures of recovery inadequately represent the dynamic state of brain development in children. It is not enough to target treatment and recovery to preinjury baseline in a child, as "the baseline function of normal peers has already moved on" (10). Injury to functional brain areas that are not yet developed may falsely mask the severity of injury until months to years later, when the child shows impairment in executive function, higher-level cognitive function, and school performance compared with his or her peers. Thus, unlike in adult patients, the full effects of a pediatric TBI may not be fully apparent at the time of injury (5,10).

The Central Role of the *N*-Methyl-D-Aspartic Acid Receptor

Only recently has a potential mechanistic explanation emerged for this paradoxic response to injury in children. A role for glutamate in posttraumatic neurotoxicity has been identified in adults. Mechanical disruption of cell membranes,

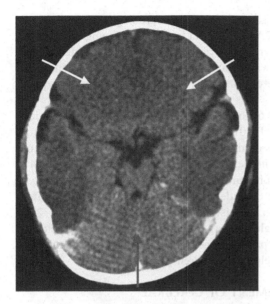

Figure 1 Noncontrast CT of a six-month-old female showing diffuse global hypodensity of the cerebral hemispheres (*solid arrows*). Imaging was performed less than two hours after initial evaluation for nonaccidental injury. By contrast, the cerebellum is relatively spared (*open arrows*). This radiographic pattern of so-called "black brain" syndrome is known as the "cerebellar-reversal" sign *Abbreviation*: CT, computer tomography.

with secondary alteration in energy-dependent cell transport (due either to hypoxia or hypotension or to both) may release toxic doses of glutamate into the extracellular space, damaging surrounding neurons (11,12). Discovery of glutamate excitotoxicity in TBI also provided a therapeutic target, leading to multiple subsequent clinical trials of N-methyl-D-aspartic acid (NMDA) receptor and glutamate antagonists (13–17). Despite promising data using such compounds in animal models of TBI, they have largely failed in clinical trials.

Moreover, NMDA blockade appears to worsen outcomes after TBI in children (10,18,19). This deleterious effect may result from interference by these drugs with normal developmental events that occur in the immature brain. The temporal control of excitatory pathways during the development of hippocampus and motor, sensory, and visual cortices appears to depend on differential expression of subunits of the NMDA receptor. Two major subunits, NR2A and NR2B, exhibit differential affinity for glutamate and ion channel opening. Little expression of NR2A occurs during the early neonatal period, but its relative concentrations compared to NR2B increase dramatically during cortical development, peaking during somatosensory cortex organization and ocular dominance column formation (18). Although neuroprotective in adults, blockade of the NMDA receptor in developing cortex results in significant neuronal apoptosis (18,20–23). NR2A-receptor activation may inhibit pruning, while administration of pharmacologic NMDA antagonists may lead to "overpruning." Injury-induced reductions in the expression of NR2A receptors in injured developing cortex may also result in overpruning (18). Overpruning of developing cortex due to lack of glutamate signaling in NR2A pathways may outweigh the potentially beneficial effect of blocking direct glutamate excitotoxicity in children and result in poor recovery of function.

In theory, selective blockade of the NR2B subunit by the later generation glutamate antagonist traxoprodil (CP-101606) could block glutamatergic neurotoxicity without deleterious effects on developing cortex. However, because of regulatory difficulties associated with performing clinical trials in children (24), pediatric patients were excluded from current trials of traxoprodil (17). Pharmacologic targeting of the apoptotic cascade, especially the caspases and mitochondrial cytochrome c, has shown promise in the treatment of TBI (5,25–27). However, because apoptosis, like glutamatergic neurotransmission, is crucial to the normal development of cortical pathways, nonselective inhibition of apoptosis could also be more harmful than helpful in children (5).

DEVELOPMENT AND MANAGEMENT OF CEREBRAL EDEMA AND ITS SEQUELAE

Diffuse cerebral swelling early after injury in pediatric patients is a significant clinical problem and a source of secondary injury because of resultant brain ischemia and herniation. Clinical management targeted at reducing brain edema led to the first robust improvements in morbidity and mortality for pediatric trauma patients (5,28–30). Research into the mechanism of severe cerebral edema in children incited the establishment of pediatric TBI as a unique area of experimentation and expertise. Although diffuse cerebral edema is up to five times more common in infants and children than in adults, it is unclear why this difference exists and how best to treat it (5,31,32).

Reaction of the Developing Brain

Four major types of reactive edema occur in the brain: vasogenic, cytotoxic, osmotic, and interstitial. The latter two are specific to particular disorders, such as a syndrome of inappropriate antidiuretic hormone and hydrocephalus, while the former two are most relevant to discussion of TBI. Furthermore, edema (leakage of protein-rich exudate into the extravascular space and/or accumulation of excess intracellular water) should be distinguished from *brain swelling* due to vascular engorgement (i.e., hyperemia, the dilation of resistance arterioles, resulting in an absolute increase in the blood volume component of the intracranial compartment) (33). While hyperemia may play a significant clinical role in a minority of pediatric patients with TBI (see below), edema is responsible for the majority of traumatic brain swelling in most patients. For example, clinical MR imaging has recently demonstrated that vascular engorgement is responsible for only 1% to 20% of increasing brain volume after TBI, whereas edema (vasogenic + cytotoxic) is responsible for 80% to 99% of traumatic brain swelling (34).

Vasogenic Edema

Breakdown of the blood-brain barrier (BBB) may been seen after trauma because of direct mechanical disruption of the endothelial tight junctions or, more commonly, because of release of vasoactive/inflammatory cytokines that result in increased permeability of the capillary membrane. True vasogenic edema is characterized by increased albumin and other high-molecular weight plasma proteins in the extracellular compartment, where they typically do not occur (33,35). While BBB opening has been documented in experimental models of TBI as early as three hours postinjury, it is usually seen only when ischemia/hypoxia is added to the mechanical injury (33,36). Furthermore, clinical imaging has failed to show alteration of the BBB permeability during the first 24 hours after injury, even in the presence of focal and diffuse edema (37,38). Thus, recent clinical studies suggest that vasogenic edema is not responsible for the majority of diffuse edema seen in TBI.

Cytotoxic Edema

Cytotoxic edema, which occurs regardless of the status of the BBB, is due to a pathologic accumulation and sequestration of water in the intracellular space. It is characterized by a breakdown of ion gradients across the cell membrane, with rapid influx of Na^+, Cl^-, Ca^{2+}, and H^+ and influx of water down its osmotic gradients. This cellular swelling can be initiated by glutamate excitotoxicity, which affects both neurons and astrocytes, and may occur as early as four hours after injury (33). As Kimelberg and Unterberg pointed out, "(since) neurons are outnumbered 20:1 by astrocytes in humans, and (astrocytes) can swell to five times their normal size, it is *obvious* that glial swelling is the main mediator of brain edema" (33,39).

Restoration of ion and water gradients is dependent on active transport. Once initiated, cytotoxic edema is augmented and sustained by the energy failure that often accompanies TBI. Characteristically, this failure may be initiated by ischemia and/or hypoxia and is sustained by mitochondrial dysfunction due to inflammation and/or Ca^{2+}-mediated activation of cell-death pathways (33,40). This dysfunction can persist for up to 14 days after injury and is responsible for a significantly larger proportion (100:1) of cell death than excitotoxicity (23,41).

Role of Mitochondria in Pediatric Response to Injury

In addition to the production of adenosine triphosphate to maintain cellular activity, mitochondria also play a critical role in Ca^{2+} sequestration from the cytosol (limiting activation of apoptotic cascades) and in the activation of programmed cell death via release of cytochrome c. Animal models of TBI are characterized by reduced cellular respiration and impaired ability to sequester calcium as early as one hour postinjury, even in areas far removed from a focal impact (41). Immature brains harbor three times the number of mitochondria per cell than do adults, and these mitochondria have a reduced ability to sequester Ca^{2+}. More importantly, mitochondria in immature brains release cytochrome c more vigorously in response to injury than do mature brains (27). Thus, differences in mitochondrial number and function might contribute to the exaggerated diffuse edema response in childhood injury compared with adults. In support of this hypothesis, cerebrospinal fluid (CSF) levels of *bcl-2, Hsp-60,* and cytochrome c (all markers of mitochondria dysfunction) have been shown to correlate with severity of injury and outcome in pediatric patients (27,42–44). Promising results were shown in preclinical trials that therapeutically targeted mitochondrial function or adopted a so-called "mitoprotective" strategies, including calcium-channel blockade, administration of antioxidant free radical scavengers, and administration of cyclosporine A, which blocks the mitochondrial inner membrane transport pore (27). Although calcium-channel blockade has not been similarly effective in patients, other agents have not yet been tested in clinical trials.

Role of Inflammation in Pediatric Response to Injury

Inflammatory responses to injury may also play a unique role in the diffuse cerebral edema characteristic of the immature brain. Neutrophil influx in response to injury and excitotoxicity (as modeled by glutamate injection) is more pronounced in immature than in mature rat brain (45,46). Similarly, clinical studies demonstrate increased levels of interleukin-6 (IL-6), IL-8, and IL-10 in CSF from children with TBI, in whom increased CSF levels of IL-8 and IL-10 are directly correlated with mortality (45,47,48). These cytokines increase BBB permeability, which results in vasogenic edema, and act as chemotaxins for neutrophils, which elaborate free radicals, alter membrane permeability, impair cellular equilibrium, and result in cytotoxic edema (45).

The inflammatory response to brain injury can be pharmacologically blunted, resulting in a reduction in late edema formation. Postinjury delivery of FK-506 (tacrolimus) to rodents reduces inflammatory markers in CSF but only inhibits edema formation in the nonimpacted hemisphere (49). Inhibition of calcineurin, a protein phosphatase activated by inflammation, may mediate the effect of FK-506 (50). Indirect benefits of FK-506 administration include inhibition of glial-derived proinflammatory cytokines (IL-1, IL-6, tumor necrosis factor α), inhibition of astrocyte proliferation and hypertrophy (glial scarring), and release of brain-derived growth factor.

Nevertheless, preclinical studies show worse long-term outcome in injured animals treated with immunosuppressants (51). Immunosuppressants may impair neuronal plasticity and regeneration in a manner similar to nonspecific blockade of glutamate. Thus, nonspecific inhibition of inflammation may be more harmful than beneficial in recovery from pediatric TBI (45,51).

ACUTE MANAGEMENT OF ELEVATED INTRACRANIAL PRESSURE IN THE PEDIATRIC PATIENT

Modern management of severe TBI aims to prevent the occurrence of secondary injury due to hypoxia, ischemia, and brain herniation. Central to this pursuit is accurate measurement of intracranial pressure (ICP) and avoidance of intracranial hypertension. The acute management of intracranial hypertension, in turn, revolves around manipulation of the individual "incompressible structures" within a fixed intracranial vault (blood, CSF, and brain parenchyma), according to the doctrine introduced by Monroe and Kelly nearly 200 years ago (52). A second set of strategies seeks to reduce the impact of relative ischemia (due to intracranial hypertension) by temporarily lowering cerebral metabolic demand.

For example, sedation and analgesia may serve both (*i*) to modify cerebral blood flow (CBF) (either directly or indirectly) and thus the cerebral blood volume and (*ii*) to reduce the cerebral metabolic demand component. Hyperventilation also reduces CBF but relies on an intact cerebral autoregulation pathway. Ventriculostomy and lumbar drainage directly reduce the volume of CSF, whereas hyperosmolar therapy serves to reduce parenchymal water volume and improve CBF rheology. Each intervention is thus designed to reduce the volume of the intracranial contents (reducing pressure) or at least to ameliorate the effects of intracranial hypertension by reducing cerebral metabolic demand.

By contrast, decompressive craniectomy aims to control intracranial hypertension by increasing the size of the intracranial compartment itself. Craniectomy, when used, is generally reserved for patients in whom medical therapy for cerebral swelling has failed.

While The Guidelines propose a critical pathway for the management of severe TBI, all of its elements represent treatment options with Class III evidence (6). Early outcome studies from implementation of the adult guidelines describe improvements in all secondary indicators of outcome (such as outcome scores, length of stay, and cost of care). However, the impact of implementing The Guidelines has not been formally studied (53).

Monitoring the Pediatric Patient

A randomized controlled trial has not been conducted to evaluate the impact of invasive ICP monitoring on the management and outcome of TBI (6). ICP monitoring by ventriculostomy or fiberoptic strain gauge remains the single most common monitoring technology used in pediatric TBI, even though the editors of The Guidelines found evidence for its use only at the level of a treatment option (6). Ventriculostomy allows for the simultaneous measurement of ICP and treatment of intracranial hypertension by ventricular CSF drainage (6). The risk of procedural complication of ventriculostomy in children is approximately four times greater than that for placement of a fiberoptic monitor. Nearly 18% of external ventricular drain placements are associated with radiographic hemorrhagic complications compared with 6.5% for fiberoptic monitors (54).

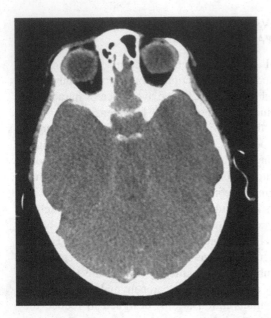

Figure 2 Abnormal CT imaging in a four-year-old male with a GCS score of 4 shows diffuse edema with bilateral cisternal effacement. This patient underwent bifrontal decompressive craniectomy in addition to intracranial pressure monitoring. *Abbreviations*: CT, computer tomography; GCS, Glasgow Coma Scale.

ICP monitoring is recommended in all children with severe TBI: Glasgow Coma Scale (GCS) score of less than or equal to 8 and an abnormal CT (edematous brain, presence of a mass lesion, etc.) (Fig. 2). ICP monitoring also serves as the primary guide to implementation of nonsurgical therapies. Unfortunately, only one-third of children younger than two years who meet criteria for ICP monitoring receive a monitor (55). The Guidelines indicate that "the presence of an open fontanel and/or open sutures ... does not preclude the development of intracranial hypertension or negate the utility of ICP monitoring" (6,56).

Even when utilized, ICP monitoring poses a number of technical challenges. Bolt-style ICP monitors drift approximately 0.95 mmHg/day in 87.4% of cases (57). Bolt monitors do not work well in children whose calvarial plates are less than 5-mm thick and/or are still largely cartilaginous. In adults, dislocation of the bolt occurs in 1.5% of cases, with dislocation of the probe in less than 1.5% (57). This complication rate is anecdotally higher in infants and young children. Alternatively, parenchymal monitors that can be introduced by tunneling without a bolt may be more resilient in infants and young children.

CBF and Cerebral Perfusion Pressure

CBF, which determines the actual delivery of oxygen and vital nutrients to the parenchyma, remains an elusive parameter to measure and treat in pediatric (and

Table 1 Age-Related Norms for Cerebral Blood Flow and Cerebral Perfusion Pressure

Age	CBF (mL/100 g/min)	Age	CPP (mmHg) goal
0–6 mo	40		
3–4 yr	108	2–6 yr	>53
9 yr	71	7–10 yr	>63
>18 yr	40–50	11–16 yr	>66

Abbreviations: CBF, cerebral blood flow; CPP, cerebral perfusion pressure.

adult) TBI. Cerebral perfusion pressure (CPP), which provides the driving force for blood flow, has been used as a validated surrogate for CBF and is easily calculated by subtracting ICP from mean arterial pressure. To a degree, the focus of pediatric TBI management has shifted from the avoidance of intracranial hypertension per se to the maximization of CBF, according to its surrogate measure, CPP.

The Guidelines recommend a minimum CPP of greater than 40 mmHg (6). Cytotoxic edema develops when CBF drops below 10 mL/100 g/min, which corresponds to energy failure and breakdown of ion exchange (33). This finding is borne out in clinical studies that demonstrate poor outcomes in association with CBF below 20 mL/100 g/min (45,58). Similarly negative outcomes are observed in children with TBI when mean CPP falls below 40 to 45 mmHg (59,60). Since publication of The Guidelines, additional data on the age dependence of CBF and CPP have emerged. Maintenance of CPP at greater than 53 mmHg for children aged 2 to 6 years, greater than 63 mmHg for ages 7 to 10 years, and greater than 66 mmHg for ages 11 to 16 years may more accurately predict improved outcome; these levels also reflect known age-related differences in baseline CBF during development (32,61) (Table 1).

Although commonly used in clinical practice, CPP is only an indirect measurement of overall organ perfusion and does not accurately reflect either global or regional variations in CBF seen after TBI. For example, focal contusions are characterized by a rim of relative hypoperfusion, with a larger area of surrounding hyperemia (33). Furthermore, CPP–targeted therapy is based on the inaccurate assumption that cerebrovascular autoregulation is intact. In fact, autoregulation is impaired in 40% to 45% of children with initial GCS score of less than 12 (62).

A more fundamental problem with "CPP management" may result from its lack of a clear operational definition (63). In essence, CPP management incorporates three distinct therapies:

- *Hypotension avoidance* (which is a standard and widely accepted component of trauma management).
- *Permissive intracranial hypertension* (i.e., allowing the ICP to rise above the traditionally accepted level of 20 mmHg without treatment, as long as CPP is within the recommended range).

- *Induced systemic hypertension* (i.e., treatment of inadequate CPP with pharmacologically induced systemic hypertension instead of traditional ICP-lowering therapies such as osmotic diuretics).

Because most early reports of CPP–directed therapy in children incorporate an unspecified conglomeration of the latter two techniques, it is difficult to establish the safety and efficacy of either (63).

Whether management of severe TBI is directed toward ICP control or optimization of CPP, avoidance of severe intracranial hypertension is necessary to prevent cerebral herniation. When it occurs, herniation generally leads to widespread secondary injury or death. Therefore, avoidance of severe intracranial hypertension (>30–35 mmHg) remains a cardinal principle in all strategies of TBI management.

Hyperosmolar Therapy

Mannitol has remained a cornerstone of the management of intracranial hypertension since its introduction to clinical use in 1961 (64). Mannitol lowers ICP by two distinct mechanisms. It causes a rapid onset (single circulatory cycle) and transient (<75 minutes) improvement in the rheostatic properties of blood. In the setting of an intact cerebral autoregulation, decreased blood viscosity is matched by a reflex vasoconstriction, which decreases the cerebral blood volume while maintaining flow and substrate delivery. There is also a slow onset (15–30 minutes) and durable (6 hours) decrease in the water volume of the cerebral parenchyma. This effect requires an intact BBB and relies on osmotic flow of water from the parenchyma to the intravascular space. In areas with an impaired BBB, a reverse-osmotic shift may occur, paradoxically increasing ICP. This shift is more often seen when mannitol is administered continuously, and when it is administered during the secondary phase of cerebral edema. Therefore, mannitol administration is currently recommended as a bolus (0.25–1.0 mg/kg), limited by maximum serum osmolarity of 320 mOsm/L (6). More recent studies in adult patients suggest that high-dose mannitol (1.4 mg/kg/bolus) is more effective at reducing both ICP and mortality. The effect of these doses has not been tested in children (65).

In 1919, hypertonic saline was first reported as a treatment for cerebral edema (66). Hypertonic saline shares the same rheostatic properties and effect on total brain water as mannitol and similarly relies on an intact BBB. Higher serum osmolarity (>350 mOsm/L) is tolerated, especially in children. Hypertonic saline also has beneficial effects on cardiac output and resuscitation from shock, thereby reducing secondary insults in the form of ischemia/hypoxia (45). The Guidelines recommend an infusion of 0.1 to 1.0 mL/kg/hr of 3% hypertonic saline for children, titrated to the minimum rate necessary to keep ICP at less than 20 mmHg. Both retrospective and prospective studies have shown reduced morbidity and mortality when elevated ICP is treated with hypertonic saline (6). Of potential interest is the role of higher concentrations of saline (e.g., 7.5% or 23.4%), which have yet to be systematically evaluated in pediatric patients.

Care should be taken during hyperosmolar therapy to maintain homeostatic intravascular volume by using adequate normal or hypertonic fluid replacement. Dehydration, decreased intravascular volume, and hypotension may catastrophically complicate management of severe TBI (6).

Sedation and Analgesia

Adequate sedation and analgesia are routinely employed in the management of critically ill patients, especially children. These agents play important roles in analgesia, ventilator management, and the avoidance of intracranial hypertension due to agitation. Their effect on ICP and outcome after pediatric TBI is unlikely to be tested in a randomized trial. However, the relative risks and benefits of particular agents continue to be examined, mostly in the form of retrospective studies.

A number of considerations particular to pediatric patients deserve mention. Propofol infusion, commonly utilized in adult patients, is absolutely contraindicated in children because of the risk of irreversible lactic acidosis, rhabdomyolysis with acute renal failure, and cardiovascular collapse (67). Benzodiazepines, which are preferred in children, have been shown to reduce cerebral metabolic rate of oxygen consumption ($CMRO_2$) by up to 25% without inducing hypotension (unlike barbiturate therapy, see below) (6). Short-acting opiates (fentanyl, remifentanil) are often used in children despite the lack of a systematic examination of their effects. Increases in ICP of up to 15 mmHg have been reported with the use of sufentanil; its use in children with head injury is contraindicated (68). Remifentanil is the only short-acting opiate to consistently reduce ICP (69).

Barbiturate Therapy

Barbiturate therapy for intracranial hypertension has been used in children who are refractory to first-line therapy with diuretics, sedation, and analgesia. A randomized trial of barbiturate therapy for intracranial hypertension in children has never been conducted. Small series suggest that induction of barbiturate coma in children refractory to other measures may reduce ICP to less than 20 mmHg in over 50% of patients (70). Nevertheless, recent meta-analysis by the Cochrane group for all age groups found no evidence to support the use of barbiturates in head-injured patients. No significant difference was observed in pooled risk of death (relative risk, RR, 1.09; 95% confidence interval, CI, 0.81–1.47), only a trend toward lower ICP (RR, 0.81; 95% CI, 0.62–1.06) and a significant incidence of hypotension, which required pressor therapy (RR, 1.8; 95% CI, 1.19–2.70) (71). The Guidelines consider barbiturate therapy an option among second-tier therapies (6).

Barbiturates lower ICP by two distinct but interrelated mechanisms: suppression of metabolic activity and decreased vascular tone. This class of agents has been shown to reduce $CMRO_2$ by 50% at doses that resulted in electro-encephalographic burst suppression (72). When cerebrovascular autoregulation is intact (often not the case), a coupled reduction in CBF and volume occurs because of the reduced metabolic need for oxygen. Barbiturates also confer a theoretical advantage by acting as free radical scavengers, inhibiting lipid peroxidation and blunting the inflammatory and excitotoxic responses (6).

Thiopental and pentothal, both short-acting barbiturates, are the preferred agents for inducing a barbiturate coma. In children, thiopental is administered as a loading dose of 10 to 20 mg/kg, and a maintenance infusion of 3 to 5 mg/kg/hr. Pentobarbital is administered as a loading dose of 10 mg/kg over 30 minutes, boluses of 5 mg/kg every hour for an additional three hours, and then maintenance of 1 mg/kg/hr (70,71,73). While serum levels may correlate with incidence of side effects (most importantly hypotension, seen in up to 90% of children), they do not correlate well with suppression of cerebral metabolic activity (73). Barbiturates are generally utilized only when adequate cerebrovascular and neurologic monitoring is available (such as Swan-Ganz or PiCCO catheters and continuous electroencephalographic monitoring). Barbiturate infusions are typically titrated to produce burst suppression (4–5 bursts/min) on electroencephalogram (74). One newer option, titration of barbiturates to a bispectral index of 0 to 10 and suppression ratios of greater than 85%, has been demonstrated in small numbers of pediatric patients to be safe and effective and to correlate well with electroencephalogram burst suppression (75,76).

Hyperventilation

Hyperventilation, which results in hypocapnia and constriction of resistance arterioles, was one of the earliest cornerstones in modern management of intracranial hypertension. On the basis of the assumption that diffuse cerebral edema in children with TBI was because of hyperemia, hyperventilation offered a potentially beneficial reduction in the cerebral blood volume. Nevertheless, both the adult and pediatric guidelines caution against prophylactic hyperventilation to $PaCO_2$ of less than 35 mmHg. Temporary hyperventilation may be considered a second-tier treatment option for refractory elevation of ICP, generally while other therapeutic measures are instituted (6). The detrimental effects of long-term hyperventilation include iatrogenic ischemia (both by reduction of CBF and left shift of the oxyhemoglobin dissociation curve) and depletion of cerebral interstitial bicarbonate (with resultant hyperreactivity of the resistance arterioles to subsequent changes in $PaCO_2$) (77). Iatrogenic hyperventilation in children has been shown to significantly increase the incidence of regional ischemia (CBF < 20 mL/100g/min) (78).

Although untested, a minority of children who suffer from severe TBI may have an idiosyncratic dysfunction of cerebral vascular regulation, which results in clinically significant hyperemia (62). It remains to be determined how to identify such children clinically and how to most effectively guide and monitor hyperventilation therapy for them to avoid secondary complications. Without accurate CBF monitoring, hyperventilation should be avoided.

Therapeutic Hypothermia

Few, if any, novel interventions for TBI carry more theoretical promise than hypothermia. It may be the most "consistently positive therapy in experimental models" (5). Induction of hypothermia has improved outcomes after experimental TBI, hypoxic-ischemic injury, stroke, and cardiac arrest. Hypothermia may intervene on a number of pathophysiologic levels: reduction of CBF, reduction of $CMRO_2$, blunting of excitotoxicity, blunting of the inflammatory response, inhibition of necrosis from primary injury, and prevention of apoptosis from secondary injury.

Nevertheless, experimental data that support the safety and efficacy of induced hypothermia are limited in adults and nearly nonexistent in children. A recent Cochrane review for all ages concluded that no evidence supports the use of hypothermia in TBI, noting trends toward reduced death and disability (odds ratio, OR, 0.75; 95% CI, 0.56–1.00) but significantly increased risk of pneumonia (OR, 1.95; 95% CI, 1.18–3.23) (79). When the Guidelines were formulated, the conclusion drawn from the two extant studies of hypothermia in children (the most recent from 1973) was the need for further study. Indeed, a multicentered trial of induced hypothermia for severe TBI in children has recently been approved and funded (Adelson, PD personal communication).

Induced hypothermia may be complicated by a high incidence of morbidity due to shivering, coagulopathy, increased blood viscosity, arrhythmia, sepsis, and pneumonia. Analysis of both laboratory and clinical data suggests that benefit-to-risk ratios may be idealized utilizing core temperature targets from 34°C to 35°C (80). Most clinical studies, including the two randomized safety trials that have emerged since publication of The Guidelines, now target cooling to approximately 32°C (6,79,81). Animal studies suggest that peak cerebral protection and reduced neurologic morbidity occur with cooling to 30°C to 32°C within 60 minutes of injury. Delayed cooling (i.e., reaching target temperature within 6 hours of injury) confers benefit only when continued for at least 48 hours, with the optimal duration unknown (80).

In children, no benefit of induced hypothermia for TBI has been proven. Two recent trials demonstrate favorable, although modest, reduction in ICP from cooling for 48 hours, beginning within 6 hours of injury (82,83). Both trials also describe rebound intracranial hypertension during rewarming and recommend passive rewarming of 1°C over 4 hours, with a goal of reaching a core temperature of greater than 36.5°C. Rebound intracranial hypertension may be due to changes in cerebral blood volume and increased inflammation, as optimal biologic temperature is achieved. Inhibition of the inflammatory response with FK-506 also confers axonal protection during rewarming in animal models of hypothermia (84). Given the variable responses of different age groups to injury, it is likely that the therapeutic targets for core temperature and the duration of cooling and rewarming are age dependent.

A corollary to therapeutic hypothermia is the avoidance of hyperthermia in brain-injured patients. The deleterious effects of fever in children with severe TBI are well described (6). Fever should be aggressively treated as appropriate with acetaminophen and/or active cooling.

Nutrition

Little evidence exists regarding the specific nutritional needs of mechanically ventilated children with severe TBI (6). Children may suffer from a specific vulnerability to hyperglycemia, which has been shown in experimental models to worsen secondary brain injury in immature animals (85). In the absence of additional clinical evidence, it may be prudent to monitor for and avoid hyperglycemia in children with severe TBI who are receiving supplemental nutrition.

Antiepileptic Drugs

The Guidelines recommend, as a standard of care, the avoidance of antiepileptic drugs as prophylaxis for late posttraumatic seizures. However, the role of antiepileptic drugs in preventing early posttraumatic seizures is more controversial (6,86). Undetected generalized seizures in a sedated or pharmacologically paralyzed patient may directly injure the brain and/or lead to acutely exacerbated intracranial hypertension, brain herniation, and death. Prophylaxis with anticonvulsants may be considered for such patients during the days after injury when cerebral edema is worst and ICP management most critical, particularly in those who harbor contusions of epileptogenic cortex in the basal frontal and temporal lobes.

Decompressive Craniectomy

Decompressive craniectomy has been used since the early 20th century to control intractable intracranial hypertension. Craniectomy represents the definitive surgical intervention for patients who fail medical management. The first decompression was reportedly performed in 1874 (for an adult patient with tumor) (87). Decompression for trauma came into practice in the 1960s (88). The Guidelines recommend decompressive craniectomy as a treatment option for children who have failed first-line medical management of intracranial hypertension. A single randomized controlled trial (representing Class III data due to issues with study design and power) demonstrated reduced ICP and trends toward reduced mortality (RR, 0.54; 95% CI, 0.17–1.72) and disability (RR, 0.54; 95% CI, 0.29–1.01) after decompressive craniectomy (89).

Analysis of larger adult trials and smaller pediatric case series suggests that children reap the greatest benefit from decompressive craniectomy. Decompression may benefit children who suffer from TBI due to nonaccidental trauma (5,45). The optimal timing for decompression is still unknown. Nevertheless, decompression is generally reserved for patients who present with a GCS score of greater than 3 and who experience secondary deterioration in the first 48 hours after injury despite best medical management (6). Decompression at the time of hematoma evacuation is left to the discretion and experience of individual surgeons. No studies have been conducted to prove the benefit of one technique over another, and review of specific surgical options is beyond the scope of this chapter. However, case reports and series indicate that wide decompressions that include the temporal fossae may be more effective in preventing uncal-transtentorial herniation and in avoiding incarceration of potentially salvageable brain at the craniectomy edges.

CONCLUSION AND FUTURE DIRECTIONS

The responses of the developing and mature nervous systems to traumatic injury differ significantly. Similar differences characterize the responses of children and adults to therapeutic intervention in TBI. Injury and treatment also vary dramatically by age subgroup within the pediatric population and according to mechanism (e.g., nonaccidental trauma).

Some themes emerge from the evolution of management of severe TBI in children. First, because of the relatively high cerebral-to-intracranial volume ratio in children and the apparent propensity of the developing brain for edema formation in response to trauma, children appear to be at greater risk than adults for sudden, massive, and catastrophic secondary injury. Second, a number of historically "standard" but nonhomeostatic treatments for severe TBI in children, such as iatrogenic dehydration, sustained hyperventilation, and prolonged prophylactic anticonvulsant medication administration, may in many cases have been potentially harmful to neurologic recovery.

Much current therapy (both evidence-based and non–evidence-based) is directed toward maintenance of homeostasis in blood pressure, ventilation, core body temperature, nutrition, etc., in an attempt to avoid secondary injury during the time of maximum vulnerability due to cerebral edema. An important additional component of therapy is the avoidance of brain herniation, which catastrophically worsens survival and neurologic outcome when it occurs. Many programs utilize predominantly surgical means to achieve the latter goal (i.e., CSF drainage and/or decompressive craniectomy), while continuing to direct medical therapy toward prohomeostatic goals. The benefits of this strategy are also untested. Nevertheless, new nonhomeostatic interventions (such as induced systemic hypertension as part of "CPP management" or iatrogenic hypothermia) should not be routinely adopted until their efficacy is evaluated using prospective randomized trials that measure both survival and neurologic outcome.

The consistent application of a systems-based management protocol and goal-directed therapy and inclusion of age-based parameters are essential for management of TBI in children. The evolution of clinical science in this area and the application of growing subspecialty and pediatric trauma center expertise will advance these goals and ultimately improve outcomes for children who suffer from this devastating disease.

REFERENCES

1. Langlois JA, Rutland-Brown W, Thomas KE. Traumatic brain injury in the United States: emergency department visits, hospitalizations, and deaths. Atlanta, Georgia: Centers for Disease Control and Prevention, National Center for Injury Prevention and Control 2006.
2. Schneier AJ, Shields BJ, Hostetler SG, et al. Incidence of pediatric traumatic brain injury and associated hospital resource utilization in the United States. Pediatrics 2006; 118(2):483–492.
3. Brener I, Harman JS, Kelleher KJ, et al. Medical costs of mild to moderate traumatic brain injury in children. J Head Trauma Rehabil 2004; 19(5):405–412.
4. Sobocki P, Lekander I, Berwick S, et al. Resource allocation to brain research in Europe (RABRE). Eur J Neurosci, 2006; 24(10):2691–2693.
5. Kochanek PM. Pediatric traumatic brain injury: quo vadis? Dev Neurosci 2006; 28(4–5):244–255.
6. Guidelines for the acute medical management of severe traumatic brain injury in infants, children, and adolescents. J Trauma 2003; 54(suppl 6):S235–S310.
7. Levin HS, Aldrich EF, Saydjari C, et al. Severe head injury in children: experience of the Traumatic Coma Data Bank. Neurosurgery 1992; 31(3):435–443 (discussion 443–444).
8. Ichord RN, Naim M, Pollock AN, et al. Hypoxic-ischemic injury complicates inflicted and accidental traumatic brain injury in young children: The role of diffusion-weighted imaging. J Neurotrauma 2007; 24(1):106–118.
9. Steinbok P, Singhal A, Poskitt K, et al. Early hypodensity on computed tomographic scan of the brain in an accidental pediatric head injury. Neurosurgery 2007; 60(4):689–694 (discussion 694–695).
10. Giza CC, Prins ML. Is being plastic fantastic? Mechanisms of altered plasticity after developmental traumatic brain injury. Dev Neurosci 2006; 28(4–5):364–379.
11. Faden AI, Demediuk P, Panter SS, et al. The role of excitatory amino acids and NMDA receptors in traumatic brain injury. Science 1989; 244(4906):798–800.
12. Mark LP, Prost RW, Ulmer JL, et al. Pictorial review of glutamate excitotoxicity: fundamental concepts for neuroimaging. AJNR Am J Neuroradiol 2001; 22(10):1813–1824.
13. Morris GF, Bullock R, Marshall SB, et al. Failure of the competitive N-methyl-D-aspartate antagonist Selfotel (CGS 19755) in the treatment of severe head injury: Results of two phase III clinical trials. The Selfotel Investigators. J Neurosurg 1999; 91(5):737–743.
14. Wagstaff A, Teasdale GM, Clifton G, et al. The cerebral hemodynamic and metabolic effects of the noncompetitive NMDA antagonist CNS 1102 in humans with severe head injury. Ann N Y Acad Sci 1995; 765:332–333.
15. Wood PL. The NMDA receptor complex: a long and winding road to therapeutics. Drugs 2005; 8(3):229–235.
16. Wood PL, Hawkinson JE. N-methyl-D-aspartate antagonists for stroke and head trauma. Expert Opin Investig Drugs 1997; 6(4):389–397.
17. Yurkewicz L, Weaver J, Bullock MR, et al. The effect of the selective NMDA receptor antagonist traxoprodil in the treatment of traumatic brain injury. J Neurotrauma 2005; 22(12):1428–1443.
18. Giza CC, Maria NS, Hovda DA. N-methyl-D-aspartate receptor subunit changes after traumatic injury to the developing brain. J Neurotrauma, 2006; 23(6):950–961.

19. Lea PM IV, Faden AI. Traumatic brain injury: developmental differences in glutamate receptor response and the impact on treatment. Ment Retard Dev Disabil Res Rev 2001; 7(4):235–248.

20. Bittigau P, Sifringer M, Pohl D, et al. Apoptotic neurodegeneration following trauma is markedly enhanced in the immature brain. Ann Neurol 1999; 45(6):724–735.

21. Ikonomidou C, Bosch F, Miksa M, et al. Blockade of NMDA receptors and apoptotic neurodegeneration in the developing brain. Science 1999; 283(5398):70–74.

22. Ikonomidou C, Turski L. Prevention of trauma-induced neurodegeneration in infant and adult rat brain: glutamate antagonists. Metab Brain Dis 1996; 11(2):125–141.

23. Pohl D, Bittigau P, Ishimaru MJ, et al. N-Methyl-D-aspartate antagonists and apoptotic cell death triggered by head trauma in developing rat brain. Proc Natl Acad Sci U S A 1999; 96(5):2508–2513.

24. Caldwell PH, Butow PN, Craig JC. Parents' attitudes to children's participation in randomized controlled trials. J Pediatr 2003; 142(5):554–559.

25. Bittigau P, Sifringer M, Felderhoff-Mueser U, et al. Neuropathological and biochemical features of traumatic injury in the developing brain. Neurotox Res 2003; 5(7):475–490.

26. Gilman CP, Mattson MP. Do apoptotic mechanisms regulate synaptic plasticity and growth-cone motility? Neuromolecular Med 2002; 2(2):197–214.

27. Robertson CL. Mitochondrial dysfunction contributes to cell death following traumatic brain injury in adult and immature animals. J Bioenerg Biomembr 2004; 36(4):363–368.

28. Bruce DA, Alavi A, Bilaniuk L, et al. Diffuse cerebral swelling following head injuries in children: the syndrome of "malignant brain edema". J Neurosurg 1981; 54(2):170–178.

29. Bruce DA, Raphaely RC, Goldberg AI, et al. Pathophysiology, treatment and outcome following severe head injury in children. Childs Brain 1979; 5(3):174–1791.

30. Raphaely RC, Swedlow DB. Downes, JJ, et al. Management of severe pediatric head trauma. Pediatr Clin North Am 1980; 27(3):715–727.

31. Lang DA, Teasdale GM, Macpherson P, et al. Diffuse brain swelling after head injury: more often malignant in adults than children? J Neurosurg 1994; 80(4):675–680.

32. Zwienenberg M, Muizelaar JP. Severe pediatric head injury: the role of hyperemia revisited. J Neurotrauma 1999; 16(10):937–943.

33. Unterberg AW, Stover J, Kress B, et al. Edema and brain trauma. Neuroscience 2004; 129(4):1021–1029.

34. Marmarou A, Fatouros PP, Barzo P, et al. Contribution of edema and cerebral blood volume to traumatic brain swelling in head-injured patients. J Neurosurg 2000; 93(2):183–193.

35. Betz AL, Iannotti F, Hoff JT. Brain edema: a classification based on blood-brain barrier integrity. Cerebrovasc Brain Metab Rev 1989; 1(2):133–154.

36. Avery S, Crockard HA, Russell RR. Evolution and resolution of oedema following severe temporary cerebral ischaemia in the gerbil. J Neurol Neurosurg Psychiatry 1984; 47(6):604–610.

37. Kawamata T, Katayama Y, Aoyama N, et al. Heterogeneous mechanisms of early edema formation in cerebral contusion: diffusion MRI and ADC mapping study. Acta Neurochir Suppl 2000; 76:9–12.

38. Maeda T, Katayama Y, Kawamata T, et al. Ultra-early study of edema formation in cerebral contusion using diffusion MRI and ADC mapping. Acta Neurochir Suppl 2003; 86:329–331.

39. Kimelberg H.K. Current concepts of brain edema. Review of laboratory investigations. J Neurosurg 1995; 83(6):1051–1059.
40. Amara SG, Fontana AC. Excitatory amino acid transporters: keeping up with glutamate. Neurochem Int 2002; 41(5):313–318.
41. Xiong Y, Gu Q, Peterson PL, et al. Mitochondrial dysfunction and calcium perturbation induced by traumatic brain injury. J Neurotrauma 1997; 14(1):23–34.
42. Clark RS, Kochanek PM, Adelson PD, et al. Increases in bcl-2 protein in cerebrospinal fluid and evidence for programmed cell death in infants and children after severe traumatic brain injury. J Pediatr 2000; 137(2):197–204.
43. Lai Y, Stange C, Wisniewski SR, et al. Mitochondrial heat shock protein 60 is increased in cerebrospinal fluid following pediatric traumatic brain injury. Dev Neurosci 2006; 28(4–5):336–341.
44. Satchell MA, Lai Y, Kochanek PM, et al. Cytochrome c, a biomarker of apoptosis, is increased in cerebrospinal fluid from infants with inflicted brain injury from child abuse. J Cereb Blood Flow Metab 2005; 25(7):919–927.
45. Bayir H, Kochanek PM, Clark RS. Traumatic brain injury in infants and children: mechanisms of secondary damage and treatment in the intensive care unit. Crit Care Clin 2003; 19(3):529–549.
46. Bolton SJ, Perry VH. Differential blood-brain barrier breakdown and leucocyte recruitment following excitotoxic lesions in juvenile and adult rats. Exp Neurol 1998; 154(1):231–240.
47. Bell MJ, Kochanek PM, Doughty LA, et al. Interleukin-6 and interleukin-10 in cerebrospinal fluid after severe traumatic brain injury in children. J Neurotrauma 1997; 14(7):451–457.
48. Whalen MJ, Carlos TM, Kochanek PM, et al. Interleukin-8 is increased in cerebrospinal fluid of children with severe head injury. Crit Care Med 2000; 28(4): 929–934.
49. Stover JF, Schoning B, Sakowitz OW, et al. Effects of tacrolimus on hemispheric water content and cerebrospinal fluid levels of glutamate, hypoxanthine, interleukin-6, and tumor necrosis factor-alpha following controlled cortical impact injury in rats. J Neurosurg 2001; 94(5):782–787.
50. Singleton RH, Stone JR, Okonkwo DO, et al. The immunophilin ligand FK506 attenuates axonal injury in an impact-acceleration model of traumatic brain injury. J Neurotrauma 2001; 18(6):607–614.
51. Lenzlinger PM, Morganti-Kossmann MC, Laurer HL, et al. The duality of the inflammatory response to traumatic brain injury. Mol Neurobiol 2001; 24(1–3): 169–181.
52. Kelly G. An account of the appearances observed in the dissection of two of three individuals presumed to have perished in the storm of the 3rd, and whose bodies were discovered in the vicinity of the Leith on the morning of the 4th of November 1821, with some reflections on the pathology of the brain. Trans Med Sci Edinb 1824; 1:84–169.
53. Fakhry SM, Trask AL, Waller MA, et al. Management of brain-injured patients by an evidence-based medicine protocol improves outcomes and decreases hospital charges. J Trauma 2004; 56(3):492–499 (discussion 499–500).
54. Anderson RC, Kan P, Klimo P, et al. Complications of intracranial pressure monitoring in children with head trauma. J Neurosurg 2004; 101(suppl 1):53–58.
55. Keenan HT, Nocera M, Bratton SL. Frequency of intracranial pressure monitoring in infants and young toddlers with traumatic brain injury. Pediatr Crit Care Med 2005; 6(5):537–541.

56. Cho DY, Wang YC, Chi CS. Decompressive craniotomy for acute shaken/impact baby syndrome. Pediatr Neurosurg 1995; 23(4):192–198.
57. Gelabert-Gonzalez M, Ginesta-Galan V, Sernamito-Garcia R, et al. The Camino intracranial pressure device in clinical practice. Assessment in a 1000 cases. Acta Neurochir (Wien) 2006; 148(4):435–441.
58. Adelson PD, Clyde B, Kochanek PM, et al. Cerebrovascular response in infants and young children following severe traumatic brain injury: A preliminary report. Pediatr Neurosurg 1997; 26(4):200–207.
59. Pfenninger J, Santi A. Severe traumatic brain injury in children—are the results improving? Swiss Med Wkly 2002; 132(9–10):116–120.
60. Downard C, Hulka F, Mullins RJ, et al. Relationship of cerebral perfusion pressure and survival in pediatric brain-injured patients. J Trauma 2000; 49(4):654–658 (discussion 658–659).
61. Chambers IR, Stobbart L, Jones PA, et al. Age-related differences in intracranial pressure and cerebral perfusion pressure in the first 6 hours of monitoring after children's head injury: association with outcome. Childs Nerv Syst 2005; 21(3): 195–199.
62. Vavilala MS, Lee LA, Boddu K, et al. Cerebral autoregulation in pediatric traumatic brain injury. Pediatr Crit Care Med 2004; 5(3):257–263.
63. Selden NR. CPP or ICP? J Neurosurg 2005; 102(suppl 1):134–135 (author reply 135).
64. Wise BL, Chater N. Use of hypertonic mannitol solutions to lower cerebrospinal fluid pressure and decrease brain bulk in man. Surg Forum 1961; 12:398–399.
65. Wakai A, Roberts I, Schierhout G. Mannitol for acute traumatic brain injury. Cochrane Database Syst Rev 2007(1):CD001049.
66. Weed LH, McKibben PS. Pressure changes in the cerebro-spinal fluid following intravenous injection of solutions of various concentrations. Am J Physiol 1919; 48(1):512–530.
67. Okamoto MP, Kawaguchi DL, Amin AN. Evaluation of propofol infusion syndrome in pediatric intensive care. Am J Health Syst Pharm 2003; 60(19):2007–2014.
68. Albanese J, Viviand X, Potie F, et al. Sufentanil, fentanyl, and alfentanil in head trauma patients: a study on cerebral hemodynamics. Crit Care Med 1999; 27(2): 407–411.
69. Tipps LB, Coplin WM, Murry KR, et al. Safety and feasibility of continuous infusion of remifentanil in the neurosurgical intensive care unit. Neurosurgery 2000; 46(3): 596–601; discussion 601–602.
70. Pittman T, Bucholz R, Williams D. Efficacy of barbiturates in the treatment of resistant intracranial hypertension in severely head-injured children. Pediatr Neurosci 1989; 15(1):13–17.
71. Roberts I. Barbiturates for acute traumatic brain injury. Cochrane Database Syst Rev 2000(2):CD000033.
72. Piatt JH Jr., Schiff SJ. High dose barbiturate therapy in neurosurgery and intensive care. Neurosurgery 1984; 15(3):427–444.
73. Kasoff SS, Lansen TA, Holder D, et al. Aggressive physiologic monitoring of pediatric head trauma patients with elevated intracranial pressure. Pediatr Neurosci 1988; 14(5):241–249.
74. Kassell NF, Hitchon PW, Gerk MK, et al. Alterations in cerebral blood flow, oxygen metabolism, and electrical activity produced by high dose sodium thiopental. Neurosurgery 1980; 7(6):598–603.

75. Grindstaff RJ, Tobias JD. Applications of bispectral index monitoring in the pediatric intensive care unit. J Intensive Care Med 2004; 19(2):111–116.

76. Jaggi P, Schwabe MJ, Gill K, et al. Use of an anesthesia cerebral monitor bispectral index to assess burst-suppression in pentobarbital coma. Pediatr Neurol 2003; 28(3): 219–222.

77. Muizelaar JP, Marmarou A, Ward JD, et al. Adverse effects of prolonged hyperventilation in patients with severe head injury: a randomized clinical trial. J Neurosurg 1991; 75(5):731–739.

78. Skippen P, Seear M, Poskitt K, et al. Effect of hyperventilation on regional cerebral blood flow in head-injured children. Crit Care Med 1997; 25(8):1402–1409.

79. Alderson P, Gadkary C, Signorini DF. Therapeutic hypothermia for head injury. Cochrane Database Syst Rev, 2004(4):CD001048.

80. Fritz HG, Bauer R. Secondary injuries in brain trauma: effects of hypothermia. J Neurosurg Anesthesiol 2004; 16(1):43–52.

81. Hutchison J, Ward R, Lacroix J, et al. Hypothermia pediatric head injury trial: the value of a pretrial clinical evaluation phase. Dev Neurosci 2006; 28(4–5):291–301.

82. Adelson PD, Ragheb J, Kanev P, et al. Phase II clinical trial of moderate hypothermia after severe traumatic brain injury in children. Neurosurgery 2005; 56(4): 740–754.

83. Biswas AK, Bruce DA, Sklar FH, et al. Treatment of acute traumatic brain injury in children with moderate hypothermia improves intracranial hypertension. Crit Care Med 2002; 30(12):2742–2751.

84. Suehiro E, Singleton RH, Stone JR, et al. The immunophilin ligand FK506 attenuates the axonal damage associated with rapid rewarming following posttraumatic hypothermia. Exp Neurol 2001; 172(1):199–210.

85. Kinoshita K, Kraydieh S, Alonso O, et al. Effect of posttraumatic hyperglycemia on contusion volume and neutrophil accumulation after moderate fluid-percussion brain injury in rats. J Neurotrauma 2002; 19(6):681–692.

86. Statler KD. Pediatric posttraumatic seizures: epidemiology, putative mechanisms of epileptogenesis and promising investigational progress. Dev Neurosci 2006; 28(4–5): 354–363.

87. Spiller W, Frazier C. Cerebral Decompression. Palliative operations in the treatment of tumor in the brain, based on the observation of fourteen cases. JAMA 1906; 1(47): 679–683.

88. Sahuquillo J, Arikan F. Decompressive craniectomy for the treatment of refractory high intracranial pressure in traumatic brain injury. Cochrane Database Syst Rev, 2006(1):CD003983.

89. Taylor A, Butt W, Rosenfeld J, et al. A randomized trial of very early decompressive craniectomy in children with traumatic brain injury and sustained intracranial hypertension. Childs Nerv Syst 2001; 17(3):154–162.

7

Decompressive Hemicraniectomy for Large Hemispheric Infarctions

Eric Jüttler, MD

Department of Neurology, University of Heidelberg, Heidelberg, Germany

Alfred Aschoff, MD, PhD, Associate Professor

Department of Neurosurgery, University of Heidelberg,
Heidelberg, Germany

Stefan Schwab, Professor Doctor, Director

Department of Neurology, University of Erlangen, Erlangen, Germany

For decades, the treatment of large space-occupying cerebral infarctions has been one of the major unsolved problems in neurointensive care medicine. As more and more young patients suffer from brain infarction, finding an optimal treatment solution has made this a most urgent topic in stroke medicine.

Subtotal or complete infarctions of the middle cerebral artery (MCA) territory, including the basal ganglia, occasionally with additional infarction of the anterior cerebral artery (ACA), the posterior cerebral artery (PCA), or both, are found in 1% to 10% of patients with supratentorial infarcts and are commonly associated with serious brain swelling, which usually manifests itself between the second and fifth days after stroke onset (1–9). These massive cerebral infarctions are life-threatening events with poor prognosis. Mass effect with raised intracranial pressure (ICP) leads to the destruction of formerly healthy brain tissue and, in severe cases, to extensive brain tissue shifts, resulting in transtentorial or uncal herniation and brain death (4,5,10). These complications are responsible for the rapid neurologic deterioration seen in these patients and account for more than two-thirds of deaths during the first week (1). In intensive care-based prospective series, the case-fatality rate of these patients was approximately 80% despite maximal medical therapy (5,11,12). Therefore, for these catastrophic cerebral infarcts the term *malignant MCA infarction* was introduced by Hacke et al. in 1965.

Only a few years ago these massive cerebral infarctions were regarded as an untreatable disease with fatal outcome. The introduction of decompressive surgery (hemicraniectomy) has completely changed this point of view. Extensive literature is available regarding hemicraniectomy in malignant ischemic brain infarction. However, until recently most of the reports were retrospective with low number of patients. Only a few prospective trials compared decompressive surgery with conservative treatment. However, the control groups in these studies consisted of patients with higher ages, more comorbidity, and more frequent lesions in the dominant hemisphere than those in the surgical groups. In particular, in most studies, information on long-term outcome is insufficient. Because of the lack of conclusive evidence of efficacy from clinical trials, controversy over the benefit of hemicraniectomy continued among neurologists and neurosurgeons, leading to large regional differences in the application of these procedures. Finally, data from randomized trials were reported in 2006. This chapter includes an integrated view on the current status of hemicraniectomy in malignant ischemic brain infarction on the basis of available data of clinical trials, also including the latest results from randomized trials. Alternative treatment options and major unsolved problems in this field of ischemic brain injury are also discussed.

DIAGNOSIS OF MALIGNANT BRAIN INFARCTION

Although the term "malignant brain infarction" was introduced in 1996, 10 years later, the field still did not have a generally accepted definition of this condition. As much consistency as possible in defining this term should be used to make studies from different institutions comparable. The following criteria are based on the inclusion criteria of the randomized trials on malignant stroke and may be given for clinical routine use (3,5,13–15).

The diagnosis of a malignant brain infarction is based on (i) the clinical syndrome with typical neurologic findings and a typical clinical course and (ii) typical neuroimaging findings (Figs. 1 and 2):

1. Clinically, patients with malignant infarctions of the MCA present with dense hemiplegia, head and eye deviation, multimodal hemineglect, and global aphasia when the dominant hemisphere is involved. It should be noted that the National Institute of Health Stroke Scale (NIHSS) score underestimates the severity of nondominant infarction (16). Therefore, the NIHSS score is typically greater than 20 when the dominant hemisphere

is involved and greater than 15 when the nondominant hemisphere is involved. Furthermore, patients show an impaired level of consciousness (LOC), with a score of greater than or equal to 1 in item 1a. (LOC) of the NIHSS (5,16) and a progressive deterioration of consciousness over the first 24 to 48 hours, frequently including a reduced ventilatory drive (5).

2. Neuroimaging shows definite infarction of at least two-thirds of the MCA territory, including the basal ganglia, with or without additional infarction of the ipsilateral ACA or the PCA territories when CT is used (14,17). Measurement of infarct volume in stroke using MRI with diffusion-weighted imaging (DWI) has shown that an infarct volume of greater than 145 cm^3 has a highly predictive value for the development of malignant brain infarction and may be used for very early diagnosis in these patients instead of CT findings (18). This finding was recently evaluated and confirmed in a randomized trial that used infarct volume on DWI as inclusion criterion (13).

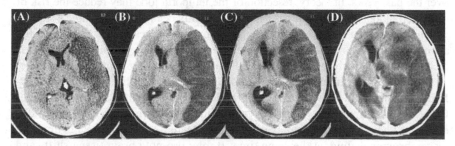

Figure 1 From left to right: Malignant MCA infarction (**A**) two days, (**B**) three days, (**C**) four days, and (**D**) five days after symptom onset, resulting in transtentorial herniation. *Abbreviation*: MCA, middle cerebral artery.

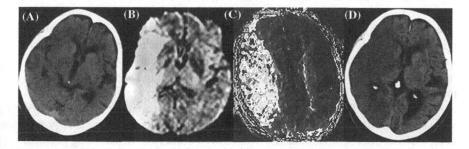

Figure 2 From left to right: (**A**) Malignant MCA infarction, (**B**) CT three hours after symptom onset, (**C**) MRI (diffusion-weighted and perfusion imaging) three hours after symptom onset, and (**D**) CT 30 hours later. *Abbreviations*: MCA, middle cerebral artery; CT, computer tomography; MRI, magnetic resonance imaging.

DECOMPRESSIVE SURGERY

Decompressive Surgery (Hemicraniectomy)—Surgical Techniques

Decompressive surgery is based on mechanical thinking: The rationale is to remove a part of the neurocranium, thereby creating space to accommodate the swollen brain, normalize ICP, avoid ventricular compression, and revert brain tissue shifts. Another concept to support decompressive surgery is that by decreasing ICP cerebral blood flow will be restored, which may allow for better perfusion and brain tissue oxygenation of remaining healthy brain tissue, reducing the infarct volume (19,20) and preventing secondary mechanical and ischemic tissue damage (10,21). Decompressive surgery in large ischemic stroke is not new. In fact, it dates back to 1935 (22). Two techniques are used: external (removal of the cranial vault and duraplasty) and internal (removal of nonviable, i.e., infarcted tissue) decompression. Both techniques can be combined (23,24).

The extent of surgical decompression and the need for tissue removal (i.e., in the case of malignant MCA infarction, temporal lobectomy) have been controversial over the past years. In theory, resection of the temporal lobe may reduce the risk of uncal herniation; however, this has never consistently been proven by clinical studies, which show similar results as series using external decompression (25,26). Currently, at most institutions, external decompressive surgery is performed because this technique is relatively simple and can be performed in every neurosurgical center.

Resection of infarcted tissue is not only more complicated, it is also difficult to distinguish between already infarcted and potentially salvageable tissue. Other surgical approaches such as ventriculostomy have not shown beneficial effects. Although ventriculostomy may help to decrease ICP by allowing drainage of cerebrospinal fluid, at the same time, it may promote brain tissue shifts and may therefore be detrimental.

A broad consensus exists among neurosurgeons regarding the recommended procedure. In short, external decompressive surgery consists of a large hemicraniectomy and a duraplasty. A large (reversed) question mark-shaped skin incision based at the ear is made. A bone flap with a diameter of at least 12 cm (including the frontal, parietal, temporal, and parts of the occipital squama) is removed (Fig. 3). Additional temporal bone is removed so that the floor of the middle cerebral fossa can be explored. The dura is then opened, and an augmented dural patch that consists of homologous periost and/or temporal fascia is inserted (the size may vary; usually a patch of 15–20 cm in length and 2.5–3.5 cm in width is used). The dura is fixed at the margin of the craniotomy to prevent epidural bleeding. The temporal muscle and the skin flap are then reapproximated and secured. Infarcted brain tissue usually is not resected. During this procedure, a sensor for registration of ICP can easily be inserted. In surviving patients, cranioplasty is performed after at least six weeks (usually 6–12 weeks), using the stored bone flap or an artificial bone flap. Only few complications after hemicraniectomy for massive cerebral infarction have been reported. Postoperative epidural and subdural hemorrhage and hygromas occurred in a few cases (23,27).

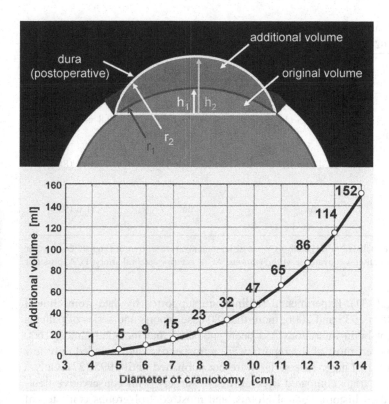

Figure 3 Relation between the diameter of craniotomy and the volume gain.

Other complications may include wound and bone flap infections. All of these can easily be recognized and handled and usually do not contribute to perioperative mortality. A far more important and more common complication is insufficient hemicraniectomy, which may lead to herniation through the craniectomy defect (28). The proportion of brain tissue to be allowed to shift outside the skull is closely related to the diameter of the bone flap, which is removed. The additional volume can be estimated using the following formula:

$$\text{Volume} = \frac{\pi \times h_2^2}{3} \times \frac{\pi \times h_1^2}{3} \times (3 \times r_1 - h_1)$$

Decompressive Surgery (Hemicraniectomy) in Malignant Hemispheric Brain Infarction: Results from Experimental and Observational Clinical Studies

In animal studies, decompressive surgery significantly reduces mortality and infarct size and improves regional blood flow and histologic and functional

Table 1 Summary of Baseline Data of All Available Nonrandomized Studies and Reports on Malignant Hemispheric Infarction

	All patients (n = 1597)	Conservative treatment (n = 512)	Hemicraniectomy (n = 1085)
Age (mean; yr)	57.0 (1465)	64.6 (449)	53.7 (1016)
Dominant vs. nondominant hemisphere (%)	35.5 vs. 64.5 (1196)	54.4 vs. 45.6 (241)	30.8 vs. 69.2 (955)
Additional infarction of the ACA/PCA (%)	28.4 (1200)	25.3 (356)	29.7 (844)
Mean time to surgery (hr)	na	na	51.6 (926)

Publications were included in this analysis when at least an abstract written in English, German, or French, or in translation was available. *Abbreviations*: ACA, anterior cerebral artery; PCA, posterior cerebral artery.

outcome (19,29–31). Experimental findings are supported by data from clinical reports. Between 1935 and 2006, more than 80 case reports and series of patients with malignant brain infarctions had been published that included almost 1600 patients. However, most of the reports were retrospective and included only few patients (Table 1). Larger case series were not published until 1995 (27). Only a few prospective trials compared decompressive surgery with conservative treatment. Some used historic control groups, and most control groups consisted of patients with higher ages, more comorbidity, and mostly lesions in the dominant hemisphere (25,32–35). Data from randomized trials were lacking until 2006.

Mortality Data

All available data are summarized in Table 2. Comparative data from non-randomized clinical studies suggest that hemicraniectomy reduces mortality in hospital from 60% to 100% in controls to 0% to 29% in surgically treated patients and reduces long-term mortality from 83% to 100% to 33%, respectively (32,36). In a review that analyzed all available individual patient data from 138 patients, overall mortality rate after hemicraniectomy after a period of 7 to 21 months was 24% (37). Some of these studies aimed to identify risk factors for an increased risk of mortality after hemicraniectomy. In another study, Glasgow Coma scale (GCS) on admission and coronary artery disease were identified as risk factors for case fatality, whereas age, NIHSS score on admission, CT findings, and other underlying diseases such as diabetes, atrial fibrillation, and hypertension were not associated with early mortality (35). Another group found that increased age (>50 years) and additional infarction of the ACA or PCA territory represent independent risk factors for increased mortality after decompressive surgery. As compared with an overall six-month (1 year) mortality of

Table 2 Summary of Mortality Data of All Available Nonrandomized Studies and Reports on Malignant Hemispheric Infarction

	Mortality in hospital (%) (n)	Mortality up to 3 mo (%) (n)	Mortality up to 6 mo (%) (n)	Mortality up to 12 mo (%) (n)
All patients	37.6 (1175)	34.2 (584)	33.1 (528)	32.7 (452)
Conservative treatment	66.5 (471)	72.7 (165)	55.8 (138)	66.7 (84)
Decompressive surgery	18.3 (704)	19.1 (419)	25.1 (390)	25.0 (368)

38% (44%), mortality rate in patients without these risk factors was 20% (22%), whereas the presence of one risk factor or both risk factors increased mortality to 41% (55%) and 60% (67%), respectively (38).

Functional Outcome

Various trials suggest that decompressive surgery reduces poor outcomes and increases favorable or independent functional outcomes (23,25,33,36,39). On the other hand, several studies doubt these results, especially in patients with increased age and with additional infarction of the ACA or PCA territory (34,35,38,40,41). Other predictors that have been proposed to predict unfavorable outcome are preoperative midline shift, low preoperative GCS, presence of anisocoria, early clinical deterioration, and internal carotid artery occlusion (42,43). In a meta-analysis in the review cited above, age was the only prognostic factor for poor outcome, whereas time to surgery, the presence of brain stem signs prior to surgery, or additional infarction of the ACA or PCA territory was not associated with the outcome (37). Available data are summarized in Table 3. According to the review, functional outcome was classified as (*i*) independent outcome (modified Rankin Scale, mRS, 0–1 or Glasgow Outcome Score, GOS, 5; Barthel Index, ≥90), (*ii*) mild-to-moderate disability (mRS, 2–3

Table 3 Summary of Functional Outcome Data of All Available Nonrandomized Studies and Reports on Malignant Hemispheric Infarction

	Mean time to follow-up, mo (n)	Independent outcome, %	Mild-to-moderate disability, %	Severe disability, %	Death, %
All Patients	12.2 (616)	4.7	22.7	43.8	28.7
Conservative treatment	5 (98)	1.0	11.2	37.8	50.0
Decompressive surgery	13.7 (518)	5.4	24.9	45.0	24.7

or GOS, 4; Barthel Index, 60–85), (*iii*) severe disability (mRS, 4 or 5 or GOS, 2–3; Barthel Index, <60), and (*iv*) death (37). In cases in which more than one outcome scale was given, outcomes were classified according to the following priority: mRS, GOS, Barthel Index. Studies that reported mean values of the Barthel Index, GOS, or mRS were not considered for this analysis.

Quality of Life

Data are scarce regarding the quality of life of patients after hemicraniectomy for malignant cerebral infarction. Data from five smaller trials show that most of the survivors had an average quality of life compared with other stroke patients (44–48). Some of the surgically treated patients were even able to return to work (44,45). One trial revealed a more profound reduction in the quality of life (49). Depression is a common finding in patients who survive malignant hemispheric infarction after hemicraniectomy: more than 50% suffer from severe depression, which is rarely treated in these patients (47). Interpretation of these findings is limited by the fact that no data are available regarding the quality of life of patients who survived a malignant hemispheric infarction and were treated conservatively.

Decompressive Surgery (Hemicraniectomy) in Malignant Hemispheric Brain Infarction: Results from Randomized Clinical Trials

With the promising results of nonrandomized studies, decompressive surgery for large space-occupying infarction has increasingly been incorporated in routine clinical practice. However, because of a lack of conclusive evidence of efficacy from randomized controlled clinical trials, experts continue to debate its benefit. This dilemma could only be answered by randomized trials. Great efforts have been taken in the past to develop appropriate study protocols that were accepted by both neurosurgeons and neurologists. Since 2000, five randomized trials have been conducted, with largely similar eligibility criteria and outcome measures: the American *Hemicraniecomy And Durotomy upon Deterioration From Infarction Related Swelling Trial* (HeADDFIRST) was completed in 2003, but had not been published at the time of this writing. The German *DEcompressive Surgery for the Treatment of malignant INfarction of the middle cerebral arterY* (DESTINY) trial and the French *DEcompressive Craniectomy In MALignant middle cerebral artery infarcts* (DECIMAL) trial were completed in 2006, and their results were reported at international stroke conferences in 2006. Two other trials are ongoing: the Dutch *Hemicraniectomy After Middle cerebral artery infarction with Life-threatening Edema Trial* (HAMLET) and the Philippinian *Hemicraniectomy For Malignant Middle cerebral artery Infarcts* (HeMMI) trial. In addition, a prospectively planned pooled analysis of the three European trials was recently published (13–15,50,51).

DESTINY was an open, controlled, prospective, multicentered randomized trial. Patients were randomized either to surgical and conservative treatment or to conservative treatment alone. The maximum time from symptom onset to treatment start was 36 hours. All patients were treated in an intensive care unit (ICU) and were intubated and ventilated. DESTINY was based on a sequential design, with mortality after 30 days as the first end point; randomization was planned to go on until statistical significance for this end point was reached. Thereafter, patient enrollment would be interrupted until the six-month functional outcome end point (primary end point), mRS, dichotomized at a score of 0–3 versus 4–6, had been collected. Depending on the observed difference in functional outcome, the final sample size would be recalculated for a second explorative trial stage. Secondary end point included analysis of the mRS 0–4 versus 5 and 6 and the distribution of scores of the mRS at six months and at one year. After inclusion of 32 patients between February 2004 and October 2005, patient recruitment was stopped because of statistically significant results of mortality. In the Intention-to-Treat analysis, 2 of 17 (11.8%) patients treated by hemicraniectomy had died, and 7 of 15 (50.3%) patients who received maximum conservative treatment on the ICU alone had died after 30 days ($p = 0.02$). Functional outcome data after 12 months are summarized in Figure 4. Further, 47.1% of the patients in the surgical arm versus 26.7% of the patients in the conservative arm reached an mRS of 0–3 ($p = 0.23$); 76.5% in the surgical arm versus 33.3% in the conservative arm reached an mRS of 0–4 ($p = 0.01$). Analysis of the distribution of the mRS scores showed positive results in favor of surgery ($p = 0.04$). After a sample-size projection for the primary end point suggested that 94 patients should be included in each arm, the trial was stopped (14).

DECIMAL was another open, controlled, prospective, multicentered randomized trial that randomly assigned patients either to surgical and conservative treatment or to conservative treatment alone. Inclusion criteria included an infarct volume on DWI of at least 145 cm^3. Hemicraniectomy had to have been performed within 30 hours after symptom onset and within six hours after randomization. The primary end point in DECIMAL was functional outcome based on the mRS score, dichotomized 0–3 versus 4–6. A sequential design for this end point was chosen on the basis of interim analyses after every four patients. Secondary end points included survival and the mRS score at 6 and 12 months. Between December 2000 and November 2005, 38 patients were enrolled. Survival was statistically significantly different among groups, with mortality rates of 5 of 20 patients (25%) in the surgical treatment group and 14 of 18 patients (77.8%) in the conservative treatment group ($p < 0.0001$). The functional outcome data after 12 months are summarized in Figure 4. Forty percent of the patients in the surgical arm versus 22.2% of the patients in the conservative arm reached an mRS of 0–3 ($p = 0.08$) (13).

DECIMAL was prematurely stopped after the 10th interim analysis both because of ethical considerations of continuing recruitment and because of expectations of a planned pooled analysis of the three European trials: DECIMAL, DESTINY, and HAMLET. This pooled analysis of the three European randomized trials on hemiacraniectomy for malignant MCA infarction is the first

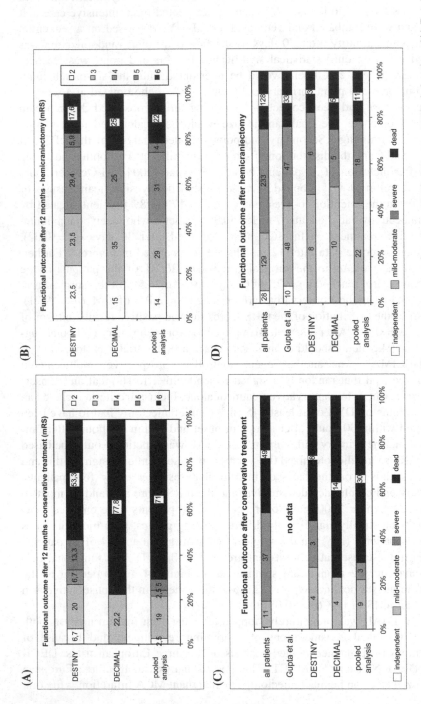

Figure 4 Functional outcome after hemicraniectomy and after conservative treatment in patients with malignant MCA infarction. (**A**) Results from randomized trials and a pooled analysis. (**B**) Results from randomized trials compared to results from all available data of nonrandomized trials and a meta-analysis of all individual patient data. *Abbreviation*: MCA, middle cerebral artery. *Source*: from Ref. 37.

instance in the field of stroke in which analyses of patient data from three different randomized trials were pooled while the trials were ongoing. For the pooled analysis, a maximum time window from stroke onset to randomization of 45 hours and 48 hours to treatment start was adopted. Outcome measures in the pooled analysis were mRS score at one year, dichotomized between 0–4 and 5–6, as well as between 0–3 and 4–6, and the case fatality at one year. All patients randomized in DECIMAL and DESTINY and 23 patients from HAMLET were eligible for the pooled analysis. Thus, 93 patients were included, of whom 51 were randomized to decompressive surgery and 42 to conservative treatment. Results demonstrated that after decompressive surgery more patients had an mRS of less than or equal to 4 (75% vs. 24%, $p < 0.0001$), with a pooled absolute risk reduction (ARR) of 51% (95% CI, 34–69). In addition, more patients had an mRS of less than or equal to 3 (43% vs. 21%, $p = 0.014$), with a pooled ARR of 23% (95% CI, 5–41). Case-fatality rate in the surgical group was 78% versus 29% in the conservative-treatment group ($p < 0.0001$), indicating a pooled ARR of 50% (95% CI, 33–67) (see Figure 4). The resulting numbers of patients needed to treat are 2 for survival with an mRS of less than or equal to 4, 4 for survival with an mRS of less than or equal to 3, and 2 for survival irrespective of outcome (51).

CONCLUSION AND FUTURE DIRECTIONS

For many years, experts did not have a consensus regarding which treatment is beneficial in patients with malignant MCA infarctions. Despite the lack of randomized, controlled trials, many specialists agreed that decompressive surgery in malignant MCA stroke is life saving. Intercessors always pointed out the benefit of survival as well as comparatively better outcome in a high proportion of surgically treated patients, substantial recovery extending at least into the second half-year and thereafter, no differences in the quality of life of patients with dominant or nondominant hemispheric infarction, and the retrospective agreement in the decision to undergo surgery in a high percentage of patients and their relatives (44,45,52,53). On the other hand, critics doubted the use of decompressive surgery, especially concerning the long-term survival and functional outcome. Their concern has always been that decompressive surgery may serve as a life-saving procedure but that the improved case-fatality rate would lead to an increased number of severely disabled patients exposed to a life of dependency, pain, and hopelessness. Consequently, neurologists and neurosurgeons had a great deal of uncertainty regarding the procedure. Some considered hemicraniectomy with duraplasty a standard procedure in large, hemispheric, ischemic infarcts and regarded withholding surgical treatment as unethical, whereas others believed that a possibly life-saving procedure is not advisable in patients with a very severe and largely irreversible neurologic deficit. Because of these issues, in some centers, hemicraniectomy has indeed become a standard procedure in space-occupying hemispheric infarct. In some patients, only conservative treatment is applied. In some cases, hemicraniectomy is only considered in young patients with lesions of the nondominant hemisphere, and in others, these patients are not treated at all.

Until recently, all of the available data came from observational studies. In 2007, for the first time, we have evidence from randomized, controlled trials that hemicraniectomy in large, hemispheric infarctions not only reduces mortality but also significantly increases the chance to survive with a moderate functional impairment and without increasing the number of completely dependent survivors.

ARE THERE ALTERNATIVES TO HEMICRANIECTOMY?

Conservative (Medical) Treatment Options

Currently, no proven conservative treatment options exist. Several conservative treatment strategies, such as artificial coma, hyperventilation, steroids, and osmotic therapy, have been proposed to reduce ICP and to limit brain tissue shifts after space-occupying ischemic stroke. Thus far, none of these therapeutic strategies to control cerebral edema formation and raised ICP is supported by adequate evidence of efficacy from experimental studies or randomized clinical trials (54–56). Several reports suggest that they are ineffective or even detrimental (5,11,57–67). To understand why medical treatment alone often fails to prevent clinical deterioration, it must be remembered that early clinical deterioration is usually not due to increases in global ICP, but is rather due to massive local swelling and shifts in brain tissue. Increases in ICP often occur secondarily. As a result, the role of therapies that focus on lowering global ICP is limited. Hofmeijer et al. (56) has published an excellent and comprehensive overview of conservative treatment strategies for increased ICP.

Mild-to-Moderate Hypothermia

Induced hypothermia is defined as physical or pharmacologic lowering of the physiologic body core temperature to 33°C to 36°C (mild hypothermia), 28°C to 32°C (moderate hypothermia), or 10°C to 28°C (deep hypothermia) (68). Hypothermia has been used in critical care medicine to achieve neuroprotection in several conditions, such as traumatic brain injury, anoxic brain injury after cardiac arrest, hepatic encephalopathy, and massive stroke. It is also well known that body temperature on admission and during the first 24 hours is associated with the extent of ischemic damage and is an independent predictor of mortality and outcome in ischemic stroke (69,70). Spontaneous hypothermia seems to reduce mortality and predict a better outcome in acute stroke (71), although these findings are still controversial (72). Presumed mechanisms of hypothermia to reduce ischemic damage include induction of ischemic tolerance by reduced brain metabolism (73,74), reduced excitatory neurotransmitter release (75,76), reduced expression of immediate early genes such as *c-fos* (77), inhibition of apoptosis (78), inhibition of metalloproteinase expression (79), reduced inflammatory response (80,81), and inhibition of blood-brain barrier disruption, which leads to reduced brain edema (82). Although the neuroprotective effect of hypothermia has been known since the 1950s, earliest experimental findings in ischemic stroke were reported in the late 1980s (83,84). Only a few animal experiments have been conducted using moderate hypothermia in large ischemic stroke. In these studies, the effect on neuroprotection was pronounced when hypothermia was started early and continued for more than 24 hours (78,85–90). Moderate hypothermia is an invasive procedure that requires treatment in an experienced ICU, including ventilation, relaxation, and measurement of ICP. The clinical data on induced hypothermia has shown promising results that suggest that moderate cooling may reduce mortality in malignant ischemic brain infarction to 17% to 50% (91–94) (Table 4). Only one study compared hypothermia and hemicraniectomy and showed less than promising results for hypothermia, with mortality rates of 47% versus 12% (95).

Hypothermia in these studies was associated with a high rate of complications, the most frequent being pneumonia, severe bradycardia, and heart insuffiency, with severe hypotonia, thrombocytopenia, and coagulopathy. Especially in the rewarming phase, a high percentage of patients developed severe increases in ICP. Compared with hemicraniectomy, hypothermia seems to be far less effective in reducing mortality. Therefore, because of possible severe side effects and the lack of conclusive data from randomized trials, this procedure cannot be readily incorporated in neurointensive care routine use as a standard treatment and is restricted to selected patients treated in experienced centers. A promising approach may be the combination of hemicraniectomy with mild hypothermia (96).

Table 4 Summary of Available Studies on Hypothermia in Malignant Hemispheric Infarction

Author(s), (yr)	n	Target temperature	Time to induction of hypothermia	Duration of hypothermia
Schwab et al., (91) (1998)	25	33°C (external cooling)	(4–24) mean 14 ± 7 hr	48–72 hr
Schwab et al., (92) (2001)	50	32–33°C (external cooling)	(4–75) mean 22 ± 9 hr	24–72 hr
Georgiadis et al., (93) (2001)	6	33°C (endovascular cooling)	(12–58) mean 28 ± 17 hr	48–78 hr
Georgiadis et al., (95) (2002)	19	33°C (n = 8 endovascular cooling; n = 11 external cooling)	(18–24) mean 24 hr	24–116 hr
Milhaud et al., (94) (2005)	12	32–33°C (external cooling)	(4–24) mean 11 ± 7 hr	120–504 hr

REFERENCES

1. Silver SL, Norris JW, Lewis AJ, et al. Early mortality following stroke: a prospective review. Stroke 1984; 15:492–496.
2. Shaw CM, Alvord EC Jr., Berry RG. Swelling of the brain following ischemic infarction with arterial occlusion. Arch Neurol 1959; 1:161–177.
3. Ropper AH, Shafran B. Brain edema after stroke. Clinical syndrome and intracranial pressure. Arch Neurol 1984; 41:26–29.
4. Frank JI. Large hemispheric infarction, deterioration, and intracranial pressure. Neurology 1995; 45:1286–1290.
5. Hacke W, Schwab S, Horn M, et al. "Malignant" middle cerebral artery infarction. Clinical course and prognostic signs. Arch Neurol 1996; 53:309–315.
6. Ng LKY, Nimmannitya J. Massive cerebral infarction with severe brain swelling: a clinicopathological study. Stroke 1970; 1:158–163.
7. Sakai K, Iwahashi K, Terada K, et al. Outcome after external decompression for massive cerebral infarction. Neurol Med Chir 1998; 38:131–135.
8. Heinsius T, Bogousslavsky J. Van Melle G. Large infarcts in the middle cerebral artery territory. Etiology and outcome patterns. Neurology 1998; 59:341–350.
9. Wardlaw JM, Dennis MS, Lindley RI, et al. Does early reperfusion of a cerebral infarct influence cerebral infarct swelling in the acute stage or the final clinical outcome? Cerebrovasc Dis 1993; 3:86–93.
10. Schwab S, Aschoff A, Spranger M, et al. The value of intracranial pressure monitoring in acute hemispheric stroke. Neurology 1996; 47:393–398.
11. Wijdicks EFM, Diringer MN. Middle cerebral artery territory infarction and early brain swelling: progression and effect of age on outcome. Mayo Clin Proc 1998; 73:829–836.
12. Berrouschot J, Sterker M, Bettin S, et al. Mortality of space-occupying (malignant) middle cerebral artery infarction under conservative intensive care. Intensive Care Med 1998; 24:620–623.
13. Vahedi K, Vicaut E, Mateo J, et al. DECIMAL trial: a sequential design, multicenter, randomized, controlled trial of decompressive craniectomy in malignant middle cerebral artery (MCA) infarction. Int Jn Stroke 2006; 1(suppl 1):38 (abstract).
14. Jüttler E, Schwab S, Schmiedek P, et al. DESTINY: decompressive surgery for the treatment of malignant infarction of the middle cerebral artery—outcome results. Int Jn Stroke 2006; 1(suppl 1):38 (abstract).
15. Hofmeijer J, Amelink GJ, Algra A, et al. Hemicraniectomy after middle cerebral artery infarction with life-threatening edema trial (HAMLET). Protocol for a randomised controlled trial of decompressive surgery in space-occupying hemispheric infarction. Trials 2006; 7:29.
16. Krieger DW, Demchuk AM, Kasner SE, et al. Early clinical and radiological predictors of fatal brain swelling in ischemic stroke. Stroke 1999; 30:287–292.
17. Barber PA, Demchuk AM, Zhang J, et al. Computed tomographic parameters predicitng fatal outcome in large middle cerebral artery infarction. Cerebrovasc Dis 2003; 16:230–235.
18. Oppenheim C, Samson Y. Manaï R, et al. Prediction of malignant middle cerebral artery infarction by diffusion-weighted imaging. Stroke 2000; 31:2175–2181.
19. Engelhorn T, Doerfler A, Kastrup A, et al. Decompressive craniectomy, reperfusion, or a combination for early treatment of acute "Malignant" cerebral hemispheric stroke in rats: Potential mechanisms studied by MRI. Stroke 1999; 30:1456–1463.

20. Jaeger M, Soehle M, Meixensberger J. Improvement of brain tissue oxygen and intracranial pressure during and after surgical decompression for diffuse brain oedema and space occupying infarction. Acta Neurochir 2005; 95(suppl):117–118.

21. Wirtz CR, Steiner T, Aschoff A, et al. Hemicraniectomy with dural augmentation in medically uncontrollable hemispheric infarction. Neurosurgery Focus 1997; 2:1–4.

22. Greco T. Le thrombosi posttraumatiche della carotide. Arch Ital Chir 1935; 39:757–784.

23. Schwab S, Steiner T, Aschoff A, et al. Early hemicranectomy in patients with complete middle cerebral artery infarction. Stroke 1998; 29:1888–1893.

24. Mori K, Ishimaru S. Maeda M., et al. Unco-parahippocampectomy for direct surgical treatment of downward transtentorial herniation. Acta Neurochir (Wien) 1998; 140: 1239–1244.

25. Mori K, Nakao Y, Yamamoto T, et al. Early external decompressive craniectomy with duroplasty improves functional recovery in patients with massive hemispheric embolic infarction: timing and indication of decompressive surgery for malignant cerebral infarction. Surg Neurol 2004; 62:420–429.

26. Robertson SC, Lennarson P, Hasan DM, et al. Clinical course and surgical management of massive cerebral infarction. Neurosurgery 2004; 55:55–62.

27. Rieke K, Schwab S, Krieger D, et al. Decompressive surgery in space-occupying hemispheric infarction: results of an open, prospective trial. Crit Care Med 1995; 23: 1576–1587.

28. Wagner S, Schnippering H, Aschoff A, et al. Suboptimum hemicraniectomy as a cause of additional cerebral lesions in patients with malignant infarction of the middle cerebral artery. J Neurosurg 2001; 94:693–696.

29. Doerfler A, Forsting M, Reith W, et al. Decompressive craniectomy in a rat model of "malignant" cerebral hemispheric stroke: experimental support for an aggressive therapeutic approach. J Neurosurg 1996; 85:853–859.

30. Forsting M, Reith W, Schaebitz WR, et al. Decompressive craniectomy for cerebral infarction: an experimental study in rats. Stroke 1995; 26:259–264.

31. Hofmeijer J, Schepers J, Veldhuis WB, et al. Delayed decompressive surgery increases apparent diffusion coefficient and improves peri-infarct perfusion in rats with space-occupying cerebral infarction. Stroke 2004; 35:1476–1481.

32. Holtkamp M, Buchheim K, Unterberg A, et al. Hemicraniectomy in elderly patients with space occupying media infarction: improved survival but poor functional outcome. J Neurol Neurosurg Psychiatry 2001; 70:226–228.

33. Cho DY, Chen TC, Lee HC. Ultra-early decompressive craniectomy for malignant middle cerebral artery infarction. Surg Neurol 2003; 60:227–232.

34. Maramattom BV, Bahn MM, Wijdicks EMF. Which patient fares worse after early deterioration due to swelling from hemispheric stroke? Neurology 2004; 63:2142–2145.

35. Wang KW, Chang WN, Ho JT, et al. Factors predictive of fatality in massive middle cerebral artey territory infarction and clinical experience of decompressive hemicraniectomy. Eur J Neurol 2006; 13:765–771.

36. Delashaw JB, Broaddus WC, Kassell NF, et al. Treatment of right hemispheric cerebral infarction by hemicraniectomy. Stroke 1990; 21:874–881.

37. Gupta R, Connolly ES, Mayer S, et al. Hemicraniectomy for massive middle cerebral artery territory infarction. A systemiatic review. Stroke 2004; 35:539–543.

38. Uhl E, Kreth FW, Elias B, et al. Outcome and prognostic factors of hemicraniectomy for space occupying cerebral infarction. J Neurol Neurosurg Psychiatry 2004; 75: 270–274.

39. Kastrau F, Wolter M, Huber W, et al. Recovery from aphasia after hemicraniectomy for infarction of the speech-dominant hemisphere. Stroke 2005; 36:825–829.

40. Yao Y, Liu W, Yang X, et al. Is decompressive caniectomy for malignant middle cerebral artery territory infarction of any benefit for elderly patients? Surg Neurol 2005; 64:165–169.

41. Harscher S, Reichart R, Terborg C, et al. Outcome after decompressive craniectomy in patients with severe ischemic stroke. Acta Neurochir (Wien) 2006; 148:31–37.

42. Kilincer C, Asil T, Utku U, et al. Factors affecting the outcome of decompressive craniectomy for large hemispheric infarctions: a prospective cohort study. Acta Neurochir (Wien) 2005; 147:587–594.

43. Rabinstein AA, Mueller-Kronast N, Maramottom BV, et al. Factors prediciting prognosis after decompressive hemicraniectomy for hemispheric infarction. Neurology 2006; 76:891–893.

44. Walz B, Zimmermann C. Böttger S, et al. Prognosis of patients after hemicraniectomy in malignant middle cerebral artery infarction. J Neurol 2002; 249:1183–1190.

45. Woertgen C, Erban P, Rothoerl RD, et al. Quality of life after decompressive craniectomy in patients suffering from supratentorial brain ischemia. Acta Neurochir (Wien) 2004; 146:691–695.

46. Curry WT, Sethi MK, Ogilvy CS, et al. Factors associated with outcome after hemicraniectomy for large middle cerebral artery infarction. Neurosurgery 2005; 56: 681–692.

47. Erban P, Woertgen C, Luerding R, et al. Long-term outcome after hemicraniectomy for space occupying right hemispheric MCA infarction. Clin Neurol Neurosurg 2005; 1431:1–4.

48. Vahedi K, Benoist L, Kurtz A, et al. Quality of life after decompressive craniectomy for malignant middle cerebral artery infarction. J Neurol Neurosurg Psychiatry 2005; 76: 1181–1182.

49. Foerch C, Lang JM, Krause J, et al. Functional impairment, disability, and quality of life outcome after decompressive hemicraniectomy in malignant middle cerebral artery infarction. J Neurosurg 2004; 101:248–254.

50. Frank JI, Krieger D, Chyatte D, et al. Hemicraniectomy and durotomy upon deterioration from massive hemispheric infarction: a proposed multicenter, prospective, randomized study. Stroke 1999; 30:243.

51. Vahedi K, Hofmeijer J, Juettler E, et al. Early decompressive surgery in malignant middle cerebral artery infarction: a pooled analysis of three randomised controlled trials. Lancet Neurology 2007; 6:215–222.

52. Leonhardt G, Wilhelm H, Doerfler A, et al. Clinical outcome and neuropsychological deficits after right decompressive hemicraniectomy in MCA infarction. J Neurol 2002; 249:1433–1440.

53. Matsuura D, Inatomi Y, Yonehara T, et al. Decompressive craniectomy for ischemic stroke. No To Shinkei 2006; 58:305–310 (abstract).

54. Bereczki D, Liu M, do Parado GF, et al. Mannitol for acute stroke. Cochrane Database Syst Rev 2004; CD001153.

55. Righetti E, Celani MG, Cantisani T, et al. Glycerol for acute stroke. Cochrane Database Syst Rev 2000; CD000096.

56. Hofmeijer J, van der Worp HB, Kappelle LJ. Treatment of space-occupying cerebral infarction. Crit Care Med 2003; 31:617–625.

57. Miuzelaar JP, Marmarou A, Ward JD, et al. Adverse effects of prolonged hyperventilation in patients with severe head injury: a randomized clinical trial. J Neurosurg 1991; 75:731–739.

58. Kaufmann AM, Cardoso ER. Aggravation of vasogenic cerebral edema by multiple-dose mannitol. J Neurosurg 1992; 77:584–589.

59. Adams HP, Brott TG, Crowell RM, et al. Guidelines for the management of patients with acute ischemic stroke: a statement for healthcare professionals from a special writing group of the Stroke Council, American Heart Association. Stroke 1994; 25: 1901–1914.

60. Schwab S, Spranger M, Schwarz S, et al. Barbiturate coma in severe hemispheric stroke: Useful or obsolete? Neurology 1997; 48:1608–1613.

61. Schwarz S, Schwab S, Bertram M, et al. Effects of hypertonic saline hydroxyethyl starch solution and mannitol in patients with increased intracranial pressure after stroke. Stroke 1998; 29:1550–1555.

62. Schwarz S, Bertram M, Aschoff A, et al. Indomethacin for brain edema following stroke. Cerebrovasc Dis 1999; 9:248–250.

63. Schwarz S, Georgiadis D, Aschoff A, et al. Effects of body position on intracranial pressure and cerebral perfusion in patients with large hemispheric stroke. Stroke 2002; 33:497–501.

64. Schwarz S, Georgiadis D, Aschoff A, et al. Effects of induced hypertension on intracranial pressure flow velocities of the middle cerebral arteries in patients with large hemispheric stroke. Stroke 2002; 33:998–1004.

65. Schwarz S, Georgiadis D, Aschoff A, et al. Effects of hypertonic (10%) saline in patients with raised intracranial pressure after stroke. Stroke 2002; 33:136–140.

66. Van der Worp HB, Kappelle LJ. Complications of acute ischaemic stroke. Cerebrovasc Dis 1998; 8:124–132.

67. Wijdicks EFM. Management of massive hemispheric cerebral infarct: Is there a ray of hope? Mayo Clin Proc 2000; 75, 945–952.

68. Bernard SA, Buist M. Induced hypothermia in critical care medicine: a review. Crit Care Med 2003; 31:2041–2051.

69. Castillo J, Davalos A, Marrugat J, et al. Timing for fever-related brain damage in acute ischemic stroke. Stroke 1998; 29:2455–2460.

70. Wang Y, Lim LL, Levi C, et al. Influence of admission body temperature on stroke mortality. Stroke 2000; 31:404–409.

71. Reith J, Jorgensen HS, Pedersen PM, et al. Body temperature in acute stroke: relation to stroke severity, infarct size, mortality, and outcome. Lancet 1996; 347:422–425.

72. Boysen G, Christensen H. Stroke severity determines body temperature in acute stroke. Stroke 2001; 32:413–417.

73. Berntman L, Welsh FA, Harp JR. Cerebral protective effect of low-grade hypothermia. Anesthesiology 1981; 55:495–498.

74. Yager JY, Asselin J. Effect of mild hypothermia on cerebral energy metabolism during the evolution of hypoxic-ischemic brain damage in the immature rat. Stroke 1996; 27:919–925.

75. Nakashima K, Todd MM. Effects of hypothermia on the rate of excitatory amino acid release after ischemic depolarization. Stroke 1996; 27:913–918.

76. Huang FP, Zhou LF, Yang GY. Effects of mild hypothermia on the release of regional glutamate and glicine during extended transient focl cerebral ischemia in rats. Neurochem Res 1998; 23:991–996.

77. Mancuso A, Derugin N, Hara K, et al. Mild hypothermia decreases the incidence of transient ADC reduction detected with diffusion MRI and expression of c-fos and hsp70 mRNA during acute focal ischemia in rats. Brain Res 2000; 887:34–45.
78. Maier CM, Ahern K, Cheng ML, et al. Optimal depth and duration of mild hypothermia in a focal model of transient cerebral ischemia: Effects on neurologic outcome, infarct size, apoptosis, and inflammation. Stroke 1998; 29:2171–2180.
79. Wagner S, Nagel S, Kluge B, et al. Topographically graded postischemic presence of metalloproteinases is inhibited by hypothermia. Brain Res 2003; 984:63–75.
80. Toyoda T, Suzuki S, Kassell NF, et al. Intraischemic hypothermia attenuates neutrophil infiltration in the rat neocortex after focal ischemia-reperfusion injury. Neurosurgery 1996; 39:1200–1205.
81. Deng H, Han HS, Cheng D, et al. Mild hypothermia inhibits inflammation after experimental stroke and brain inflammation. Stroke 2003; 34:2495–2501.
82. Karibe H, Zarow GJ, Graham SH, et al. Mild intraischemic hypothermia reduces postischemic hyperperfusion, delayed postischemic hypoperfusion, blood-brain barrier disruption, brain edema, and neuronal damage volume after temporary focal cerebral ischemia in rats. J Cereb Blood Flow Metab 1994; 14:620–627.
83. Busto R, Dietrich D, Globus MYT, et al. The importance of brain temperature in cerebral ischemic injury. Stroke 1989; 20:1113–1114.
84. Busto R, Dietrich WD, Globus MY, et al. Small differences in intraischemic brain temperature critically determine the extent of ischemic neuronal injury. J Cereb Blood Flow Metab 1987; 7:729–738.
85. Corbett D, Thornhill J. Temperature modulation (hypothermic and hyperthermic conditions) and its influence on histological and behavioural outcomes following cerebral ischemia. Brain Pathol 2000; 10:145–152.
86. Rajek A, Greif R, Sessler DI, et al. Core cooling by central venous infusion of ice-cold (4 degrees and 20 degrees C) fluid: isolation of core and peripheral thermal compartments. Anesthesiology 2000; 93:629–637.
87. Berger C. Schäbitz WR, Georgiadis D, et al. Effects of hypothermia on excitatory amino acids and metabolism in stroke patients: a microdialysis study. Stroke 2002; 33:519–524.
88. Kollmar R, Frietsch T, Georgiadis D, et al. Early effects of acid-based management during hypothermia on cerebral infarct volume, edema, and cerebral blood flow in acute focal cerebral ischemia in rats. Anesthesiology 2002; 97:868–874.
89. Kollmar R, Schäbitz WR, Heiland S, et al. Neuroprotective effect of delayed moderate hypothermia after focal cerebral ischemis: An MRI study. Stroke 2002; 33:1899–1904.
90. Doerfler A, Schwab S, Hoffmann TT, et al. Combination of decompressive craniectomy and mild hypothermia ameliorates infarction volume after permanent focal ischemis in rats. Stroke 2001; 32:2675–2681.
91. Schwab S, Schwarz S, Spranger M, et al. Moderate hypothermia in the treatment of patients with severe middle cerebral artery infarction. Stroke 1998; 29:2461–2466.
92. Schwab S, Georgiadis D, Berrouschot J, et al. Feasibility and safety of moderate hypothermia after massive hemispheric infarction. Stroke 2001; 32:2033–2035.
93. Georgiadis D, Schwarz S, Kollmar R, et al. Endovascular cooling for moderate hypothermia in patients with acute stroke: first results of a novel approach. Stroke 2001; 32:2550–2553.

94. Milhaud D, Thouvenot E, Heroum C, et al. Prolonged moderate hypothermia in massive hemispheric infarction: clinical experience. J Neurosurg Anesthesiol 2005; 17:49–53.
95. Georgiadis D, Schwarz S, Aschoff A, et al. Hemicraniectomy and moderate hypothermia in patients with severe ischemic stroke. Stroke 2002; 33:1584–1588.
96. Els T, Oehm E, Voigt S, et al. Safety and therapeutical benefit of hemicraniectomy combined with mild hypothermia in comparison with hemicraniectomy alone in patients with malignant ischemic stroke. Cerebrovasc Dis 2006; 21:79–85.

8

Anticoagulation in Ischemic Stroke

Carolyn A. Cronin, MD, PhD, Resident

*Department of Neurology, The Johns Hopkins University School of Medicine,
Baltimore, Maryland, U.S.A.*

Robert J. Wityk, MD, FAHA, Associate Professor

*Department of Neurology, The Johns Hopkins University School of Medicine
and Cerebrovascular Division, The Johns Hopkins Hospital,
Baltimore, Maryland, U.S.A.*

INTRODUCTION

Anticoagulation has been used as a treatment for acute ischemic stroke for decades. A case series published in 1958 described 58 patients treated with anti-coagulation (either heparin or coumadin), some in the acute setting and some in the long-term, and 37 nonrandomly selected "similar" patients who were not anticoagulated (1). On anticoagulation, 28 of 29 patients who had previously been experiencing frequent transient ischemic attacks (TIAs) had cessation of attacks; similarly, 11 of 14 patients who were having stepwise decline in function had cessation of the decline and some improvement. In contrast, no improvement was seen in patients who had fully developed stroke at the time of anticoagulation. The patients who were not treated with anticoagulation had either persistence of TIAs or progression to stroke during the period of observation.

In the following years, heparin became more widely used in the acute stroke setting. Use of anticoagulation in the acute stroke setting has been thought to decrease or reverse initial deficits, prevent the progression of strokes in evolution, or prevent acute recurrent strokes. However, use of anticoagulation brings with it the risk of increased rate of serious bleeding, both systemic bleeding and intra-cranial hemorrhage, that can be catastrophic. Data from a series of trials conducted in the last decade that examined this issue showed that, for the majority of stroke patients, anticoagulation in the acute setting is not beneficial; consequently, the use of anticoagulation has declined (2–4). A review of the charts of 763 consec-utive stroke patients with atrial fibrillation seen between 1996 and 2002 found that anticoagulation as the first-prescribed antithrombotic agent declined from 70% to 22% and that antiplatelet prescription increased from 27% to 78% (5). The American Heart Association/American Stroke Association Guidelines (2005 update) for the early management of the general population of patients with ischemic stroke states, "Current data do not provide evidence in support of the efficacy of early anticoagulation in improving outcomes after acute ischemic stroke" (6). This chapter will provide a review of the literature that guides current anticoagulation treatment decisions and identify areas in which further study may be warranted.

TRIALS OF UNFRACTIONATED HEPARIN FOR ACUTE ISCHEMIC STROKE

The largest of the trials of anticoagulation in acute ischemic stroke was the International Stroke Trial (IST) (7) in which 19,435 patients were randomized within 48 hours of symptom onset to either (*i*) subcutaneous heparin in two doses (medium dose, 12,500 units b.i.d. and low dose, 5000 units b.i.d.) or (*ii*) no heparin, with treatment continued for 14 days or until discharge. The medium dose was used to achieve anticoagulation of the patient, whereas the low dose was used primarily to prevent deep venous thrombosis. These groups were further divided to receive aspirin, 300 mg daily, or no aspirin. The analysis of events at 14 days showed that heparin decreased the rate of recurrent ischemic stroke by approximately 1%, but at the expense of increasing the rate of intra-cerebral hemorrhage (ICH) also by approximately 1%, so that the total rates of second stroke (ischemic or hemorrhagic) within 14 days were not different (Table 1). In addition, no significant difference was seen in the rate of death at 14 days (9.0% with heparin vs. 9.3% without heparin). However, when the two doses of heparin were further subdivided, the medium-dose (12,500 units b.i.d.)

Table 1 International Stroke Trial Results: Events Within 14 Days

	All[a] Heparin	All[b] Avoid heparin	Afib[b] Heparin	Afib[b] Avoid heparin
Recurrent ischemic stroke	2.9%	3.8%	2.3%	4.9%
Hemorrhagic stroke	1.2%	0.4%	2.8%	0.4%
Total	4.1%	4.2%	5.1%	5.3%

All[a], All patients.
Afib[b], Atrial fibrillation.
Source: From Ref. 7.

heparin group had more deaths and nonfatal strokes at 14 days compared with the low-dose (5000 units b.i.d.) heparin group (medium dose, 12.6%; low dose, 10.8%; $p = 0.007$). The medium-dose heparin group also had a trend for more ICHs (medium dose, 1.8%; low dose, 0.7%) and for a higher rate of transfused or fatal extracranial hemorrhage (medium dose, 2.0%; low dose, 0.6%). The rates of recurrent ischemic stroke were not significantly different between the two doses (medium dose, 3.2%; low dose, 2.6%), although low-dose heparin trended toward being more effective at preventing recurrent ischemic stroke.

Aspirin, on the other hand, had a small but statistically significant effect of decreasing the rate of recurrent ischemic stroke (3.9–2.8%, $p < 0.001$) and had no change in the very low rate of ICH (0.8–0.9%). The conclusion from the study was that aspirin, but not heparin, was beneficial in the acute stroke setting and that if heparin is used, it should be limited to low-dose administration for prevention of deep venous thrombosis. An advantage of this study was that the simple protocol allowed enrollment of a large number of patients, leading to the ability to detect small differences in groups. Criticisms of this study include the fact that no coagulation tests were performed in the heparin group so that data are nonexistent on whether the patients were therapeutically anticoagulated (or overanticoagulated).

LOW-MOLECULAR-WEIGHT HEPARINS IN ACUTE ISCHEMIC STROKE

In addition to unfractionated heparin, low-molecular-weight heparins (LMWHs) have also been studied as a treatment for acute ischemic stroke. Unfractionated heparin primarily acts by activating antithrombin III, which subsequently inhibits thrombin and, to a lesser extent, activated factor X. LMWHs are derived from unfractionated heparin and differ in their mode of action, preferentially inhibiting factor Xa rather than thrombin. Trials of LMWH versus unfractionated heparin for the treatment of venous thromboembolism (8) and for acute coronary syndrome (9) suggest that LMWH is more efficacious without increasing the risk of bleeding. The hope was that LMWH might have the same beneficial effect in ischemic stroke, thus shifting the risk-benefit analysis toward treatment with anticoagulation.

In a trial of LMWH, 312 patients were randomized to subcutaneous high-dose nadroparin (4100 IU b.i.d.), low-dose nadroparin (4100 IU q.d.), or placebo (10). Treatment was started within 48 hours of stroke onset and continued for 10 days. In the high-dose nadroparin group, a decreased rate of death or dependency was seen at six months, but curiously, no benefit was seen at the three-month assessment in this group. This result has not been repeated in any other trial. Other studies with LMWH in acute ischemic stroke include the Heparin in Acute Embolic Stroke Trial (HAEST) with dalteparin (11), the Therapy of Patients with Acute Stroke (TOPAS) trial with certoparin (12), and the Tinzaparin in Acute Ischemic Stroke Trial (TAIST) with tinzaparin (13). None of these other studies of LMWH found a benefit to treatment.

The largest of the stroke trials with LMWH was Trial of ORG 10172 in Acute Stroke Treatment (TOAST), which enrolled 1281 patients (14). Patients were treated for seven days with IV ORG 10172 or placebo given as a bolus within 24 hours of symptom onset, and the infusion rate was adjusted on the basis of anti-factor Xa activity. Of note, during the course of the study, patients with large strokes (National Institutes of Health Stroke Scale, NIHSS > 15) were excluded following an increased rate of ICH seen early in the study. Within 10 days of treatment, patients treated with ORG 10172 had more serious intracranial hemorrhages than placebo-treated patients (14 vs. 4 patients, $p < 0.05$), suggesting that, unlike the positive safety results in the cardiac literature, in stroke patients, LMWH is still associated with an increased rate of systemic and intracranial hemorrhage. At seven days, patients who received LMWH had a higher rate of "very favorable" outcome (defined as a Glasgow Outcome Scale score of 1 and Barthel Index score of 19 or 20) (33.9% vs. 27.8%, $p = 0.01$), but this was not a prespecified end point. In contrast, no difference was observed between the groups in "favorable outcome" at seven days, and no difference was observed in any outcome measure at three months. Therefore, the conclusion was that treatment with ORG 10172 in acute ischemic stroke had no benefit.

EARLY ANTICOAGULATION FOR CARDIOEMBOLIC STROKE

Subgroups of patients who may benefit from early anticoagulation are those with cardioembolic strokes as it may be possible to prevent early recurrent embolic strokes. Evidence certainly suggests that anticoagulation is beneficial in the secondary prevention of stroke in patients with a variety of cardiac sources of embolism, such as atrial fibrillation or prosthetic heart valves. The continuing question is how soon to start anticoagulation in a patient with a high-risk cardiac source of embolism who has just had an acute ischemic stroke. One of the first attempts to answer this question comes from the Cerebral Embolism Study Group (CESG) trial published in 1983 (15). In this study, 45 patients with presumed cardioembolic stroke were randomized within 48 hours of stroke onset to IV heparin for 14 days or to no immediate anticoagulation. Two patients had recurrent embolism and two patients had asymptomatic hemorrhagic infarcts, all in the nonanticoagulated group. The trial was stopped early because of these findings, which suggested a benefit of early anticoagulation. This approach was also supported by other prospective and retrospective case series at the time (16–18).

For example, in one study of 54 consecutive patients with embolic strokes, 7 of 29 patients who were not immediately anticoagulated had recurrent brain emboli in the first seven days, while none of the 25 patients who were immediately anticoagulated had recurrence during that time, and only one patient (in the anticoagulated group) had asymptomatic cerebral hemorrhage (16). This study included no random assignment of treatment, and the use of heparin was left up to the patient's personal physician. A retrospective chart review (published in the same issue as the prior study) of 44 patients with embolic strokes found that 11 patients not treated with anticoagulation had recurrent embolic strokes (4 within the first 14 days), while 16 patients were anticoagulated in the first 48 hours with no adverse events (18). These studies and their own initial results led the CESG to conclude that the rate of recurrent embolism was 14% to 22%, that immediate anticoagulation would reduce that rate, and that immediate anticoagulation was well tolerated. The authors recommended immediate anticoagulation of embolic strokes, except for patients with large infarcts, for whom a delay of one week was recommended on the basis of a concern for a higher rate of hemorrhagic infarction.

More recently, several large trials have found the risk of recurrent stroke from atrial fibrillation within 14 days to be much lower than had earlier been assumed; between 5% and 8% in the IST (7), the HAEST (12), and the Chinese Acute Stroke Trial (CAST) (19). When the subgroup of patients with atrial fibrillation from the IST was analyzed, the rate of recurrent ischemic stroke was indeed higher than the general population (4.9% vs. 3.8%, Table 1) (20). However, the rate of hemorrhagic stroke with anticoagulation was also higher (2.8 vs. 1.2). Therefore, for patients with atrial fibrillation, as was the case for the total stroke population, the combined rate of recurrent ischemic stroke with symptomatic intracranial hemorrhages was not different (5.1% with heparin vs. 5.3% without heparin). A similar conclusion was reached in a meta-analysis of randomized controlled trials of anticoagulant treatment in all types of acute cardioembolic stroke (21). However, it bears noting that many of the trials performed to this point were deficient in two aspects: (*i*) the initiation of anticoagulation was often delayed and rarely occurred before six hours from onset of acute ischemic stroke and (*ii*) hematologic monitoring of the effect of the drug (to avoid over- or underanticoagulation) was often not performed (22).

The increased rate of hemorrhagic conversion in patients with atrial fibrillation compared with the general stroke population may solely be a result of anticoagulation therapy, or alternatively it may reflect an increased proportion of large cortical strokes in the atrial fibrillation group. It is believed that these larger strokes could be more prone to symptomatic hemorrhagic conversion and that this difference may be exacerbated by anticoagulation, an explanation that is supported by a retrospective study from the CESG in which the charts of 30 cases of cardiogenic brain embolism with either asymptomatic hemorrhagic infarction or symptomatic hemorrhagic infarction or intracerebral hematoma were analyzed (23). Of the eight patients with symptomatic bleeding, seven were receiving anticoagulation and six of those had large infarcts [>3 cm of hypodensity on computed tomography (CT)], suggesting that patients with the combination of large infarcts and anticoagulation are more prone to symptomatic hemorrhage.

A similar finding is seen in trials of thrombolytic therapy for acute ischemic stroke. In the European Cooperative Acute Stroke Study II (ECASS II) trial, an increased rate of parenchymal hematoma was seen in patients with initial CT changes of greater than one-third of the middle cerebral artery territory compared with patients with no changes on initial CT or changes in less than one-third the middle cerebral artery territory (24).

It is worth noting that results from the IST (discussed above) provide evidence against the notion that symptomatic hemorrhage is more prevalent in patients with atrial fibrillation even in the absence of anticoagulation as it was only with the administration of heparin that the rate of hemorrhagic stroke increased in patients with atrial fibrillation compared with the total population (Table 1). This finding again suggests that embolic etiology of stroke (likely with a higher proportion of large infarcts, although this was not defined) was not enough to increase the rate of hemorrhage. Thus, the combination of large infarct and anticoagulation seems to be the group most at risk for hemorrhagic stroke.

If instead of atrial fibrillation as the source of emboli, patients have a more thrombogenic source (such as mechanical heart valves) (25), the balance of the risk-benefit equation might favor anticoagulation, which may be especially true in those patients in whom the ischemic infarct volume is small and thus at lower risk for hemorrhagic infarction. Similarly, it is not uncommon for acute stroke patients to also have other compelling reasons for systemic anticoagulation (e.g., deep venous thrombosis or pulmonary embolism). These systemic factors likely do not change the risk of hemorrhagic cerebral infarction but would favor early anti-coagulation because of the higher risk of withholding treatment. Unfortunately, no clinical trials have been published that might provide guidance as to when these specific risk factors are present; therefore, the decision to anticoagulate becomes one of estimating the risk-benefit ratio and of clinical judgment (26).

EARLY ANTICOAGULATION IN OTHER STROKE TYPES

As described above, the trials with anticoagulation for acute ischemic stroke have not shown a benefit for the stroke population as a whole or for a subgroup of patients with atrial fibrillation. A further question is whether patients with other stroke types would benefit from early anticoagulation. Two recent trials have enrolled only patients determined to have nonlacunar ischemic strokes with the rationale being that as lacunar strokes are thought to be secondary to lipohyalinosis of small perforator arteries caused by uncontrolled hypertension, they are unlikely to be helped by anticoagulation. In a recent Italian trial, patients with presumed nonlacunar hemispheric cerebral infarctions were treated with IV heparin or saline started within three hours of symptom onset (27). (At the time of the study, thrombolytic therapy for acute ischemic stroke had not yet been approved in Italy). Among 418 patients studied, the heparin group had more functionally independent patients at 90 days (38.9 % vs. 28.6%, $p = 0.025$). This encouraging result was offset by the fact that the heparin group also had more symptomatic brain hemorrhages (6.2% vs. 1.4%, $p = 0.008$) and a trend for higher rates of major extracranial bleeding (2.9% vs. 1.4%). Nonetheless, a trend toward fewer deaths in the heparin group (16.8% vs. 21.9%, not statistically significant) was observed. This result suggests that acute anticoagulation may be beneficial for specific populations of patients if it is started in the hyperacute ($<$3 hours) time period, but for that further study is needed.

The increasingly widespread use of various types of thrombolytic therapy within the three to six-hours window after stroke onset makes further investigation of ultra-early heparin therapy unlikely. This dilemma was demonstrated in the Rapid Anticoagulation Prevents Ischemic Damage (RAPID) trial, which attempted to treat patients with nonlacunar stokes with heparin or aspirin within 12 hours of stroke onset, but was terminated early as a result of poor enrollment (67 patients in 30 months) (28).

Heparin is still commonly used in the acute setting in other subgroups of patients, including patients with symptomatic critical carotid stenosis awaiting surgical intervention, severe posterior circulation stenosis, and cerebral artery dissection. Patients with basilar artery thrombosis, for example, often present with stuttering that progresses over hours to days, perhaps because of propagation of clot in a region of atherosclerotic stenosis. It is appealing to consider the combined use of heparin and antiplatelet agents to limit this process. Unfortunately, no large trials have been conducted in well-defined subgroups of ischemic stroke patients to determine the efficacy of this practice.

Many of the patients who were reported in 1958 to have benefited from anticoagulation were likely patients with critical large-artery stenosis (1). Patients were described to have stereotyped TIAs with the recurrent ones in the same vascular distribution. With modern imaging techniques, patients with critical carotid stenosis are frequently identified at the time of their first TIA and subsequently sent for surgical intervention. If surgery is not recommended, patients are treated with cholesterol-lowering agents to target the underlying etiology of the atherosclerosis. The author envisioned the process as follows:

> If advance or worsening of the clinical picture is related to progression of the thrombotic process, the use of anticoagulant substances would have a rational basis. However, since they probably do not influence atherosclerotic deposition, it might be anticipated that, as the plaques enlarge, a time will be reached when anticoagulant action will no longer postpone cerebral ischemia. (1)

The question remains as to whether anticoagulation could be a bridge therapy until the time of surgical intervention or a long-term therapy for those patients who are not surgical candidates. Analysis of the subgroup of patients from the TOAST trial who had ischemic stroke in the cerebral hemisphere ipsilateral to an occlusion or a stenosis of more than 50% of the internal carotid artery, as identified by carotid ultrasound, suggested that anticoagulation did provide a significant benefit with danaparoid versus placebo, with favorable outcome at seven days (64 of 119, 53.8% vs. 41 of 108, 38.0%; $p < 0.05$) and at three months (68.3% vs. 53.2%; $p < 0.05$) (29). This finding warrants confirmation by other studies.

Internal carotid artery dissection (ICAD) is also a situation in which anticoagulation is used in the acute stroke setting. The possible mechanisms of infarction in ICADs include thromboembolism from the hematoma located in the dissected vessel wall and development of hemodynamic compromise from luminal narrowing by the intramural hematoma. A survey of imaging studies from 131 patients with ICAD found that all the patients had territorial infarcts and that 5% also had border-zone infarcts (30). This result indicates that thromboembolism, and not hemodynamic compromise, is the main stroke mechanism in internal carotid dissection and suggests that anticoagulation may be beneficial in preventing recurrent thromboembolism. However, a study of 20 patients treated with heparin for ICAD found that 5 patients had delayed occlusion of the internal carotid artery during treatment and 1 of these 5 patients had associated neurologic worsening (31). These 5 patients had significantly higher activated partial thromboplastin time ratios (2.6 ± 0.4 vs. 2.0 ± 0.5). The authors suggested that while anticoagulation may be helpful in decreasing the rate of recurrent thromboembolism, it may contribute to an enlargement of the intramural hematoma and secondarily worsen hemodynamic compromise.

Most neurologists currently favor the use of anticoagulation in patients with acute cervical artery dissection, except in patients with large hemispheric infarcts or in patients who may have extension of the dissection into the intra-cranial space (and thus be at risk of subarachnoid bleeding). A clinical trial would be extremely useful in answering this question.

Other Anticoagulants

Development of new anticoagulant pharmaceuticals continues to raise the hope that an anticoagulant can be found that is antithrombotic but has a lower risk of hemorrhagic complications than heparin or LMWH.

Ancrod is a protease derived from the venom of the Malaysian pit viper; it degrades circulating fibrinogen and interferes with maturation of fibrin cross-linking. An early study in 1994 found its use was safe in acute ischemic stroke and had some promise for improved outcome in patients who could quickly achieve a target fibrinogen level (32). Unfortunately, a recent large randomized clinical trial of 1222 subjects found no functional benefit at three months with the use of ancrod (33).

Direct thrombin inhibitors are a new class of drugs that may be able to replace heparin and have theoretical advantages over heparin. Bivalirudin has been used as an adjunct in percutaneous coronary intervention but has not been studied in ischemic stroke (34). Argatroban has been found safe in acute ischemic stroke patients (35) and has an acceptable safety profile in a small study that uses the drug in combination with IV tissue plasminogen activator (36). Studies that show efficacy have yet to be published.

CONCLUSION

The current clinical trial data do not support the routine use of anticoagulation in patients with acute ischemic stroke. However, dosing, dose-response, and ultra-early use of heparin or LMWH have not been studied in as much detail as other stroke treatments, such as thrombolytic therapy. Early anticoagulation may have a role in subsets of patients with a high-risk potential for recurrent stroke (e.g., left ventricular thrombus, prosthetic heart valves, and perhaps, large artery stenosis), but the optimal timing of anticoagulation and the risk-benefit ratio for each of these subgroups of patients await further study.

REFERENCES

1. Fisher CM. The use of anticoagulants in cerebral thrombosis. Neurology 1958; 8:311–333.
2. Dobkin BH. Heparin for lacunar stroke in progression. Stroke 1983; 14:421–423.
3. Duke RJ, Bloch RF, Turpie AGG, et al. Intravenous heparin for the prevention of stroke progression in acute partial stable stroke: a randomized trial. Ann Intern Med 1986; 105:825–828.
4. Haley EC, Kassell NF, Torner JC. Failure of heparin to prevent progression in progressing ischemic infarction. Stroke 1988; 19:10–14.
5. Cordonnier C, Leys D, Deplanque D, et al. Antithrombotic agents' use in patients with atrial fibrillation and acute cerebral ischemia. J Neurol 2006; 253:1076–1082.
6. Adams H, Adams R, Zoppo GD, et al. Guidelines for the early management of patients with ischemic stroke. 2005 guidelines update. Stroke 2005; 36:916–921.
7. International Stroke Trial Collaborative Group. The International Stroke Trial (IST): a randomized trial of aspirin, subcutaneous heparin, both, or neither among 19435 patients with acute ischemic stroke. Lancet 1997; 349:1569–1581.
8. Leizorovicz A, Simonneau G, Decousus H, et al. Comparison of efficacy and safety of low molecular weight heparins and unfractionated heparin in initial treatment of deep venous thrombosis: a meta-analysis. BMJ 1994; 309:299–304.
9. Cohen M, Demers C, Gurfinkel EP, et al. A comparison of low-molecular-weight heparin with unfractionated heparin for unstable coronary artery disease. N Engl J Med 1997; 337:447–452.
10. Kay R, Wong KS, Yu YL, et al. Low-molecular-weight heparin for the treatment of acute ischemic stroke. N Engl J Med 1995; 333:1588–1593.
11. Berge E, Abdelnoor M, Nakstad PH, et al. Low molecular-weight heparin versus aspirin in patients with acute ischaemic stroke and atrial fibrillation: A double-blind randomised study. Lancet 2000; 355:1205–1210.
12. Diener HC, Ringelstein EB, von Kummer R, et al. Treatment of acute ischemic stroke with the low-molecular-weight heparin certoparin: results of the TOPAS trial. Stroke 2001; 32:22–29.
13. Bath PM, Lindenstrom E, Boysen G, et al. Tinzaparin in acute ischaemic stroke (TAIST): a randomised aspirin-controlled trial. Lancet 2001; 358:702–710.
14. The Publications Committee for the Trial of ORG 10172 in Acute Stroke Treatment (TOAST) Investigators. Low-molecular-weight heparinoid, ORG 10172 (danaparoid), and outcome after acute ischemic stroke: a randomized controlled trial. JAMA 1998; 279:1265–1272.
15. Cerebral Embolism Study Group. Immediate anticoagulation of embolic stroke: a randomized trial. Stroke 1983; 14:668–676.
16. Furlan AJ, Cavalier SJ, Hobbs RE, et al. Hemorrhage and anticoagulation after nonseptic embolic brain infarction. Neurology 1982; 32:280–282.

17. Hart RG, Coull BM, Hart D. Early recurrent embolism associated with nonvalvular atrial fibrillation: a retrospective study. Stroke 1983; 14:688–693.
18. Koller RL. Recurrent embolic cerebral infarction and anticoagulation. Neurology 1982; 32:283–285.
19. CAST (Chinese Acute Stroke Trial) Collaborative Group. CAST: randomized, placebo-controlled trial of early aspirin use in 20000 patients with acute ischemic stroke. Lancet 1997; 349:1641–1649.
20. Saxena R, Lewis S, Berge E, et al. Risk of early death and recurrent stroke and effect of heparin in 3169 patients with acute ischemic stroke and atrial fibrillation in the international stroke trial. Stroke 2001; 32:2333–2337.
21. Paciaroni M, Agnelli G, Micheli S, et al. Efficacy and safety of anticoagulant treatment in acute cardioembolic stroke: a meta-analysis of randomized controlled trials. Stroke 2007; 38:423–430.
22. Chamorro A. Immediate Anticoagulation for Acute Stroke in Atrial Fibrillation? Yes. Stroke 2006; 37(12):3052–3053.
23. Cerebral Embolism Study Group. Immediate anticoagulation of embolic stroke: brain hemorrhage and management options. Stroke 1984; 15:779–789.
24. Dzialowski I, Hill MD, Coutts SB, et al. Extent of early ischemic changes on computed tomography (CT) before thrombolysis: prognostic value of the Alberta stroke program early CT score in ECASS II. Stroke 2006; 37:973–978.
25. Cannegieter SC, Rosendaal FR, Briet E. Thromboembolic and bleeding complications in patients with mechanical heart valve prostheses. Circulation 1994; 89:635–641.
26. Moonis M, Fisher M. Considering the role of heparin and low-molecular-weight heparins in acute ischemic stroke. Stroke 2002; 33:1927–1933.
27. Camerlingo M, Salvi P, Belloni G, et al. Intravenous heparin started within the first 3 hours after onset of symptoms as a treatment for acute nonlacunar hemispheric cerebral infarctions. Stroke 2005; 36:2415–2420.
28. Chamorro A, Busse O, Obach V, et al. The rapid anticoagulation prevents ischemic damage study in acute stroke—final results from the writing committee. Cerebrovasc Dis 2005; 19:402–404.
29. Adams HP Jr., Bendixen BH, Leira E, et al. Antithrombotic treatment of ischemic stroke among patients with occlusion or severe stenosis of the internal carotid artery: a report of the Trial of Org 10172 in Acute Stroke Treatment (TOAST). Neurology 1999; 53:122–125.
30. Benninger DH, Georgiadis D, Kremer C, et al. Mechanism of ischemic infarct in spontaneous carotid dissection. Stroke 2004; 35:482–485.
31. Dreier JP, Lurtzing F, Kappmeier M, et al. Delayed occlusion after internal carotid artery dissection under heparin. Cerebrovasc Dis 2004; 18:296–303.
32. The Ancrod Stroke Study Investigators. Ancrod for the treatment of acute ischemic brain infarction. Stroke 1994; 25:1755–1759.
33. Hennerici MG, Kay R, Bogousslavsky J, et al. Intravenous ancrod for acute ischaemic stroke in the European Stroke Treatment with Ancrod Trial: a randomized, controlled trial. Lancet 2006; 368:1871–1878.
34. Exaire JE, Butman SM, Ebrahimi R, et al. Provisional glycoprotein IIb/IIIa blockade in a randomized investigation of bivalirudin versus heparin plus planned glyco-protein IIb/IIIa inhibition during percutaneous coronary intervention: predictors and outcome in the randomized evaluation in percutaneous coronary intervention Linking

Angiomax to Reduced Clinical Events (REPLACE)-2 trial. Am Heart J 2006; 152:157–163.

35. LaMonte MP, Nash ML, Wang DZ, et al. Argatroban anticoagulation in patients with acute ischemic stroke (ARGIS-1): a randomized, placebo-controlled safety study. Stroke 2004; 35:1677–1682.

36. Sugg RM, Pary JK, Uchino K, et al. Argatroban tPA stroke study: study design and results in the first treated cohort. Arch Neurol 2006; 63:1057–1062.

9

Angioplasty and Stenting of Cervical Carotid, Intracranial, and Vertebral Arteries

Aclan Dogan, MD, Assistant Professor
Bryan Petersen, MD, Associate Professor
David Lee, MD, Assistant Professor
Gary Nesbit, MD, Associate Professor
Lindsay Wenger
Stanley L. Barnwell, MD, Associate Professor

Department of Radiology, Oregon Health & Science University,
Portland, Oregon, U.S.A.

Carotid artery angioplasty and stenting (CAS) has evolved into one of the most common approaches to treatment of cervical carotid atherosclerotic disease. The approach was first described by Kerber and colleagues in 1980 (1). In the same decade, reports on at least two other small series of patients were published that showed high technical success rates and low complication rates (2–4). The approach was greatly popularized beginning in the early 1990s, and by 2000, CAS procedures dramatically increased (5,6). Between 1996 and 1999, at least 11 carotid stent series that included more than 1300 patients were published (3,7). All of these studies demonstrated high technical success rates and acceptably low complication rates.

CAS developed as a less invasive alternative to the standard surgical carotid endarterectomy (CEA) approach, which had been shown to be a safe and effective procedure to reduce the risk of stroke in patients with carotid atheromatous disease, both symptomatic and asymptomatic (8,9). Within this group of patients with carotid atheromatous disease, subsets exist that are clearly at higher risk for complications from surgery. The benefit of CEA in the low surgical risk population generally is eliminated if the combined 30-day stroke and death rates exceed 5% to 7% for symptomatic patients, and 3% for asymptomatic patients. Numerous other reports have detailed the complication rate of surgery based on patient selection (10–14). It was in this group of patients that constituted a "high surgical risk" that CAS was developed as an alternative. As experience was gained, this technique was used to treat a much larger pool of patients who were not necessarily at higher risk for surgery. The procedure became so commonplace that the Centers for Medicare and Medicaid issued revised guidelines that restricted reimbursement for this procedure to high-risk patients or those involved in category B Investigational Device Exemption studies and post approval studies at qualified centers. In addition, the Centers for Medicare and Medicaid insisted that centers that offer this service undergo a certification process demonstrating their ability to perform this procedure safely and effectively.

The main issues regarding CAS relate to its relative safety and efficacy compared with surgical CEA, rates of restenosis within arteries treated with a stent, management of restenosis if it does occur after CAS, effect of advanced age (>80 years) on outcome, and the need for distal filter protection to reduce embolic complications from this procedure. Many issues related to performance of CAS have been largely resolved over the past 20 years. As an example, some of the first carotid stents that were placed were not self-expanding but were deployed by expanding them with a balloon. These stents were easily crushed, and if that occurred, they would not reexpand (15,16).

TECHNICAL CONSIDERATIONS FOR CERVICAL CAROTID ARTERY ANGIOPLASTY AND STENTING

Preoperative Care and Evaluation

Antiplatelet Therapy

Experience has clearly shown the need for dual antiplatelet treatment prior to placing stents in the cervical carotid arteries (16). In most trials, dual antiplatelet therapy is started five days before the procedure and includes aspirin (325 mg) and clopidogrel (75 mg) daily. In cases in which pretreatment has not been administered, alternative regimens include aspirin (325 mg) and a load of clopidogrel (600 mg) at least four hours before the procedure. Some centers are evaluating the pharmacologic response to antiplatelet therapy administered immediately before performing these procedures, although this is not a universal practice.

Anticoagulation

The procedures are performed with full heparin anticoagulation. Among most of the protocol studies, an activated clotting time of greater than 250 seconds is required. Typically, a bolus of 5000 units of heparin is given, followed by additional 1000- to 3000-units increments based on the activated clotting time level.

Blood Pressure Control

Early experience demonstrated that uncontrolled hypertension could result in intracerebral hemorrhage after CAS has been performed (16,17). The scenario was particularly a problem with a critical stenosis in the setting of contralateral carotid artery occlusion. Generally, most study protocols require a systolic blood pressure be maintained at less than 180 mmHg.

The decision to perform CAS depends on a combination of clinical indications and preoperative evaluation of the cervical carotid arteries, which can be accomplished by carotid duplex ultrasound, MR angiography, CT angiography, or conventional angiography. The final decision regarding proceeding with the actual carotid artery angioplasty and stent procedure, however, depends on the angiographic evaluation. Anywhere along the treatment chain, problems can be encountered that may prohibit performance of the procedure, including access difficulty in the femoral artery at the groin, as well as excessive tortuosity or atherosclerotic occlusion of the iliac arteries, aorta, or origins of the great vessels. Significant tortuosity of the aortic arch or the cervical carotid arteries may also prohibit safe performance of a CAS procedure. The access devices have some rigidity to them and may not be able to navigate through extremely tortuous anatomy. While some of these issues may be resolved on the preoperative studies, some may not be apparent until the actual CAS procedure has begun.

Procedure

The CAS procedure is performed with the patient under moderate sedation, 1 to 4 mg of midazolam and 100 to 400 mcg of fentanyl typically being administered during the course of a procedure. In a straightforward case, the operative time is less than one hour. Each CAS procedure begins with a diagnostic angiogram. A study of the aortic arch is performed to evaluate the type of arch involved as well as to look for atheromatous disease at the origins of the great vessels that may prohibit safe passage of subsequent catheters and guidewires. Each carotid artery is then selectively catheterized, with visualization of both the cervical region and the intracranial circulation. Evaluation of the cervical carotid artery involves looking for the presence of acute thrombus, significant calcification, degree of stenosis, the normal arterial diameter, and excessive tortuosity. The intracranial circulation is examined for tandem lesions affecting intracranial blood vessels.

The diagnostic catheters generally have a very small inner diameter and must be exchanged for larger sheaths. The sheaths have much larger inner diameters and allow passage of the variety of stents and balloons necessary for this procedure. Typically, a 6 French sheath is exchanged for the diagnostic catheter and extends from the femoral artery in the leg up into the affected cervical common carotid artery. The large inner diameter sheath, because of its rigidity,

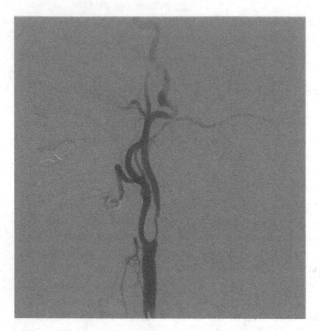

Figure 1 Cervical carotid artery angiogram, RAO projection, pretreatment. *Abbreviation*: RAO, right anterior oblique.

also allows stability for subsequent passage of devices and for injecting contrast and imaging of the carotid arteries during the course of angioplasty and stenting.

Carotid artery angioplasty is performed using continuous fluoroscopy so that the operator can monitor the position and movement of the devices. In addition, a technique called *roadmapping* allows an image of a blood vessel to be portrayed on the video screen in real time. Using the combination of road-mapping and fluoroscopy, the devices used in this procedure can be navigated through tortuous anatomy and severe stenoses in a safe and effective fashion.

With a large inner diameter sheath in place and a roadmap image of the blood vessel portrayed on the video screen, a very small guidewire is then navigated through the guide sheath into the carotid artery, and across the stenotic lesion distally into the high cervical internal carotid artery (Fig. 1). This microguidewire is typically very thin (0.014″) and has a shapeable tip. The shape at the tip allows torque to occur at the distal end of the guidewire when the proximal end outside the body at the groin is turned, allowing the micro-guidewire to be navigated through tortuous anatomy and severe stenoses.

An embolic protection device, also known as a filter device, is then navigated through the sheath, into the carotid artery, across the lesion, and then deployed much above the lesion in the high cervical internal carotid artery. In most instances, the filter device is attached to the microguidewire. Some device manufacturers separate the microguidewire from the filter device. Once the micro-guidewire is delivered across the lesion and above, the filter device is delivered. As the filter device is initially navigated through the artery, it is confined inside of a delivery tube. Once it is navigated distal to the lesion, it is opened up in a similar fashion to an umbrella and remains in place throughout the procedure. The filter device typically has a pore size of approximately 100 μm that allows blood flow distally to the intracranial circulation, but will capture any significant embolic debris larger than 100 μm that break loose during the course of the procedure.

With the filter device in place, the lesion is typically first treated with what is termed *prestent angioplasty*. In most instances, the stenotic lesion is so tight that passing the larger-diameter stents through the lesion may be difficult. Prestent angioplasty allows for partial opening of the lesion to facilitate advancement of the stent. Typically, a balloon 4 mm in diameter is used in the cervical carotid arteries for prestent angioplasty, and it opens up the stenotic lesion sufficiently to allow the stent to be navigated across the lesion. This prestent angioplasty balloon is then removed.

Dilation of the lesion at the cervical carotid artery bifurcation with even a 4-mm prestent angioplasty balloon can cause significant effects on both heart rate and blood pressure. Significant sinus bradycardia or complete block may result as the balloon is inflated but generally always reverses within seconds as the balloon is deflated. In an effort to lessen this effect, pretreatment with atropine (1 mg) may be given. However, this approach is not universal.

The prestent angioplasty typically allows much easier passage of the stent. As the stent is introduced into the sheath in the groin, it is constrained within a catheter. The sheath has a low profile and typically crosses the stenotic lesion in the cervical carotid artery without much difficulty. Once it is centered over the lesion, it is uncovered and expands. All stents currently used extracranially are self-expanding. This feature allows for reexpansion if the stent is compressed for any reason, such as if the patient pushes on his/her neck or during ultrasonography.

The stents come in a variety of lengths, diameters, and as either straight or tapered. The length of the stent used is determined by the length of the lesion to be treated. Stent lengths are chosen to extend beyond the lesion, both proximally and distally, by at least 1 cm to ensure full coverage of the stenotic lesion. The diameter of the stent is chosen on the basis of the largest diameter of the carotid artery in which the stent will be placed and is generally at least 1 mm greater than the normal diameter of the artery so that it is stable and will not move once it is deployed. More recently, tapered stents have been developed to account for the difference in the diameter between the common carotid artery and the more distal internal carotid artery.

After the stent has been deployed, residual stenosis may occur at the lesion. While the stent has some self-expanding radial outward force, it is not typically sufficient to open up the stenotic lesion by itself. To reverse the stenosis, post-stent angioplasty is typically performed. A second balloon is navigated inside the stent and then expanded to the normal diameter of the artery. For most cervical internal carotid artery stenotic lesions, a post-stent angioplasty is performed using either a 5.0- or 5.5-mm dilation balloon, which usually allows the artery to achieve normal diameter with no residual stenosis. For lesions of the cervical carotid artery bifurcation, significant bradycardia and hypotension very frequently occur with the dilation. If atropine had not been given before, it is typically given before the final balloon angioplasty is performed.

After the stent has been deployed and postdilated, the filter is removed. Angiographic analysis is first made to ensure that an adequate result has been achieved. In addition, the filter is evaluated to assess whether any significant embolic debris has been captured. It is extremely rare to see any angiographic evidence of debris in the filter. A filter recovery sheath is navigated up to the filter, and the filter is recaptured and removed, along with any embolic debris. Visual inspection of the filter seldom demonstrates significant embolic matter.

Postoperative Care

Generally, patients spend one night in the ICU. Blood pressure control is carefully monitored after this procedure. Balloon angioplasty and stenting of the carotid bifurcation occasionally result in prolonged hypotension, a problem that generally responds to fluids; however, occasionally, vasopressors are given for a period (up to 24 hours), while the baroreceptor reflex equilibrates. Most patients are discharged the following day.

Anticoagulation is stopped at the end of the procedure but not reversed. Antiplatelet therapy is continued after the procedure. Typically, aspirin (325 mg) is continued indefinitely. Plavix is continued for 30 days on most trial protocols. Patients may return to normal activity shortly after discharge, with no restrictions in their activity. The only caveat would be to avoid chiropractic manipulation of the neck. Clinical follow up with ultrasound is performed at 30 days. Angiographic follow up is not generally performed.

Comparing CAS with CEA requires separating the patient populations into those with high-risk features for surgery and those with no particular risk factors for surgery. Most of the available literature relates to CAS in populations at high surgical risk, but trials that compare CAS with surgery in patients at low surgical risk have been conducted (18,19).

The literature is replete with multiple series that show varying degrees of safety and efficacy of carotid stenting (16,17). It has only been in the last 10 years that a number of carefully designed and controlled trials have been performed that compare CAS with CEA or evaluate the results of CAS in patients at high risk for surgery. Previous comparison trials in which distal protection was not used and the technical issues such as antiplatelet therapy were not standardized have much less relevance today (20).

THE SECURITY REGISTRY TRIAL

The SECuRITY Registry Trial (21) was a prospective, multicentered (30 sites), nonrandomized safety and efficacy study of a distal filter protection device and a CAS in 305 pivotal patients and 93 lead-in patients with carotid artery disease. These patients were considered at high risk for surgery. The primary end points were (*i*) the incidence of major adverse events (MAEs), defined as death, stroke, or myocardial infarction (MI) (Q wave and non–Q wave) at 30 days postprocedure for the stent and a distal filter protection device, termed "Emboshield," and (*ii*) MAEs at 30 days postprocedure in the incidence of ipsilateral stroke at one year for the Xact stent. Secondary end points were the incidence of vascular complications other than in the MAEs at 30 days and restenosis and/or target lesion revascularization at six months and one year postprocedure.

At 30 days following the study procedure, 92.5% of the treated patients were free of MAEs. The primary end point of the study was a composite rate of the 30-day MAEs and ipsilateral strokes at one year. The composite rate of occurrence for the primary end point at 12 months was 8.5%. Acute success in effectively treating the target lesion was demonstrated in 96.7% of the patients who underwent the study procedure. At 12 months, long-term durability of the procedure was also demonstrated by 99.3% of the treated patients being free from repeat revascularization. Additionally, at 6 months and 12 months postprocedure, restenosis was demonstrated in only a small percentage of the patient population—4.9% and 4.1%, respectively.

The primary objective of the SECuRITY Registry Trial was met, demonstrating that the carotid stenting with the Xact stent is noninferior to CEA, based on results of historical controls. The clinical results of this study indicate that the Xact carotid stent system, when used in conjunction with the Emboshield embolic protection system, provides a safe, effective, and durable method for the treatment of carotid stenosis in patients at high risk for CEA.

THE CABERNET TRIAL

The Carotid Artery Stenting Trial (CABERNET) was a prospective, nonrandomized, multicentered registry of 454 patients that used 21 carefully selected centers in both the United States and Europe (22). The patients were either symptomatic with greater than 50% stenosis by Doppler ultrasound and angiogram, or asymptomatic with 80% stenosis by Doppler ultrasound or with 60% stenosis as determined by angiogram without any neurologic symptoms. The trial objective was to evaluate the safety and efficacy of the Boston Scientific carotid stent and delivery system and their distal filter protection device, the FilterWire, by assessing the outcomes of patients with CAS who were at high risk for CEA. The primary end points were a composite MAE rate, including all death, stroke, and MI at up to 30 days, plus ipsilateral stroke, including any death-related ipsilateral stroke, from 31 to 365 days. The other primary end point was all death, all strokes, and all MIs at one year.

The 30-day primary end point MAE rate (death, stroke, or MI within 30 days) was 3.9%. The 30-day all stroke rate was 3.4%, but only 1.3% of these were defined as major. Ipsilateral major stroke only occurred in 1.1%, and non-ipsilateral stroke occurred in 0.7%. The one-year MAE rates were 4.7%, including death in 0.5% (nonneurologic), stroke in 4.2%, and MI in 0.2%. The one-year end point MAE rate for all death, stroke, and MI was 11.9%. Restenosis of greater than 80% was found to be only 0.9% at up to six months and 2.7% at one year. At one year, only 2% of the patients had target vessel revascularization procedures.

The primary end points of the trial were met. These findings demonstrated that carotid stenting using the Boston Scientific NexStent Carotid Stent with the FilterWire system was comparable to CEA in the high-surgical-risk study population. The restenosis rates were extremely low, as was the need for target vessel revascularization.

THE ARCHER TRIAL

The ACCULINK for Revascularization of Carotids in High-Risk Patients) (ARCHeR) Trial (23) consisted of three separate trials. The ARCHeR Trial 1 included 158 patients who were treated with the AccuLink carotid stent system, mostly in the United States and at some carefully selected sites in Europe and Argentina. The ARCHeR Trial 2 included 278 patients treated with the Accu-Link stent and the Accunet distal filter embolic protection system. The ARCHeR Trial 3 involved 145 patient treated with a new version of the AccuLink stent and Accunet filter. The control was historical high-risk CEA data.

The combined primary end point of death, stroke, and MI in the first 30 days plus ipsilateral stroke between 31 days and 1 year was 8.3%, 10.2% in ARCHeR Trial 2, and 8.3% during the first 30 days in ARCHeR Trial 3. The historical control group showed a 14.5% incidence rate. At 30 days, the rates of major stroke were: ARCHeR Trial 1, 3.8%; ARCHeR Trial 2, 2.5%; and ARCHeR Trial 3, 2.8%. In conclusion, CAS was safer compared to historical control CEA in high-risk patients.

THE BEACH TRIAL

The Boston Scientific EPI-A Carotid Stenting Trial for High Risk Surgical Patients (BEACH) Trial (24) enrolled 747 patients at high risk for surgery, with 480 being in the pivotal trial performed in the United States. The purpose was to evaluate the outcomes of patients with CAS at high risk for CEA using the carotid Wallstent and the FilterWire EZ distal protection system. These patients have been followed for two years. The stroke risk in the first 30 days was 3.1%, which reduced to 2.3% between 31 days and 1 year, and to 0.9% at between one and two years. In regard to restenosis, the rates were extremely low and no revascularization was required. In conclusion, this study demonstrated both safety of the procedure and the protection from stroke that stenting offers with a two-year follow-up. No significant restenosis was noted.

These four trials directly compare CAS with CEA.

THE CARESS TRIAL

The purpose for the Carotid Revascularization Using Endarterectomy or Stenting Systems (CARESS) trial (25,26) was to determine if protected carotid stenting is equivalent to CEA in patients with carotid stenosis. It was a prospective, multicentered trial performed in the United States. The patients encompassed a broad range of risks. The primary outcome was mortality and nonfatal stroke at 30 days. The secondary outcome was a composite of total mortality, stroke, and MI at 30 days. The trial enrolled 439 patients. More than 90% of patients had greater than 75% stenosis; approximately 68% were asymptomatic. The 30-day composite rate of mortality in stroke was statistically insignificant at 2% in both groups. The secondary end point of all mortality, stroke, and MI was 3% in the CEA group and 2% in the CAS group—also statistically insignificant.

In a follow-up assessment at one year, the CARESS phase I study suggested that the 30-day and 1-year risk of death, stroke, or MI with CAS is equivalent to that with CEA in symptomatic and asymptomatic patients with carotid stenosis. No significant differences were noted between CEA and CAS patients in the secondary end points of restenosis (CEA, 3.6%, vs. CAS, 6.3%) or carotid revascularization (CEA, 1.0% vs. CAS, 1.8%). In conclusion, this study suggests that the 30-day risk of stroke or death following carotid stenting with cerebral protection is equivalent to standard CEA in a broad-risk population of patients with carotid stenosis. The need for revascularization at one year was extremely low in both groups and not statistically different.

THE SPACE TRIAL

The Stent-Supported Percutaneous Angioplasty of the Carotid Artery versus Endarterectomy (SPACE) trial (27) compared the safety and efficacy of stent-protected percutaneous angioplasty of the carotid artery and CEA against stroke and other vascular events in patients with symptomatic carotid stenosis. Only sites in Germany, Austria, and Switzerland were included. Enrollment was completed of 1214 randomized patients in February 2006.

SPACE failed to show one method over another as being safer or a more effective prophylactic method at 6- or 30-day end points. The rate of the primary end point was 6.84% with CAS and 6.34% with CEA, and the one-sided p-value for noninferiority is 0.09. There were no significant differences for the secondary end points of stroke (7.51% vs. 6.16%), ipsilateral disabling stroke or death (4.67% vs. 3.77%), or procedural failure (3.17% vs. 2.05%) at 30 days. Further end points will be collected at 6, 12, and 24 months (27).

In conclusion, at 30 days, both procedures seemed equivalent. Additional data from this trial will be forthcoming.

THE SAPPHIRE TRIAL

The pivotal Stenting and Angioplasty with Protection in Patients at High Risk for Endarterectomy (SAPPHIRE) trial was a multicentered, prospective, randomized, triangular, sequential trial that compared patients at increased risk for adverse events from CEA who received a stent to a surgical CEA control (28). The primary objective of the SAPPHIRE trial was to compare the safety and effectiveness of the Cordis PRECISE stent system, used in conjunction with the ANGIOGUARD distal filter protection guidewire, to CEA in the treatment of carotid artery disease in patients at increased risk for adverse events from CEA. Study hypotheses examined whether the MAE rate of randomized inpatients was not inferior to randomized CEA patients. The primary end point was a composite of the MAEs (defined as death, any stroke, or MI, Q wave or non–Q wave) in the first 30 days following treatment and death or ipsilateral stroke between 31 days and 12 months.

A total of 747 patients were enrolled in the Sapphire study at 29 centers in the United States. The randomized population included 334 patients (167 stent/ 167 CEA), 310 of whom were treated per protocol. The one-year MAE rate at 30 days and death or ipsilateral stroke from 31 days to 360 days was 12.0% for the randomized stent patients, compared with 19.2% for the control CEA group. Cranial nerve injury occurred in 4.2% of the patients who underwent CEA and in none of the patients who underwent CAS. Targeted lesion revascularization at one year was necessary in 4.3% of the CEA patients and in only 0.6% of the CAS patients. The cumulative percent of MAEs at one year was 12.2% in the CAS patients and 20.1% in the CEA patients.

These results demonstrate noninferiority ($p = 0.004$) of CAS to CEA. The number of patients who required revascularization because of stenosis was lower in patients who underwent CAS. The overall incidence of MAEs was less at one year in CAS patients, compared to CAE patients.

THE EVA-3S TRIAL

The Symptomatic Severe Carotid Stenosis (EVA-3S) Trial was a multicentered, randomized, noninferiority trial (29) performed in France that compared stenting with endarterectomy in patients with symptomatic carotid artery stenosis of at least 60%. The primary end point was the incidence of any stroke or death within 30 days after treatment. The entry criteria for the interventionalists was much less than other trials.

The trial was stopped prematurely after the inclusion of 527 patients for reasons of both safety and futility. The 30-day incidence of any stroke or death was 3.9% after endarterectomy; the relative risk of any stroke or death after stenting was significantly higher compared with endarterectomy. The 30-day incidence of disabling stroke or death was 1.5% after endarterectomy (95% CI, 0.5 to 4.2) and 3.4% after stenting (95% CI, 1.7 to 6.7); the relative risk was 2.2 (95% CI, 0.7 to 7.2). At six months, the incidence of any stroke or death was 6.1% after endarterectomy and 11.7% after stenting ($p = 0.02$). There were more major local complications after stenting and more systemic complications (mainly pulmonary) after endarterectomy, but the differences were not significant. Cranial-nerve injury was more common after endarterectomy than after stenting (29).

The results of this trial stand out in startling contrast compared with other trials that mostly involved centers in the United States. The qualifications of the investigators who placed the stents has come under question, as noted in the editorial by Furlan (Furlan). The other studies cited above had lead-in phases, during which demonstrated safety and efficacy was required before enrolling patients. The training requirements for the investigators on the EVA-3S Trial were not as extensive as those of the other trials. A review of this issue has been reported by Qureshi (30).

The evidence currently available is that for patients at high risk for surgical CEA, CAS provides a safer alternative in regard to MAEs compared with historical controls. In the SAPPHIRE Trial, which directly compared surgery and carotid artery stenting in the United States, CAS clearly seemed favorable over the surgical approach. Surgery appeared to be a better alternative in only one study, which was conducted in France (19,29). The suggested explanation of these findings was that the surgeons had a great deal of prior experience, whereas the interventionalists had much less.

The importance of experience in performing CAS procedures and the associated learning curve have been well documented (16,31).

As experience was gained in the technique of CAS, there was a clear reduction in the incidence of neurologic complications. In a description of their early experience in this technique, Vitek et al. reported an initial complication rate of 8.2% in their series from 1994 to 1995, which was reduced to 4% in their series from 1997 to 1998 (16). Although they attributed some of the improvement to dual antiplatelet therapy, they also pointed to improvements in the technique that is in use currently.

As another example of the ramifications of the lack of experience with the CAS technique, Teitelbaum et al. in their 1998 review of the 26 CAS procedures noted a technical success of 96% but a high complication rate. At 30 days, combined death, stroke, and ipsilateral blindness occurred in 27% of patients, although only two of the ipsilateral strokes (7.7%) were directly related to the CAS procedure. It would appear that many of these patients were not pretreated with full antiplatelet therapy. In addition, over half of their stent procedures involved the use of the Palmaz stent, the use of which has largely been abandoned because of its lack of free expansion after being crushed. The experiences of these investigators in these early days and their willingness to publish them laid the groundwork for the success of the procedure today.

RESTENOSIS

Initial concerns about higher rates of restenosis after CAS have not borne out either in multiple case series or in the larger trials (17,32–34). Restenosis, defined as greater than 50% reduction in diameter, occurs in approximately 6% of patients after CEA (32,35,36). This risk may be reduced with the surgical technique of adding a patch to the surgical incision closure site. Repeat endarterectomy for restenosis is technically more difficult and is associated with an increased risk of cranial nerve palsies (36,37). Among all of the major trials, the restenosis rate after CAS was either less than or equivalent to that after CEA.

When restenosis does occur after CAS, retreatment is associated with very high technical success rates and very low complication rates (38,39). In an evaluation of this issue in 32 in-stent restenoses following CAS, complete procedural success was achieved in all patients, with no complications at 30 days (39). An additional evaluation of the embolic debris captured by the filter used in each case revealed the presence of fibrous nets and erythrocytes, leukocytes, platelets, and occasionally, hypercellular tissue fragments, rather than the fragments of plaque and acute thrombus that were seen in the filters from the original treatments (40,41). Based on these findings, it would appear that retreatment of in-stent stenosis after CAS may be technically easier and safer than the original treatment (38,39,42–44).

Many have questioned the safety of CAS in the elderly population. With CEA, increasing age may also be associated with increased risks (45–47). While it appears that CEA is generally safe in these patients if they do not have other high-risk features, issues pertinent to CAS may increase the risk compared to the surgical approach (48,49). Evidence suggests an increased risk of complication from CAS in patients who are older than 80 years (17,50,51), which may relate primarily to unfavorable anatomy or to less tolerance of the brain and other organs to any embolic or physiologic changes that occur during CAS. Of these factors, difficult arch anatomy with elongation, calcified origins, and tortuosity that occur more frequently in the elderly was thought to be the largest contributing factor (48).

The issue of the need for distal filter protection was raised early in the progress of CAS (52,53). Generally, all CAS procedures are now performed using distal filter protection devices. In the early development of carotid stenting, filter devices were not available and yet the procedure seemed very safe in regard to thromboembolic complications (16). However, the theoretical concern of emboli resulting from CAS procedures was raised, and a number of different filter protection devices were developed (54–56). While no randomized trial has been conducted to compare CAS with and without filter protection devices, the available data does clearly indicate that filter protection offers significant safety over nonprotected procedures (3,7,57–59). In a study that evaluated the role of filter protection devices in reducing ischemic complications related to CAS, investigators found a significantly lower rate of ipsilateral lesions on diffusion-weighted imaging when filters were used (59). Unprotected CAS was performed in 67 patients, and filters were used in another 139 patients. Both the number of patients with new lesions versus no lesions, and the number of lesions in patients who had lesions, were significantly higher in patients who underwent CAS without protection. Although more clinically significant ischemic complications were noted in the unprotected group than in the filter group, this difference did not reach statistical significance.

CONCLUSIONS AND FUTURE DIRECTIONS—CERVICAL CAROTID ARTERY ANGIOPLASTY AND STENTING

CAS now has a defined role in the treatment of carotid artery atheromatous disease. Over the past 20 years, catheterization techniques, antiplatelet therapy, anticoagulation, distal filter protection, and stent choices have all been refined.

The procedure is clearly preferable for patients at high risk for surgical CEA, particularly patients with restenosis after surgery or those with prior radiation therapy or other forms of "hostile" neck anatomy. For patients at low risk for surgery, most studies demonstrate equivalence and tendency for better results with CAS, compared to surgery.

The Carotid Revascularization Endarterectomy Stenting Trial (CREST), sponsored by the National Institutes of Neurological Disorders and Stroke, is ongoing as of writing this chapter. It is a prospective, randomized, multicentered US trial involving 2500 patients and has strict experience criteria for both the surgeons and interventionalists. Results from the CREST trial will provide the most useful data regarding a comparison of the two approaches in low-risk patients.

The evidence suggests that in-stent stenosis after CAS is very infrequent and that if it does occur, it is easily managed by repeating the procedure. Distal filter protection devices are now routinely used and, although unproven, seem to add safety to the procedure.

INTRACRANIAL AND VERTEBRAL ARTERY ANGIOPLASTY AND STENTING

The issues that surround intracranial and vertebral artery angioplasty and stenting relate primarily to the overall safety and efficacy of this treatment for symptomatic intracranial atheromatous disease and how they compare to medical treatment. As experience with this technique has grown, questions that have been largely answered in the field of cervical CAS remain unanswered for intracranial angioplasty and stenting; they concern overall safety, efficacy, the restenosis rate, methods by which to decrease restenosis or treat it if it occurs, and the length of antiplatelet therapy. Many questions remain about the optimal technique.

The Technique of Intracranial Angioplasty and Stenting

Preoperative care for a patient who will undergo intracranial angioplasty and stenting is virtually identical to cervical CAS procedures in regard to antiplatelet therapy, anticoagulation, and blood pressure control. These procedures are typically performed using general anesthesia. The end point is angiographic normalization of a blood vessel diameter, not an immediate clinical outcome, and the advantages of having the patient immobile outweigh being able to follow their neurologic exam during the procedure. However, this approach is not

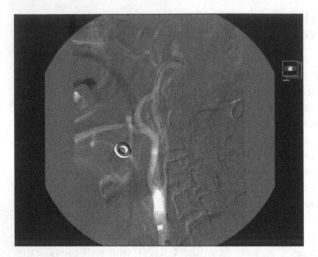

Figure 2 Cervical carotid artery angiogram, with filter protection device placed above the lesion and high cervical internal carotid artery.

universal. Angiography is performed in a fashion similar to that for CAS. The shape of the arch and the tortuosity of the cervical carotid or vertebral arteries are evaluated as part of the decision-making process as to whether an intracranial angioplasty and stenting procedure is feasible. Imaging of the intracranial arteries is performed to evaluate the normal size of the artery, the length of the narrowing, and the presence of tandem lesions. For most centers, reliance on three-dimensional angiography is necessary, as very accurate measurements of the diameter of the small arteries is important to prevent oversizing of the balloon used for prestent angioplasty, as well as possible rupture.

In a similar fashion to CAS, a large inner diameter sheath is placed in the cervical carotid arteries or vertebral arteries that provides a stiff support platform from which subsequent maneuvers are to be performed. In addition, the large inner diameter of the sheath allows for continuous angiographic imaging during the course of the procedure. Once the sheath is in place, most centers with experience in doing these procedures will first gain access by navigating a microcatheter and microguidewire across the lesion. (Fig. 2) The microcatheter is then used to place a much longer exchange microguidewire, which serves as a platform for subsequent maneuvers. The only currently approved system for intracranial angioplasty and stent is the Wingspan system. Using the approved instructions for use, the lesion is first predilated with an angioplasty balloon to just under the normal size of the artery. Once this prestent angioplasty balloon procedure has been performed, the balloon is withdrawn and the Wingspan stent system is delivered over the microguidewire across the lesion. Similar to CAS systems, the Wingspan stent system is self-expanding as it deploys across the lesion. Follow-up angiography is then performed, and if an acceptable result has

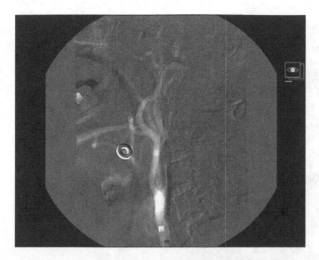

Figure 3 Cervical carotid artery road map image, oblique projection, showing 4 mm/40 mm present angioplasty balloon inflated across lesion.

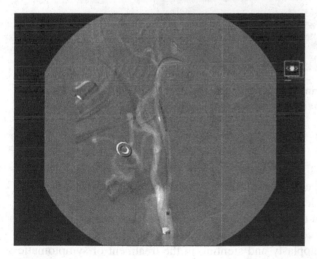

Figure 4 X ray demonstrating stent across lesion, not yet deployed, with filter protection device in high cervical internal carotid artery above the lesion and stent.

been achieved, the guidewires are removed. It is very seldom that post-stent angioplasty is performed for this procedure. Generally, whatever result is achieved with present angioplasty and the Wingspan stent system is deemed acceptable. Unlike CAS, no distal filter embolic protection devices are currently available (Figs. 3, 4, and 5).

Postoperative care is very similar to that of CAS procedures. The patient is generally extubated in the angiography suite and taken overnight to the ICU. The

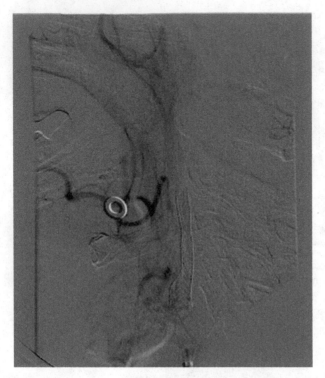

Figure 5 X ray demonstrating stent completely deployed across the lesion, with filter protection device in high cervical internal carotid artery above the lesion and stent.

heparin anticoagulation is not reversed. Aspirin (325 mg) is continued indefinitely, and because of the higher rate of restenosis, clopidogrel (plavix) generally continued for at least six months. Most patients are discharged the following day. The patient may resume normal activity without restriction within days, primarily as they recover from the general anesthetic.

The role of the angioplasty and stenting in the treatment of symptomatic intracranial atheromatous disease is evolving. Numerous early case reports and small series of cases suggested that angioplasty and stenting of intracranial arteries was both feasible and safe (60–63). Other studies clearly showed that the natural history of symptomatic intracranial atheromatous disease was very poor [extracranial-intracranial bypass (ECIC) TRIAL]. In addition, the best medical therapy still resulted in high rates of stroke or death. Studies that compared aspirin with coumadin for symptomatic intracranial atheromatous disease have not shown particular benefit of one therapy or the other (64–66). Two trials have evaluated intracranial angioplasty and stenting for symptomatic atheromatous stenoses (7) (Figs. 6, 7, and 8).

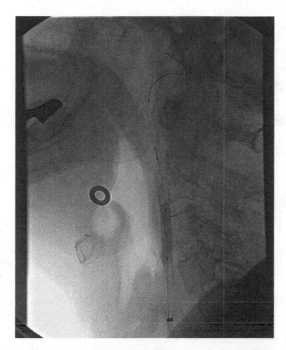

Figure 6 X ray demonstrating 5.5-mm post-stent angioplasty balloon inflated to dilate stent to remove residual stenosis.

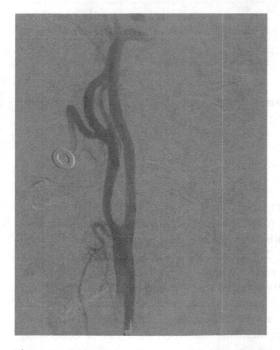

Figure 7 Cervical carotid artery angiogram, RAO and lateral projections, posttreatment, with filter protection device removed. *Abbreviation*: RAO, right anterior oblique.

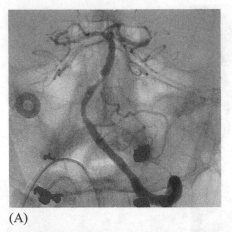

(A)

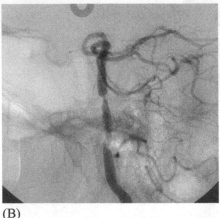

(B)

Figure 8 Left vertebral artery angiogram, anteroposterior (A) and lateral (B) projections, showing stenosis of mid-basilar artery.

SSYLVIA

The Stenting of Symptomatic Atherosclerotic Lesions in the Vertebral or Intracranial Arteries (SSYLVIA) trial involved 61 patients with both intracranial and extracranial stenotic lesions (67). This multicentered, nonrandomized, prospective trial evaluated the Neurolink intracranial stent for treatment of vertebral or intracranial arterial stenoses. The device used was the Guidant Neurolink intracranial stent, a balloon-expandable stent. All patients were symptomatic referable to a single, atherosclerotic lesion that resulted in at least a 50% narrowing of the artery. Technical success was achieved in 95% of cases. In the first 30 days, 6.6% of patients had strokes, but no mortality occurred. Between 30 days and 1 year, the stroke incidence increased to 7.3%. A concerning occurrence was a high rate of in-stent stenosis found at the six-month follow-up angiogram. Less than 3% of patients had greater than 50% stenosis immediately after the stent was placed. However, on the follow-up angiogram six months later, 37% of patients had greater than 50% narrowing. Interestingly, very few of the patients had any symptoms. While the results were very encouraging and led to approval of the device by the FDA, the company never made the stent commercially available.

WINGSPAN SYSTEM

The second trial evaluating intracranial angioplasty and stenting for intracranial atheromatous disease involved the Wingspan system (68,69). The study enrolled 45 patients from 12 European sites with intracranial atherosclerotic lesions of greater than 50%. This was the first study of a self-expanding stent for atheromatous disease in the brain. The technique used predilation of the lesion with a balloon to partly open it but not to achieve complete reversal of the stenosis. To reduce the risk of intracranial arterial rupture, predilation was only taken to 80% of the normal arterial diameter. The expectation was that the self-expanding properties of the stent would allow further opening.

Technical success was achieved in 98% of patients. The 30-day death and ipsilateral stroke rate was 4.5%, which increased to 7.1% at six months. No arterial dissections or ruptures were reported. Follow-up studies demonstrated overall no significant in-stent stenosis. In fact, immediately post stenting, the mean residual stenosis was 32%. Follow-up angiograms were performed in 40 of the 45 patients at six months, and the mean narrowing was only 28%, suggesting continued opening of some of the arteries when this self-expanding stent was used.

A trial has not been conducted to compare medical treatment of intracranial atheromatous disease with angioplasty and stenting. The two Warfarin–Aspirin Symptomatic Intracranial Disease (WASID) trials suggested that in patients who received the best medical therapy, symptomatic intracranial disease carried only a 9% to 12% annual risk of major stroke or death (7,64,65). The risk of stroke at one year was 19%, with intracranial stenosis of 70% to 99% despite treatment with aspirin or warfarin (70). The results of both the Wingspan study and the SSYLVIA study compare favorably with medical therapy (Figs. 9, 10, and 11).

RESTENOSIS AND INTRACRANIAL STENTING

With the relatively higher rates of restenosis associated with intracranial stenting as noted in the SSYLVIA trial, interest has developed in using drug-eluting stents in this setting. These stents, at least in the coronary arena, appear to be associated with much lower rates of restenosis than bare metal stents (71–74). One group treated 26 intracranial arteries with drug-eluting stents, including both the Boston Scientific Taxus stent and the Cordis Cypher stent (72). The stents were successfully delivered in 90% of cases. Twenty of these cases had follow-up angiography, and only 5% had restenosis of 50% or more. Another group reported on eight cases in which

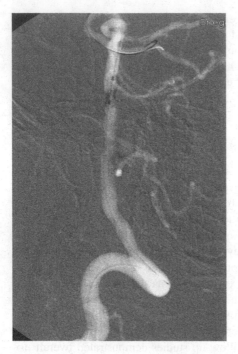

Figure 9 X ray showing 3-mm Gateway balloon straddling the stenotic lesion in the basilar artery as prestent angioplasty is being performed.

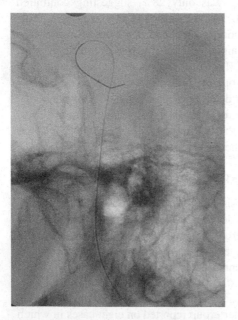

Figure 10 X ray showing Wingspan stent deployed in basilar artery over stenotic lesion.

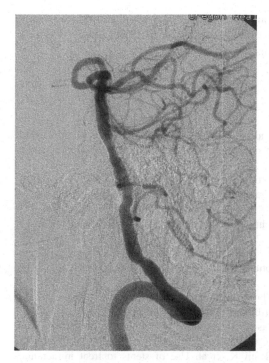

Figure 11 Left vertebral artery angiogram, lateral projections, showing reversal of stenosis in the mid-basilar artery after prestent angioplasty and deployment of Wingspan stent.

they used drug-eluting stents (71). Follow up included angiography, transcranial Doppler, and CT angiography over a mean of 11 months. None of the patients had significant stenosis or required revascularization.

CONCLUSIONS AND FUTURE DIRECTIONS—INTRACRANIAL AND VERTEBRAL ARTERY ANGIOPLASTY AND STENTING

Symptomatic intracranial atheromatous disease has a bad prognosis, even with the best medical therapy. Both balloon-expandable and self-expanding stents can be safely navigated into intracranial arteries, and reversal of the narrowing can be achieved. A significant reduction in stroke rates with this disease appears to occur after stenting. There also appears to be a problem with in-stent stenosis, although the clinical results are better. Preliminary reports suggest that drug-eluting stents may significantly reduce this occurrence. The technique is still evolving, and the optimal approach is still unclear. These issues include the choices between drug-eluting versus bare metal stents, self-expanding versus balloon-expanded stents, as well as the optimal amount of revascularization necessary to achieve reduction of stenosis while ensuring patient safety and avoidance of arterial rupture. Antiplatelet regimens are similar to CAS procedures. The higher restenosis rates suggest that dual antiplatelet therapy may be continued for longer periods of time, generally six months to more than one year, similar to cardiology regimens (75,76).

REFERENCES

1. Kerber CW, Cromwell LD, Loehden OL. Catheter dilatation of proximal carotid stenosis during distal bifurcation endarterectomy. AJNR Am J Neuroradiol 1980; 1(4):348–349.
2. Bockenheimer SA, Mathias K. Percutaneous transluminal angioplasty in arteriosclerotic internal carotid artery stenosis. AJNR Am J Neuroradiol 1983; 4(3): 791–792.
3. Caplan LR, Meyers PM, Schumacher HC. Angioplasty and stenting to treat occlusive vascular disease. Rev Neurol Dis 2006; 3(1):8–18.
4. Theron J, Raymond J, Casasco A, et al. Percutaneous angioplasty of atherosclerotic and postsurgical stenosis of carotid arteries. AJNR Am J Neuroradiol 1987; 8(3): 495–500.
5. Wholey MH, Al-Mubarek N, Wholey MH. Updated review of the global carotid artery stent registry. Catheter Cardiovasc Interv 2003; 60(2):259–266.
6. Wholey MH, Wholey M, Mathias K, et al. Global experience in cervical carotid artery stent placement. Catheter Cardiovasc Interv 2000; 50(2):160–167.
7. Meyers PM, Schumacher HC, Tanji K, et al. Use of stents to treat intracranial cerebrovascular disease. Annu Rev Med 2007; 58:107–122.
8. Beneficial effect of carotid endarterectomy in symptomatic patients with high-grade carotid stenosis. North American Symptomatic Carotid Endarterectomy Trial Collaborators. N Engl J Med 1991; 325(7):445–453.
9. Endarterectomy for asymptomatic carotid artery stenosis. Executive Committee for the Asymptomatic Carotid Atherosclerosis Study. JAMA 1995; 273(18):1421–1428.
10. Abbott AL, Chambers BR, Stork JL, et al. Embolic signals and prediction of ipsilateral stroke or transient ischemic attack in asymptomatic carotid stenosis: a multicenter prospective cohort study. Stroke 2005; 36(6):1128–1133.
11. Biller J, Feinberg WM, Castaldo JE, et al. Guidelines for carotid endarterectomy: a statement for healthcare professionals from a Special Writing Group of the Stroke Council, American Heart Association. Circulation 1998; 97(5):501–509.
12. McCrory DC, Goldstein LB, Samsa GP, et al. Predicting complications of carotid endarterectomy. Stroke 1993; 24(9):1285–1291.
13. Rothwell PM, Slattery J, Warlow CP. A systematic comparison of the risks of stroke and death due to carotid endarterectomy for symptomatic and asymptomatic stenosis. Stroke 1996; 27(2):266–269.
14. Wennberg DE, Lucas FL, Birkmeyer JD, et al. Variation in carotid endarterectomy mortality in the Medicare population: trial hospitals, volume, and patient characteristics. JAMA 1998; 279(16):1278–1281.
15. Mathur A, Dorros G, Iyer SS, et al. Palmaz stent compression in patients following carotid artery stenting. Cathet Cardiovasc Diagn 1997; 41(2):137–140.
16. Vitek JJ, Roubin GS, Al-Mubarek N, et al. Carotid artery stenting: technical considerations. AJNR Am J Neuroradiol 2000; 21(9):1736–1743.

17. Roubin GS, New G, Iyer SS, et al. Immediate and late clinical outcomes of carotid artery stenting in patients with symptomatic and asymptomatic carotid artery stenosis: a 5-year prospective analysis. Circulation 2001; 103(4):532–537.

18. Hobson RW II. CREST (Carotid Revascularization Endarterectomy versus Stent Trial): background, design, and current status. Semin Vasc Surg 2000; 13(2):139–143.

19. Mas JL, Chatellier G, Beyssen B, et al. Endarterectomy versus stenting in patients with symptomatic severe carotid stenosis. N Engl J Med 2006; 355(16):1660–1671.

20. Endovascular versus surgical treatment in patients with carotid stenosis in the Carotid and Vertebral Artery Transluminal Angioplasty Study (CAVATAS): a randomised trial. Lancet, 2001; 357(9270):1729–1737.

21. SECuRITY Registry Trial. Available at: http://www.fda.gov/cdrh/mda/docs/p040038. html. Accessed September 6, 2005.

22. The CABERNET Trial. Available at: http://www.carotid.com/clinical_trials.html. Accessed September 12, 2007.

23. The ARCHeR Trial. Available at: http://www.strokecenter.org/trials/trialDetail. aspx?tid=100&search_string=carotid%20stent. Accessed September 13, 2007.

24. The BEACH Trial. Available at: http://www.strokecenter.org/trials/trialDetail.aspx? tid=544&search_string=BEACH. Accessed September 13, 2007.

25. Carotid revascularization using endarterectomy or stenting systems (CARESS): phase I clinical trial. J Endovasc Ther 2003; 10(6):1021–1030.

26. Carotid Revascularization Using Endarterectomy or Stenting Systems (CaRESS) phase I clinical trial: 1-year results. J Vasc Surg 2005; 42(2):213–219.

27. Ringleb PA, Allenberg J, Bruckmann H, et al. 30 day results from the SPACE trial of stent-protected angioplasty versus carotid endarterectomy in symptomatic patients: a randomised non-inferiority trial. Lancet 2006; 368(9543):1239–1247.

28. Yadav JS, Wholey MH, Kuntz RE, et al. Protected carotid-artery stenting versus endarterectomy in high-risk patients. N Engl J Med 2004; 351(15):1493–1501.

29. Mas JL, Chatellier G, Beyssen B. Carotid angioplasty and stenting with and without cerebral protection: clinical alert from the Endarterectomy Versus Angioplasty in Patients With Symptomatic Severe Carotid Stenosis (EVA-3S) trial. Stroke 2004; 35(1):E18–E20.

30. Qureshi AI. Carotid angioplasty and stent placement after EVA-3S trial. Stroke 2007; 38(6):1993–1996.

31. Verzini F, Cao P, De Rango P, et al. Appropriateness of learning curve for carotid artery stenting: an analysis of periprocedural complications. J Vasc Surg 2006; 44(6):1205–1211 (discussion 1211–1202).

32. Alric P, Branchereau P, Berthet JP, et al. Carotid artery stenting for stenosis following revascularization or cervical irradiation. J Endovasc Ther 2002; 9(1):14–19.

33. Cernetti C, Reimers B, Picciolo A, et al. Carotid artery stenting with cerebral protection in 100 consecutive patients: immediate and two-year follow-up results. Ital Heart J 2003; 4(10):695–700.

34. Dietz A, Berkefeld J, Theron JG, et al. Endovascular treatment of symptomatic carotid stenosis using stent placement: long-term follow-up of patients with a balanced surgical risk/benefit ratio. Stroke 2001; 32(8):1855–1859.

35. Frericks H, Kievit J, van Baalen JM, et al. Carotid recurrent stenosis and risk of ipsilateral stroke: a systematic review of the literature. Stroke 1998; 29(1):244–250.

36. Meyer FB, Piepgras DG, and Fode NC. Surgical treatment of recurrent carotid artery stenosis. J Neurosurg 1994; 80(5):781–787.

37. Melliere D, Becquemin JP, Berrahal D, et al. Management of radiation-induced occlusive arterial disease: a reassessment. J Cardiovasc Surg (Torino) 1997; 38(3): 261–269.

38. Levy EI, Hanel RA, Lau T, et al. Frequency and management of recurrent stenosis after carotid artery stent implantation. J Neurosurg 2005; 102(1):29–37.

39. Reimers B, Tubler T, de Donato G, et al. Endovascular treatment of in-stent restenosis after carotid artery stenting: immediate and midterm results. J Endovasc Ther 2006; 13(4):429–435.

40. Angelini A, Reimers B, Della Barbera M, et al. Cerebral protection during carotid artery stenting: collection and histopathologic analysis of embolized debris. Stroke 2002; 33(2):456–461.

41. Cremonesi A, Manetti R, Setacci F, et al. Protected carotid stenting: clinical advantages and complications of embolic protection devices in 442 consecutive patients. Stroke 2003; 34(8):1936–1941.

42. Chakhtoura EY, Hobson RW II, Goldstein J, et al. In-stent restenosis after carotid angioplasty-stenting: incidence and management. J Vasc Surg 2001; 33(2):220–225.

43. Lal BK, Hobson RW II, Goldstein J, et al. In-stent recurrent stenosis after carotid artery stenting: life table analysis and clinical relevance. J Vasc Surg 2003; 38(6): 1162–1168.

44. Willfort-Ehringer A, Ahmadi R, Gschwandtner ME, et al. Single-center experience with carotid stent restenosis. J Endovasc Ther 2002; 9(3):299–307.

45. Ballotta E, Renon L, Da Giau G, et al. Octogenarians with contralateral carotid artery occlusion: a cohort at higher risk for carotid endarterectomy? J Vasc Surg 2004; 39(5):1003–1008.

46. Mozes G, Sullivan TM, Torres-Russotto DR, et al. Carotid endarterectomy in SAPPHIRE-eligible high-risk patients: implications for selecting patients for carotid angioplasty and stenting. J Vasc Surg 2004; 39(5):958–965.

47. Norman PE, Semmens JB, Laurvick CL, et al. Long-term relative survival in elderly patients after carotid endarterectomy: a population-based study. Stroke 2003; 34(7): E95–E98.

48. Lam RC, Lin SC, DeRubertis B, et al. The impact of increasing age on anatomic factors affecting carotid angioplasty and stenting. J Vasc Surg 2007; 45(5):875–880.

49. Rockman CB, Jacobowitz GR, Adelman MA, et al. The benefits of carotid endarterectomy in the octogenarian: a challenge to the results of carotid angioplasty and stenting. Ann Vasc Surg 2003; 17(1):9–14.

50. Hobson RW II, Howard VJ, Roubin GS, et al. Carotid artery stenting is associated with increased complications in octogenarians: 30-day stroke and death rates in the CREST lead-in phase. J Vasc Surg 2004; 40(6):1106–1111.

51. Kastrup A, Schulz JB, Raygrotzki S, et al. Comparison of angioplasty and stenting with cerebral protection versus endarterectomy for treatment of internal carotid artery stenosis in elderly patients. J Vasc Surg 2004; 40(5):945–951.

52. Crawley F, Clifton A, Buckenham T, et al. Comparison of hemodynamic cerebral ischemia and microembolic signals detected during carotid endarterectomy and carotid angioplasty. Stroke 1997; 28(12):2460–2464.

53. Markus HS, Clifton A, Buckenham T, et al. Carotid angioplasty. Detection of embolic signals during and after the procedure. Stroke 1994; 25(12):2403–2406.

54. Muller-Hulsbeck S, Jahnke T, Liess C, et al. In vitro comparison of four cerebral protection filters for preventing human plaque embolization during carotid interventions. J Endovasc Ther 2002; 9(6):793–802.

55. Muller-Hulsbeck S, Stolzmann P, Liess C, et al. Vessel wall damage caused by cerebral protection devices: ex vivo evaluation in porcine carotid arteries. Radiology 2005; 235(2):454–460.

56. Vos JA, van den Berg JC, Ernst SM, et al. Carotid angioplasty and stent placement: comparison of transcranial Doppler US data and clinical outcome with and without filtering cerebral protection devices in 509 patients. Radiology 2005; 234(2): 493–499.

57. Hauth EA, Jansen C, Drescher R, et al. MR and clinical follow-up of diffusion-weighted cerebral lesions after carotid artery stenting. AJNR Am J Neuroradiol 2005; 26(9):2336–2341.

58. Kastrup A, Groschel K, Krapf H, et al. Early outcome of carotid angioplasty and stenting with and without cerebral protection devices: a systematic review of the literature. Stroke 2003; 34(3):813–819.

59. Kastrup A, Nagele T, Groschel K, et al. Incidence of new brain lesions after carotid stenting with and without cerebral protection. Stroke 2006; 37(9):2312–2316.

60. Connors JJ III, Wojak JC. Percutaneous transluminal angioplasty for intracranial atherosclerotic lesions: evolution of technique and short-term results. J Neurosurg 1999; 91(3):415–423.

61. Ecker RD, Levy EI, Sauvageau E, et al. Current concepts in the management of intracranial atherosclerotic disease. Neurosurgery 2006; 59(5 suppl 3):S210–S218.

62. Higashida RT, Meyers PM, Connors JJ III, et al. Intracranial angioplasty & stenting for cerebral atherosclerosis: a position statement of the American Society of Interventional and Therapeutic Neuroradiology, Society of Interventional Radiology, and the American Society of Neuroradiology. AJNR Am J Neuroradiol 2005; 26(9): 2323–2327.

63. Levy EI, Horowitz MB, Koebbe CJ, et al. Transluminal stent-assisted angiplasty of the intracranial vertebrobasilar system for medically refractory, posterior circulation ischemia: early results. Neurosurgery 2001; 48(6):1215–1221.

64. Chimowitz MI, Kokkinos J, Strong J, et al. The Warfarin-Aspirin Symptomatic Intracranial Disease Study. Neurology 1995; 45(8):1488–1493.

65. Chimowitz MI, Lynn MJ, Howlett-Smith H, et al. Comparison of warfarin and aspirin for symptomatic intracranial arterial stenosis. N Engl J Med 2005; 352(13): 1305–1316.

66. Mohr JP, Thompson JL, Lazar RM, et al. A comparison of warfarin and aspirin for the prevention of recurrent ischemic stroke. N Engl J Med 2001; 345(20): 1444–1451.

67. Stenting of Symptomatic Atherosclerotic Lesions in the Vertebral or Intracranial Arteries (SSYLVIA): study results. Stroke 2004; 35(6):1388–1392.

68. Wingspan trial. Available at: http://www.fda.gov/cdrh/pdf5/h050001c.pdf. Accessed September 13, 2007.

69. Henkes H, Miloslavski E, Lowens S, et al. Treatment of intracranial atherosclerotic stenoses with balloon dilatation and self-expanding stent deployment (WingSpan). Neuroradiology 2005; 47(3):222–228.

70. Kasner SE, Chimowitz MI, Lynn MJ, et al. Predictors of ischemic stroke in the territory of a symptomatic intracranial arterial stenosis. Circulation 2006; 113(4): 555–563.

71. Abou-Chebl A, Bashir Q, and Yadav JS. Drug-eluting stents for the treatment of intracranial atherosclerosis: initial experience and midterm angiographic follow-up. Stroke 2005; 36(12):E165–E168.

72. Gupta R, Al-Ali F, Thomas AJ, et al. Safety, feasibility, and short-term follow-up of drug-eluting stent placement in the intracranial and extracranial circulation. Stroke 2006; 37(10):2562–2566.

73. Moses JW, Leon MB, Popma JJ, et al. Sirolimus-eluting stents versus standard stents in patients with stenosis in a native coronary artery. N Engl J Med 2003; 349(14): 1315–1323.

74. Stone GW, Ellis SG, Cox DA, et al. A polymer-based, paclitaxel-eluting stent in patients with coronary artery disease. N Engl J Med 2004; 350(3):221–231.

75. Berger PB. Clopidogrel after coronary stenting. Curr Interv Cardiol Rep 1999; 1(3): 263–269.

76. Waksman R, Ajani AE, White RL, et al. Prolonged antiplatelet therapy to prevent late thrombosis after intracoronary gamma-radiation in patients with in-stent restenosis: Washington Radiation for In-Stent Restenosis Trial plus 6 months of clopidogrel (WRIST PLUS). Circulation 2001; 103(19):2332–2335.

10

Neuromonitoring in Ischemic Stroke

Kairash Golshani, MD, Senior Resident
Emun Abdu, MD, Senior Resident
*Department of Neurological Surgery, Oregon Health & Science University,
Portland, Oregon, U.S.A.*

Anish Bhardwaj, MD, FAHA, FCCM, Professor[a] and Director[b]
*[a]Neurology, Neurological Surgery, Anesthesiology & Peri-Operative Medicine,
[b]Neurosciences Critical Care Program, Oregon Health & Science University,
Portland, Oregon, U.S.A.*

INTRODUCTION

Stroke is the third most common cause of death in the United States after heart disease and cancer. It is also the leading cause of serious disability. With advances in the management of stroke with thrombolytic therapy and neurointerventional procedures, there is an effort to concentrate these treatment recourses in designated stroke centers. A meta-analysis of randomized studies in the treatment of stroke indicates improved mortality preventing one death per 50 stroke admissions per year (1), and it is expected that this trend will continue to demonstrate improvement. A critical component of these specialized stroke centers is the critical care and monitoring during the peri-ischemic period. Patients with severe stroke are not only at risk for common intensive care unit (ICU) complications such as ventilator-associated pneumonia but are also at risk for neurologic complications such as progressive ischemia because of hypotension, vessel reocclusion following thrombolysis, hemorrhagic conversion, and malignant cerebral edema. This chapter reviews the armamentarium of tools used to promptly diagnose and treat such complications. For the purposes of this discussion, these diagnostic tools are discussed under the following subheadings: components of the neurologic examination, neuroimaging, invasive tissue monitoring, and neurophysiologic monitoring.

Neurologic Examination

One of the fundamental tools in assessing and monitoring patients who have suffered ischemic stroke is the neurologic examination. Evaluation of patients often begins in the field, and identification and documentation of the time of the last normal neurologic examination is essential when assessing a patient for thrombolytic treatment. Similarly, a diligent neurologic examination must be performed and monitored for patients receiving critical care because the eligibility for intervention often depends on how quickly a change in the neurologic status is identified. It is also critical that normal and abnormal components of neurologic examination are carefully documented and passed on to each caregiver so that changes in neurologic status can be promptly noted and evaluated further.

An essential component of the neurologic examination is evaluation of the patient's level of consciousness. This is often articulated using the Glasgow Coma Scale (GCS) that has three components: opening of eyes, verbal response, and motor response. Although this examination can be performed in the field by emergency medical services personnel and has good interrater reproducibility, its utility in the setting of stroke is somewhat limited because of the incidence of aphasia in some patients. A typical patient with dominant hemispheric stroke will often have spontaneous eye opening, no spontaneous speech, and purposeful movement yielding a GCS of 10. However, the level of consciousness of such a patient is actually much less severe than a trauma patient with a similar score. Therefore, it is important to utilize descriptive terms as opposed to a single-digit scoring in such patients. In addition, the ability of the patient to repeat and name objects is critical to document serial neurologic examinations. In aphasic patients, the motor examination can also be modified when assessing the patient's ability to follow commands. Using visual cues, one can often assess a patient's ability to follow simple commands (e.g., hold up a finger or stick out the tongue). When patients are intubated and sedated, it is imperative to wean the sedation one to four times per day to assess their neurologic examination. Alternatively, patients can be left intubated with only a low-dose narcotic drip to suppress the cough reflex. This allows for constant monitoring of the neurologic status.

Along with assessment of the patient's level of consciousness, a detailed cranial nerve examination should be performed in all patients with stroke. Visual field deficits are common accompaniment of large cortical strokes, and other cranial nerve deficits are found in brain stem strokes. In addition, certain components of the cranial nerve examination (e.g., pupillary reflex, gag reflex) are crucial for early diagnosis of uncal and tonsillar herniation. The pupillary examination is essential to document for patients upon admission to determine if there are any baseline abnormalities. Often patients will have 1 to 2 mm of anisocoria, and patients who have had eye surgery or eye trauma may have an abnormal shape to the pupil. Patients suffering from brain stem strokes or spontaneous/iatrogenic dissection of the carotid artery often have a Horner's eye ipsilateral to the lesion. Once a baseline examination is completed, the ICU nurse should check the pupils on an hourly basis for any changes. Unilateral papillary dilation is often due to uncal herniation resulting from mass effect from either hemorrhagic transformation or cerebral edema. Once pupillary dilation has occurred, the patient is at risk for progressing to brain death, and therapeutic interventions such as mannitol, hyperventilation, and hemicraniectomy should be instituted emergently to prevent further injury from brain stem compression or cerebral ischemia. Patients with posterior fossa strokes may also have hemorrhagic conversion or malignant edema leading to hydrocephalus and tonsillar herniation. Patients with tonsillar herniation exhibit loss of gag and cough reflexes constituting a neurologic emergency often requiring placement of an external ventricular drain and posterior fossa decompression.

Finally, the motor and sensory examination often uncovers neurologic deficits in patients with stroke. While these deficits are often grossly obvious, subtle deficits may be found using a series of simple maneuvers. Examination of the pronator drift is very useful for detecting subtle motor weakness due to a supratentorial lesion. It is performed by asking the patient to hold both hands up with the palms facing the ceiling and then asking them to close their eyes. Patients with cortical weakness will slowly pronate and drop the weak arm when visual cues are removed. Another maneuver used to detect cortical motor deficits is examination of rapid alternating movements. This can be elicited by asking the patient to tap the thumb and index finger as widely and rapidly as possible. Alternatively, the patient can be asked to put the palms of his hands together and tap his fingers as widely and rapidly as possible. Patients with cortical weakness will often have both decreased amplitude and frequency of tapping on the affected side. Weakness otherwise should be graded on a well-established 5-point scale for each muscle group. The sensory examination not only encompasses pursuit of primary modalities (sensation to light touch, pin prick, proprioception and vibration), but also to secondary modalities (2-point discrimination, graphesthesia, and stereognosis). Patients with subtle strokes may present with deficits in the latter group of sensory modalities; however, the level of consciousness of patients with severe stroke or dominant hemispheric stroke often precludes patients from being able to reliably perform a detailed sensory examination.

Finally, examination of the patient's language function is essential not only to localize the area of ischemia but also for monitoring purposes. Evaluation of language not only includes the patient's ability to speak and follow commands but also the patient's ability to repeat, name objects, read and write.

The National Institutes of Health Stroke Scale (NIHSS) is frequently used to determine the severity of stroke prior to and following treatment. Its components include assessment of the level of consciousness, gaze, visual field, facial function, motor function, coordination, sensation, language, extinction, and inattention. NIHSS is a standardized method to evaluate patients using all the modalities mentioned above and is often used as a tool for enrollment of patients in clinical trials. The scale has good interexaminer reproducibility not only among stroke specialists but also among non–neurologist practitioners (2,3). Although the NIHSS is predictive of long-term outcome and correlates well with the Barthel Index, GOS (Glasgow Outcome Score), and the modified Rankin score (4), recent data suggest that the NIHSS may also be predictive of progression of neurologic symptoms in the acute period. In one study, NIHSS score reduction greater than 40% was highly predictive of recanalization following intravenous (IV) recombinant tissue plasminogen activator (r-tPA) administration (sensitivity of 65%, specificity of 85% at 60 minutes) (5). In another report, patients with ischemic stroke with NIHSS score greater than 7 had a significantly higher incidence of neurologic progression (65.9%) during the first 48 hours after acute stroke (6). Patients with baseline NIHSS greater than or equal to 20 for left-sided (dominant hemisphere) stroke or greater than or equal to 15 for right-sided (nondominant hemisphere) stroke had a significantly higher rate of death due to malignant cerebral edema (7). Although NIHSS is useful in predicting the risk of clinical worsening, it is not a practical tool for continuous bedside monitoring of acute stroke patients. Rather it is a useful tool in the assessment following an ischemic insult to determine patients' suitability for certain treatment protocols, predict the probability of early complications, and prognosticate long-term outcome.

Neuroimaging

Significant advances have been made in neuroimaging over the last decade. It has become a tool not only for initial assessment of stroke patients but also for monitoring in the peri-ischemic period. One of the oldest and most readily available tools for assessment of stroke patients is the noncontrast CT scan of the head. The availability of CT scans and short scanning times (under 2 minutes) have made CT scans the chest X ray of the neurointensive care unit.

The newer fourth generation CT scanners have not only become more sensitive for detecting hemorrhagic conversion and mass effect, they have also become more sensitive for detecting subtle signs of cerebral ischemia. These include wedge-shaped hypodensity in a vascular distribution, hyperdense middle cerebral artery (MCA) sign, and loss of the gray-white differentiation particularly along the basal ganglia. Other less specific signs of infarction include asymmetric focal hypoattenuation, cortical sulcal effacement, and loss of insular ribbon (obscuration of sylvian fissure). When combined, these findings have a sensitivity of 66% and a specificity of 87% for detection of early ischemic stroke (8). In addition, the risk of a poor outcome is significantly increased when these findings are present on initial CT (odds ratio 3.11). In particular, presence of two or more early ischemic signs (attenuation of lentiform nucleus, loss of insular ribbon, and hemispheric sulcal effacement) significantly increased the risk of poor outcome (68% with Rankin grade 5 or death) (9). The presence of early ischemic changes on CT were correlated with larger volume on magnetic resonance imaging diffusion-weighted imaging (MRI-DWI) scans (10).

There is some controversy regarding the association of these findings and outcome after IV r-tPA for ischemic stroke. Patients with MCA hypodensity greater than 33% are twice as likely to suffer symptomatic intracranial hemorrhage (ICH) after IV r-tPA, and patients with greater than 33% hypodensity in the MCA distribution have more than a fourfold increased risk of hemorrhage after IV r-tPA (11). However, other studies have found no correlation of these changes to the risk of ICH after IV r-tPA administration (12). Finally, there are some data that suggest that patients with a hyperdense MCA on initial CT may have better outcome with intra-arterial r-tPA than IV r-tPA (13). Beyond this, it is yet to be determined whether these early ischemic changes will guide subsequent therapy during the acute stroke period.

Although it is important to identify early signs of ischemia in stroke patients, in the critical care setting, CT is mainly used to identify presence of malignant cerebral edema or hemorrhagic conversion of stroke. Malignant cerebral edema often complicates large MCA strokes, and previous studies have demonstrated that patients with nondominant MCA strokes, who develop malignant edema, benefit from surgery (14). More recent data also indicate that a select group of young patients with dominant MCA stroke may have an improvement in recovery of aphasia after decompressive hemicraniectomy (15). These patients often begin to develop edema and mass effect during the first 24 hours that plateaus three to five days after stroke and slowly resolves over the next few weeks. Evidence of edema on CT scans includes sulcal effacement, obliteration of suprasellar and perimesencephalic cisterns, midline shift in septum pellucidum or pineal gland, and subfalcine herniation. Left untreated, these patients often progress to uncal herniation and brain death. Although studies have shown that patients taken for decompressive craniectomy and duraplasty do better when surgery is done within the first 24 hours after ictus, overaggressive management of such patients may lead to unnecessary surgery (14,16). Indications for surgery include clinical decline and progression of mass effect; therefore, in such patients, nonenhanced CT scans are often done on a scheduled basis (every 12–24 hours) to monitor the degree of mass effect. While there are no clear radiographic criteria for when these patients should be taken to surgery, most patients taken to surgery often have midline shift (in septum pellucidum) greater than 1 cm or pineal shift greater than 5 mm. However, in a univariate analysis the degree of shift at the time of surgery has no correlation with functional outcome (17). Therefore, the clinical examination and CT finding must be correlated during the evaluation of such patients.

Multimodal CT scan with IV contrast has become more readily available for evaluation of patients with stroke. This includes CT angiography (CTA) for evaluation of cerebral vasculature and CT perfusion (CTP) for quantitative evaluation of regional cerebral blood flow (CBF). CTA is a structural study of the cerebral vessels in which a bolus of IV contrast is given and a thin slice CT is performed during the arterial phase of this bolus. The quality of the scan is operator dependent, given that the timing of the scan has to be in harmony with the arterial phase of the contrast agent. This may contribute to its limited utility for evaluation. Studies have demonstrated that the sensitivity of CTA compared with the neurologic examination for the diagnosis of stroke is relatively low and there is no correlation between three-month outcome and pathologic findings on CTA (18,19). In contrast to CTA, CTP may represent a more useful tool for monitoring and evaluating stroke patients. It is performed by monitoring the transit of contrast continuously in both the arterial phase and the venous phase through a few representative slices on the CT scan. It yields regional information about cerebral blood volume (CBV) and CBF as well as hemispheric mean transit time (MTT) for flow of contrast from the arterial phase to the venous phase. An MTT of more than 2 seconds is usually indicative of hemispheric ischemia, and CBF/CBV greater than 2 standard deviations difference compared with the unaffected side is classified as abnormal. When used in combination with noncontrast CT (NCCT), it may be useful in discriminating infarction from ischemic penumbra (20). On NCCT, areas of isolated focal swelling typically have low CBF but high CBV. High CBV is also found in areas of low CBF that are normal on NCCT. Areas of parenchymal hypoattenuation have decreased CBF, most likely to progress to infarction based on 72-hour MRI-DWI scans regardless of reperfusion. On the other hand, areas of isolated focal swelling were protective against progression to infarction (OR 30.6), and areas of low CBF and CBV were highly likely to progress to infarction (OR 37.1) when compared with areas of low CBF with normal or elevated CBV. In addition, areas of low CBF and normal CBV were at higher risk for progressing to infarction than areas that demonstrated high CBV. This indicates that high CBV may be a marker for salvageable tissue in ischemic penumbra. Attempts have been made to better correlate this relationship between CBV and probability of infarction. In a retrospective study where CBV was measured in the core infarction, 5 mm inside the border of infarction and 5 mm outside the border of infarction, normalized CBV (pCBV) of 52% correlated with a 0.75 probability of infarction, a pCBV of 58% correlated with a 0.5 probability of infarction, and a pCBV of 66% correlated with a 0.25 probability of infarction (21). Unfortunately, this data has not been confirmed in prospective studies or reperfusion studies. More studies are necessary not only to determine the ability of CTP to predict size of infarction and penumbra but also whether interventions based on CTP data lead to improved functional outcome.

Recently, attempts have been made to use CTP to predict malignant cerebral edema. In a small retrospective case control study, 8 of 12 patients with CTP maps showing greater than 50% perfusion deficit in MCA territory and all patients with greater than 66% perfusion deficit developed malignant edema (22). In addition, all patients with perfusion deficits in anterior cerebral artery (ACA) or posterior cerebral artery (PCA) territories also developed malignant edema. Similarly, a 66% or greater perfusion deficit in the MCA territory had a sensitivity of 91% and specificity of 94% for malignant edema (23). However, because the number of patients in these studies is low, prospective data are necessary to determine if early intervention (hemicraniectomy) would provide a benefit over conventional therapies and practices.

Xenon-CT uses stable xenon as an inhaled contrast agent to determine regional CBF. Like CTP, it provides a high-resolution map of the brain with quantitative CBF values. Because studies in primates have shown that areas of reduced CBF (7–29 mL/100 g/min) may represent the penumbra in which injury can be reversed with reperfusion, xenon-CT and CTP may be useful in identifying patients suitable for thrombolysis even if time to presentation exceeds 6 hours (24). One study demonstrated a very narrow rim of tissue with CBF between 7 and 20 mL/100 g/min in patients with stroke (25). However, no studies have been done that demonstrate improvement in outcome when thrombolytic therapy is done on the basis of CBF measurements performed with xenon-CT, CTP, or other modalities. In addition, both the image acquisition and interpretation of xenon-CT is extremely operator dependent and often requires that the patient be mechanically ventilated and paralyzed. Although controversy still exists regarding the utility of xenon-CT for identifying volume of penumbra, other studies have shown that xenon-CT may be useful for predicting risk of ICH following recanalization as well as risk for developing malignant edema following ischemic stroke. For example, patients with mean MCA CBF greater than 13 mL/100 g/min were at a significantly higher risk of symptomatic ICH following intra-arterial r-tPA and recanalization (OR 1.58) (26). In another study, stroke patients who developed severe edema had a mean MCA CBF of 10.4 mL/100 g/min compared with 19 mL/100 g/min in patients with mild edema (27). Patients who developed clinical evidence of brain herniation had a mean MCA CBF of 8.6 mL/100 g/min. Despite these studies, use of xenon-CT has been limited to a few institutions mainly because of the difficulty in handling large amounts of xenon gas.

Positron emission tomography (PET) is another imaging tool that not only measures CBF and CBV but also yields data about oxygen consumption ($CMRO_2$), oxygen extraction (OEF), and glucose metabolism. Areas of reduced regional CBF (< 12 mL/100 g/min) or reduced $CMRO_2$ (< 65 μmon/100 g/min) correlated with infracted brain tissue on follow-up CT (28,29). However, areas of reduced CBF (12–22 mL/100 g/min) but preserved $CMRO_2$ represented tissue that can be salvaged with reperfusion. This tissue also had an oxygen extraction ratio between 80% and 100%. There is some controversy regarding threshold for infarction. A study demonstrated that 95% of tissue with CBF less than 4.8 mL/100 g/min progressed to infarction, while 95% of tissue with CBF greater than 14 mL/100 g/min remained outside the core infarction (30). However, risk of infarction for CBF between 4.8 and 14 mL/100 g/min was variable. Oxygen markers utilized for PET scans are cumbersome requiring multitracer application and arterial sampling, making its use in the clinical setting somewhat limited. Newer markers are also being tested not only for their ability to measure cerebral blood flow but also for their ability to monitor neuronal integrity. [^{11}C]flumazenil (FMZ) is a ligand that binds to the γ-aminobutyric acid (GABA) receptor. The ability of this ligand to bind to its receptor is dependent not only on CBF but also on the structural integrity of the cell in the tissue. There is a significant correlation between FMZ binding defects ($<$ 4 times the mean value of white matter) and subsequent infarction despite reperfusion (31). Therefore, this modality may be helpful in determining the volume of tissue that has been irreversibly injured due to ischemia. In addition, FMZ-PET may be useful for identifying patients at risk for malignant cerebral edema. In one study, patients who underwent a malignant course had a significantly higher volume of ischemic core ($<$ 50% CBF of contralateral hemisphere) and significantly lower volume of ischemic penumbral (defined as CBF 50–70% of contralateral hemisphere) (32). In addition, the volume of FMZ binding was also significantly higher in the malignant group (157.9 cm^3) than in the benign group (47.0 cm^3). A cutoff value of 95 cm^3 was determined for irreversible neuronal damage (using FMZ) and 105 cm^3 for ischemic core measurements (using CBF).

Like PET, single-photon emission tomography (SPECT) monitors the clearance of tracers to calculate CBF. ^{133}Xenon is the only tracer that allows quantification of CBF; however, the complexity of the data analysis and the lack of detail imaging limit the use of this modality in a clinical scenario (33). Other tracers that allow for a qualitative evaluation of CBF include ^{99m}Tc-ethyl-cysteinate-dimer (ECD), which allows not only measurement of perfusion but also of cell viability given that retention of ECD requires the presence of a cytosolic esterace present only on viable cells. Despite lack of quantifiable data, SPECT studies in the setting of stroke were able to identify hypoperfused areas relative on the contralateral side in the acute postischemic period and later (34,35). This data also correlated with long-term outcome. Further evaluation of the asymmetry between the ischemic and corresponding nonischemic hemisphere showed that tissue tracer uptake between 40% to 70% of the contralateral side during the first three to six hours after onset of symptoms is indicative of the ischemic penumbra (34,36). Severe hypoperfusion ($<$ 35% of contralateral isotope uptake) is predictive of hemorrhagic complication with reperfusion (37) or malignant cerebral edema (38). Data on postreperfusion SPECT indicates that when isotope uptake exceeds 70% of contralateral hemisphere, risk of infarction is significantly reduced regardless of the degree of recanalization (39).

The advent of DWI and perfusion-weighted imaging (PWI) has significantly enhanced the utility of MRI scans for the diagnosis and monitoring of patients with stroke. DWI images are hyperintense in areas of restricted diffusion in the brain. This corresponds to areas of cytotoxic edema where there is accumulation of intracellular water because of malfunction of the Na$^+$/K$^+$ ATP pump and other ion pumps that are reliant on an energy source. It is therefore presumed that hyperintensity on DWI is indicative of the core area of infarction and that such changes are detectable within minutes after onset of stroke (40,41). Furthermore, the volume of brain with positive signal and the apparent diffusion coefficient of water can be calculated to measure the severity of the infarction. In practice, DWI images are often dynamic and reversible in the first few hours after onset of symptoms; however, images obtained 24 hours after onset of symptoms are indicative of final infarct size. In addition, although DWI does predict early neurologic decline in patients with severe infarction involving occlusion of the MCA or ICA, studies have shown that DWI images by themselves are poor predictors of functional outcome (42,43). However, one study has demonstrated that a DWI volume greater than 145 cm^3 was 100% sensitive and 94% specific for prediction of malignant cerebral edema (44).

PWI utilizes a process similar to CT perfusion where an IV bolus of gadolinium is monitored during its transit through the brain. Like CTP, MR perfusion provides data on mean transit time, CBV, and regional perfusion; however, unlike CT perfusion, measurements of CBF are only relative to the contralateral hemisphere. Nevertheless, PWI provides a high-resolution map of areas with restricted CBF. In addition, perfusion changes precede changes detected on DWI. In fact, studies have shown that patients who have a mismatch between the severity of neurologic symptoms (NIHSS $\geq$ 8) and ischemic volume on DWI (< 25 mL) on MRI within 12 hours from symptom onset are at risk for early neurologic decline (decrease in NIHSS $\geq$ 4) and increase in size of infarction (45). Furthermore, the degree of change in size of infarction and neurologic decline was significantly greater in patients who did not receive reperfusion therapy. PWI may also allow detection of the tissue at risk for infarction (46). Tissue in the ischemic penumbra is characterized by a 73% increase in MTT and 29% increase in CBV. In one study, the volume of CBF abnormalities was greater than the volumes of DWI abnormalities and the final volume of infarction lies somewhere within these values. The final infarct volume (based on T2 images on day 7) increased in about 50% of patients and in some patients, enlargement of the infarct volume occurred after 24 hours indicating that ischemic tissue may still be at risk for infarction in the subacute period (47,48). In a previous report, the area that progressed to infarction in 24 to 72 hours after onset of symptoms and found reduced CBF (37% of contralateral side) and reduced CBV (47% of contralateral side) in comparison to the infarct core (CBF 12%, CBV 19%) (49). Comparison of MR perfusion with PET data demonstrates that areas of DWI-PWI mismatch correlate poorly with areas of increased oxygen extraction on PET images (50); however, areas with time to peak flow greater than 4 correlated best with areas of hypoperfusion (< 20 mL/100 g/min) on ^{15}O-water PET (51). Despite these limitations, a recent study in stroke patients receiving hyperdynamic therapy, a 30 mL decrease in volume of hypoperfused brain on PWI (using TTP threshold > 2.5 sec) was highly predictive of neurologic improvement (decreases in NIHSS of $\geq$ 3). The ability of MR-perfusion to identify tissue at risk for infarction in the acute and subacute period makes it a valuable tool in the management of patients in the peri-ischemic period.

Transcranial Doppler sonography (TCD) is another imaging modality used to monitor stroke patients. It is a simple test that can be done at bedside and repeated as often as necessary. Alternatively, continuous monitoring can also be accomplished by using a headband to hold a TCD probe in position. TCD does not require administration of any IV contrast agent and may therefore serve as an alternative means of monitoring in patients with renal disease. TCD yields data on CBF velocity, resistance index, and pulsatile index of major intracranial arteries. It has been used in stroke to monitor recanalization after IV r-tPA and time to recanalization has been correlated with early neurologic recovery (52,53). Continuous monitoring may also be useful in detecting reocclusion after recanalization has occurred (54). Recently, TCD has been used as a therapeutic modality to enhance clot lysis using r-tPA. Although, there was evidence of improved recanalization with TCD, the improvement in long-term outcome was not statistically significant (55). Although the therapeutic value of TCD is still yet to be determined, its use for bedside cerebral vessel monitoring makes it considerably valuable particularly in patients at risk for vessel reocclusion or embolic occlusion (e.g., patients with carotid dissection).

Invasive Monitoring

Multiple methods of invasive neuromonitoring using transcranial probes have been developed and put into use in the clinical setting. These include intracranial pressure (ICP) monitoring, jugular venous mixed oxygen monitoring, parenchymal brain tissue oxygenation (PbO_2) monitoring, and microdialysis. Even though these modalities have been studied well in the laboratory or in other clinical situations such as trauma, their use for the monitoring of stroke patients has not been standard of care.

ICP monitoring has been used for many years in the setting of traumatic brain injury (TBI); however, its use in the setting of ischemic stroke is somewhat controversial. In early studies, ICP monitors failed to reliably predict neurologic decline in stroke patients with malignant cerebral edema (56). In these studies, clinical signs of herniation preceded rise in ICP, and changes on CT scans did not correlate with changes in ICP. However, most of the patients in these studies were monitored using epidural or contralateral ICP monitors. Studies in primates shows that an interhemispheric gradient of 13.8 ± 4.3 mmHg exists 12 hours after the onset of stroke (57). In addition, given that patients experience large MCA strokes, usually a large component of temporal edema contributing to transtentorial herniation, global ICP monitoring using frontal parenchymal probes may fail to detect deterioration from focal edema in the temporal lobe. Another argument against ICP monitoring in stroke patients is that conventional ICP treatment using mannitol and hyperventilation mainly affects the normal hemisphere and does not produce long-lasting decrease in ICP (58). However, a study comparing hypertonic saline-hydroxylethyl starch solution with mannitol to treat a stroke patient whose ICP increased greater than 25 mmHg showed an 11.4 mmHg decline in ICP with the hypertonic saline (HS) and a 6.4 mmHg decline with mannitol (59). Although they were able to demonstrate effective ICP monitoring and a treatment effect with both mannitol and HS, there are no data on the effect of such a treatment on long-term outcome. In addition, 3 of the 30 ICP crisis episodes involved papillary dilation without increase in ICP.

A more recent study involving the use of 10% HS after mannitol treatment failed also showed a significant decrease in ICP (9.9 mmHg); however, the decrease in ICP was only temporary, and ICP began to rise after 35 minutes (60). Although conservative management of ICP may have limited use in the setting of ischemic stroke, it may serve as a temporizing measure for patients requiring operative intervention. ICP monitoring has not been well studied in terms of guiding the need for operative intervention; however, a recent study has indicated that patients who have undergone hemicraniectomy may further benefit from temporal lobectomy when the ICP is greater than 30 mmHg. It is interesting to note that most of these patients had evidence of stroke in multiple vascular territories (MCA ± ACA or PCA) indicating that such patients may be candidates for temporal lobectomy at the time of decompression. In these patients, ICP measurements may be more useful given that cerebral edema is more hemispheric rather than localized to the temporal lobe. Finally, a report of ICP changes in 34 patients found that ICP elevation greater than 26.6 mmHg had a high probability to progress to a malignant course (likelihood ratio 33.10, sensitivity 96%, specificity 100%) (32). Further study is necessary to determine if treatment based on ICP measurement results in long-term improvement of neurologic status.

Although the main goal of ICP monitoring is to prevent uncal herniation, a secondary goal is to prevent secondary ischemic injury due to intracranial hypertension. In this respect, bedside monitoring of cerebral oxygenation may allow identification of secondary ischemic injury. One of the older methods used for monitoring brain tissue oxygen extraction involves monitoring of mixed jugular venous oxygenation ($SjVO_2$) via a probe in the jugular bulb. A decrease in $SjVO_2$ may be secondary to a decrease in oxygen delivery (systemic hypotension or decrease in CPP) or an increase in oxygen usage (seizure). Although $SjVO_2$ monitoring has been useful in the setting of TBI, it may prove to be less useful in the setting of stroke. In TBI the injury is usually global involving both hemispheres; however, in the setting of stroke, injury is unilateral. Because venous blood from both hemispheres mixes in the sagittal sinus, it is not a practical method to monitor oxygenation in one hemisphere. In addition, in TBI cerebral autoregulation is compromised creating a direct relationship between cardiac output and oxygen delivery to the brain; however, in the setting of stroke, while autoregulation may be compromised in the ischemic penumbra, it is intact in the nonischemic brain. A mixture of venous blood from these two areas would underestimate ischemia from the penumbra. This is consistent with data demonstrating that the critical threshold used to detect secondary ischemia in patients with TBI ($SjVO_2 < 50\%$) does not extrapolate to stroke patients (61). $SjVO_2$ monitoring may be more useful in the setting of malignant cerebral edema because both ischemic and nonischemic brain may have compromised CBF because of elevated ICP; however, more studies are required to identify the threshold for ischemic injury in stroke patients. In order to more accurately measure bedside CBF, a technique similar to the Swan-Ganz catheter has been utilized (62).

Thermistor catheters were placed in the dominant jugular vein and in the thoracic aorta and ice-cold indocyanide green dye was injected on the arterial side. A temperature degradation curve was obtained, and the area under the curve was used to determine actual CBF. Although CBF was significantly lower in patients who died and ICP elevation was more often associated with low CBF in patients who died, it is unclear if treatment based on such data will improve outcome. In addition, this technique requires troubleshooting experience and is somewhat invasive with a risk for arterial dissection, stroke, and venous thrombosis.

A newer method of measuring cerebral oxygen delivery involves measuring PbO_2. Although use of this modality has been associated with improved outcome in the setting of TBI, studies on its use in the setting of stroke are lacking. Limitations of this probe include the limited volume that is being monitored, making it difficult to use as a tool to monitor the ischemic penumbra. These probes have been utilized in conjunction with ICP monitoring in patients with malignant cerebral edema associated with ischemic stroke (63). Although a correlation was found between improvement of ICP and PbO_2 during treatment with osmotic agents and hemicraniectomy, the number of patients studied was too few to create correlations between PbO_2 and outcome. However, another study demonstrated that patients with PbO_2 less than 10.5 mmHg had a high likelihood of malignant cerebral edema (sensitivity 94%, specificity 100%) (32). In addition, a recent study investigating autoregulation (changes in PbO_2 as a function of changes in CPP) in patients with large MCA infarcts showed lack of autoregulation in patients who progress to malignant cerebral edema (64). Evidence of dysregulation could be found within the first 24 hours and had a sensitivity of 85.7% and specificity of 83.3% for predicting a malignant course. Further study is necessary to determine if PbO_2 monitoring may help delineate which patients may benefit from CPP treatment and/or hemicraniectomy.

One of the invasive monitoring techniques adapted from the laboratory setting to the clinical setting is in vivo cerebral microdialysis. This technique involves intraparenchymal placement of a small catheter with a polyamide dialysis membrane that allows passage of molecules smaller than 20,000 Da. The catheter is continuously perfused with a physiologic solution (i.e., Ringers) at rates of 0.1 to 10 μL/min and dialyzate collections at regular intervals and analyzed for glucose, lactate/pyruvate (L/P) ratio, glutamate, aspartate, and glycerol. Limitations of this technique include isolated focal measurements and lack of standardized values because of use of different membrane lengths and perfusate rates in experimental studies. However, recent studies have found a good correlation between the L/P ratio and cerebral ischemia in the setting of subarachnoid hemorrhage (65). Similarly, in the setting of stroke, microdialysis has shown large elevations in levels of glutamate, aspartate, L/P ratio, and glycerol (66,67). Elevated levels of glutamate and a high L/P ratio in microdialyzates have been documented in patients who develop mass-occupying cerebral edema after MCA infarction (68). Finally, microdialysis parameters have been studied in association with ICP and PbO_2 to determine ability to predict malignant clinical progression of ischemic stroke (32). While changes in all microdialysis parameters were associated with malignant progression, the sensitivity and specificity of these changes were inferior to that of ICP, CPP, and PbO_2. In addition, changes in microdialysis did not precede changes in ICP and PbO_2 (74.2–100.6 hours after onset of stroke). However, there was a correlation between elevated ICP, decreased PbO_2 and CPP, and changes in microdialysis parameters indicating that when cerebral perfusion reaches a critical threshold (CPP 50–60 mmHg), secondary ischemia is accentuated causing more edema and malignant progression. Unfortunately, as for other invasive monitoring techniques such as ICP and PbO_2, outcome studies are necessary to determine treatment effects using these monitoring modalities.

Neurophysiologic Monitoring

Neurophysiologic monitoring mainly involves monitoring of electrical impulses in the brain. Electroencephalography (EEG) and somatosensory evoked potentials (SSEPs) are the two modalities that have been studied in the setting of stroke, and their clinical application will be briefly discussed.

EEG records the summated responses of pyramidal neurons arising from cortical layers 3, 5, and 6 from a particular region of brain via scalp electrodes. Because these pyramidal layers are exquisitely sensitive to cerebral ischemia, EEG may serve as a particularly useful monitoring modality during the peri-ischemic period. In addition, EEG is relatively inexpensive, available at most institutions, and allows for continuous noninvasive, dynamic monitoring of patients at the bedside. More recently, quantitative EEG (QEEG) has become available for detection of subtle ischemia using regional alpha-beta/theta-delta power ratios. A depression of alpha and beta activity has been associated with poor outcome in stroke (69). Previous studies have correlated QEEG activity with DWI images and 30-day NIHSS outcome (70). An EEG pattern has been identified consisting of regional attenuation of all frequencies without delta activity (RAWOD). This pattern was associated with significantly decreased CBF on xenon-CT and poor outcome (67% mortality) mainly related to severe cerebral edema (27,71). EEG may also be useful for treatment of the ischemic penumbra. Patients with ischemic stroke when treated with hypertensive hypervolemic therapy (HHT) exhibited an improvement in focal slowing corresponding with improved CBF on xenon-CT (71). However, larger studies are necessary to determine if treatment of the ischemic penumbra based on EEG patterns result in improved outcome. In addition, EEG readings are often perturbed by sedating medications used in ventilated patients in the ICU; therefore, interpretation of EEG findings in terms of cerebral ischemia must be conducted with caution.

EEG is also the standard criterion for diagnosis and detection of seizures. Between 1.8% and 15% of patients experience convulsive seizures during the peri-ischemic period; however, the prevalence of subclinical nonconvulsive seizures stroke is probably even higher (71). In addition, 2% to 9% of stroke patients experience status epilepticus. Because seizure activity increases metabolic demands, patients who experience seizures in the setting of ischemic stroke are at higher risk for poor outcome. Studies have shown increased mortality in stroke patients who experience in-hospital seizures (72). In this regard, it may be prudent to use continuous EEG monitoring for all severe stroke patients particularly in the first 24 hours where 70% to 90% of early stroke-associated seizures occur and the ischemic penumbra is most vulnerable to further injury.

Like EEG, SSEPs also undergo predictable changes with cerebral ischemia. SSEP monitoring is conducted by stimulating a motor response in a peripheral nerve and then monitoring the proprioceptive afferents as they ascend to the cortex. For instance, median nerve SSEPs are monitored at the peripheral nerve, the brachial plexus, the cervical spinal cord, the brain stem, subcortical structures (thalamus), and finally the cortex. In this respect, SSEPs may be complimentary to EEG recordings for monitoring of subcortical and brain stem structures. In addition, unlike EEG recordings, SSEPs are more resistant to the effects of sedating medications. An SSEP records both the amplitude of responses and the latency between responses along the afferent pathway. In primate models, a decrease in cortical amplitude and an increase in latency is observed when CBF is reduced to 16 mL/100 g/min (73,74). This may be indicative of the ischemic penumbra in which ischemic cells are salvageable. Although SSEP monitoring has been successfully used to predict intraoperative ischemia in the setting of carotid endartectomy and aneurysm clipping (75), outcome studies for continuous SSEP monitoring are lacking. Although initial SSEPs are predictive of functional recovery in the setting of stroke, serial examinations (performed weekly) were not of any additional value for prognostication (76,77). However, one cannot extrapolate from this data that continuous monitoring during the acute period will be of diagnostic value. Further studies are warranted to determine the value of SSEP monitoring in the acute setting.

CONCLUSION AND FUTURE DIRECTIONS

Frequent and continuous monitoring of critical variables in patients with ischemic stroke allows for rapid identification of evolution of pathophysiologic mechanisms, institute timely interventions to halt, and modify sequalae (78). The bedside neurologic examination remains an indispensable tool in monitoring critically ill patients. Other physiologic monitoring includes ICP monitoring, EEG and evoked potentials, and neurometabolic parameters utilizing cerebral microdialysis. Methodology for assessing CBF remains cumbersome. By incorporating all these techniques, continuous multimodality monitoring is being utilized in certain specialized centers and it holds promise for the future (63). However, the impact of multimodal monitoring on long-term functional outcomes remains unclear at present and requires further investigation.

REFERENCES

1. How do stroke units improve patient outcomes? A collaborative systematic review of the randomized trials. Stroke Unit Trialists Collaboration. Stroke 1997; 28: 2139–2144.
2. Wang S, Lee SB, Pardue C, et al. Remote evaluation of acute ischemic stroke: reliability of National Institutes of Health Stroke Scale via telestroke. Stroke 2003; 34:e188–e191.
3. Goldstein LB, Samsa GP. Reliability of the National Institutes of Health Stroke Scale. Extension to non-neurologists in the context of a clinical trial. Stroke 1997; 28:307–310.
4. Adams HP Jr, Woolson RF, Clarke WR, et al. Design of the Trial of Org 10172 in Acute Stroke Treatment (TOAST). Control Clin Trials 1997; 18:358–377.
5. Mikulik R, Ribo M, Hill MD, et al. Accuracy of serial National Institutes of Health Stroke Scale scores to identify artery status in acute ischemic stroke. Circulation 2007; 115:2660–2665.
6. DeGraba TJ, Hallenbeck JM, Pettigrew KD, et al. Progression in acute stroke: value of the initial NIH stroke scale score on patient stratification in future trials. Stroke 1999; 30:1208–1212.
7. Jauss M, Krieger D, Hornig C, et al. Surgical and medical management of patients with massive cerebellar infarctions: results of the German-Austrian Cerebellar Infarction Study. J Neurol 1999; 246:257–264.
8. Wardlaw JM, Mielke O. Early signs of brain infarction at CT: observer reliability and outcome after thrombolytic treatment—systematic review. Radiology 2005; 235:444–453.
9. Moulin T, Cattin F, Crépin-Leblond T, et al. Early CT signs in acute middle cerebral artery infarction: predictive value for subsequent infarct locations and outcome. Neurology 1996; 47:366–75.
10. Derex L, Nighoghossian N, Hermier M, et al. Magnetic resonance imaging: significance of early ischemic changes on computed tomography. Cerebrovasc Dis 2004; 18:232–235.
11. Tanne D, Kasner SE, Demchuk AM, et al. Markers of increased risk of intracerebral hemorrhage after intravenous recombinant tissue plasminogen activator therapy for acute ischemic stroke in clinical practice: the Multicenter rt-PA Stroke Survey. Circulation 2002;105:1679–1685.
12. Patel SC, Levine SR, Tilley BC, et al. Lack of clinical significance of early ischemic changes on computed tomography in acute stroke. JAMA 2001; 286:2830–2838.
13. Agarwal P, Kumar S, Hariharan S, et al. Hyperdense middle cerebral artery sign: can it be used to select intra-arterial versus intravenous thrombolysis in acute ischemic stroke? Cerebrovasc Dis 2004;17:182–190.
14. Robertson SC, Lennarson P, Hasan DM, et al. Clinical course and surgical management of massive cerebral infarction. Neurosurgery 2004; 55:55–61.
15. Kastrau F, Wolter M, Huber W, et al. Recovery from aphasia after hemicraniectomy for infarction of the speech-dominant hemisphere. Stroke 2005; 36:825–829.
16. Schwab S, Steiner T, Aschoff A, et al. Early hemicraniectomy in patients with complete middle cerebral artery infarction. Stroke 1998; 29:1888–1893.
17. Rabinstein AA, Mueller-Kronast N, Maramattom BV, et al. Factors predicting prognosis after decompressive hemicraniectomy for hemispheric infarction. Neurology, 2006; 67:891–893.

18. Verro P, Tanenbaum LN, Borden N, et al. Clinical application of CT angiography in acute ischemic stroke. Clin Neurol Neurosurg 2007; 109:138–145.

19. Ritter MA, Poeplau T, Schaefer A, et al. CT angiography in acute stroke: does it provide additional information on occurrence of infarction and functional outcome after 3 months? Cerebrovasc Dis 2006; 22:362–367.

20. Parsons MW, Pepper EM, Bateman GA, et al. Identification of the penumbra and infarct core on hyperacute noncontrast and perfusion CT. Neurology 2007; 68:730–736.

21. Hunter GJ, Silvennoinen HM, Hamberg LM, et al. Whole-brain CT perfusion measurement of perfused cerebral blood volume in acute ischemic stroke: probability curve for regional infarction. Radiology 2003; 227:725–730.

22. Lee SJ, Lee KH, Na DG, et al. Multiphasic helical computed tomography predicts subsequent development of severe brain edema in acute ischemic stroke. Arch Neurol 2004; 61:505–509.

23. Ryoo JW, Na DG, Kim SS, et al. Malignant middle cerebral artery infarction in hyperacute ischemic stroke: evaluation with multiphasic perfusion computed tomography maps. J Comput Assist Tomogr 2004; 28:55–62.

24. Jones TH, Morawetz RB, Crowell RM, et al. Thresholds of focal cerebral ischemia in awake monkeys. J Neurosurg 1981; 54:773–782.

25. Kaufmann AM, Firlik AD, Fukui MB, et al. Ischemic core and penumbra in human stroke. Stroke 1999; 30:93–99.

26. Gupta R, Yonas H, Gebel J, et al. Reduced pretreatment ipsilateral middle cerebral artery cerebral blood flow is predictive of symptomatic hemorrhage post-intra-arterial thrombolysis in patients with middle cerebral artery occlusion. Stroke 2006; 37: 2526–2530.

27. Firlik AD, Yonas H, Kaufmann AM, et al. Relationship between cerebral blood flow and the development of swelling and life-threatening herniation in acute ischemic stroke. J Neurosurg 1998; 89:243–249.

28. Baron JC, Rougemont D, Soussaline F, et al. Local interrelationships of cerebral oxygen consumption and glucose utilization in normal subjects and in ischemic stroke patients: a positron tomography study. J Cereb Blood Flow Metab 1984; 4:140–149.

29. Powers WJ, Grubb RL Jr, Darriet D, et al. Cerebral blood flow and cerebral metabolic rate of oxygen requirements for cerebral function and viability in humans. J Cereb Blood Flow Metab 1985; 5:600–608.

30. Heiss WD, Sobesky J, Hesselmann V. Identifying thresholds for penumbra and irreversible tissue damage. Stroke 2004; 35:2671–2674.

31. Heiss WD, Kracht L, Grond M, et al. Early [(11)C]Flumazenil/H(2)O positron emission tomography predicts irreversible ischemic cortical damage in stroke patients receiving acute thrombolytic therapy. Stroke 2000; 31:366–369.

32. Heiss WD, Dohmen C, Sobesky J, et al. Prediction of malignant course in MCA infarction by PET and microdialysis. Stroke 2003; 34:2152–2158.

33. Lassen NA. Cerebral blood flow quantitation in clinical routine studies: how far have we now come? J Nucl Med 1995; 36:2343–2344.

34. Marchal G, Bouvard G, Iglesias S, et al. Predictive value of (99m)Tc-HMPAO-SPECT for neurological Outcome/Recovery at the acute stage of stroke. Cerebrovasc Dis 2000; 10:8–17.

35. Karonen JO, Liu Y, Vanninen RL, et al. Combined diffusion and perfusion MRI with correlation to single-photon emission CT in acute ischemic stroke. Ischemic penumbra predicts infarct growth. Stroke 1999; 30:1583–1590.

36. Hanson SK, Grotta JC, Rhoades H, et al. Value of single-photon emission-computed tomography in acute stroke therapeutic trials. Stroke 1993; 24:1322–1329.
37. Ueda T, Sakaki S, Yuh WT, et al. Outcome in acute stroke with successful intra-arterial thrombolysis and predictive value of initial single-photon emission-computed tomography. J Cereb Blood Flow Metab 1999; 19:99–108.
38. Herderscheê D, Limburg M, van Royen EA, et al. Thrombolysis with recombinant tissue plasminogen activator in acute ischemic stroke: evaluation with rCBF-SPECT. Acta Neurol Scand 1991; 83:317–322.
39. Ezura M, Takahashi A, Yoshimoto T. Evaluation of regional cerebral blood flow using single photon emission tomography for the selection of patients for local fibrinolytic therapy of acute cerebral embolism. Neurosurg Rev 1996;19:231–236.
40. Hoehn-Berlage M. Diffusion-weighted NMR imaging: application to experimental focal cerebral ischemia. NMR Biomed 1995; 8:345–358.
41. Moseley ME, Cohen Y, Kucharczyk J, et al. Diffusion-weighted MR imaging of acute stroke: correlation with T2-weighted and magnetic susceptibility-enhanced MR imaging in cats. AJNR Am J Neuroradiol 1990; 11:423–429.
42. Arenillas JF, Rovira A, Molina CA, et al. Prediction of early neurological deterioration using diffusion- and perfusion-weighted imaging in hyperacute middle cerebral artery ischemic stroke. Stroke 2002; 33:2197–2203.
43. Hand PJ, Wardlaw JM, Rivers CS, et al. MR diffusion-weighted imaging and outcome prediction after ischemic stroke. Neurology 2006; 66:1159–1163.
44. Oppenheim C, Samson Y, Manaï R, et al. Prediction of malignant middle cerebral artery infarction by diffusion-weighted imaging. Stroke 2000; 31:2175–2181.
45. Dávalos A, Blanco M, Pedraza S, et al. The clinical-DWI mismatch: a new diagnostic approach to the brain tissue at risk of infarction. Neurology 2004, 62:2187–2192.
46. Sorensen AG, Tievsky AL, Ostergaard L, et al. Contrast agents in functional MR imaging. J Magn Reson Imaging 1997;7:47–55.
47. Baird AE, Benfield A, Schlaug G, et al. Enlargement of human cerebral ischemic lesion volumes measured by diffusion-weighted magnetic resonance imaging. Ann Neurol 1997; 41:581–589.
48. Sorensen AG, Buonanno FS, Gonzalez RG, et al. Hyperacute stroke: evaluation with combined multisection diffusion-weighted and hemodynamically weighted echo-planar MR imaging. Radiology 1996; 199:391–401.
49. Schlaug G, Benfield A, Baird AE, et al. The ischemic penumbra: operationally defined by diffusion and perfusion MRI. Neurology 1999; 53:1528–1537.
50. Sobesky J, Zaro Weber O, Lehnhardt FG, et al. Does the mismatch match the penumbra? Magnetic resonance imaging and positron emission tomography in early ischemic stroke. Stroke 2005; 36:980–5.
51. Sobesky J, Zaro Weber O, Lehnhardt FG, et al. Which time-to-peak threshold best identifies penumbral flow? A comparison of perfusion-weighted magnetic resonance imaging and positron emission tomography in acute ischemic stroke. Stroke 2004; 35:2843–2847.
52. Christou I, Alexandrov AV, Burgin WS, et al. Timing of recanalization after tissue plasminogen activator therapy determined by transcranial doppler correlates with clinical recovery from ischemic stroke. Stroke 2000; 31:1812–1816.
53. Karnik R, Stelzer P, Slany J. Transcranial Doppler sonography monitoring of local intra-arterial thrombolysis in acute occlusion of the middle cerebral artery. Stroke 1992; 23:284–287.

54. Rubiera M, Alvarez-Sabín J, Ribo M, et al. Predictors of early arterial reocclusion after tissue plasminogen activator-induced recanalization in acute ischemic stroke. Stroke 2005; 36:1452–1456.

55. Alexandrov AV, Molina CA, Grotta JC, et al. Ultrasound-enhanced systemic thrombolysis for acute ischemic stroke. N Engl J Med 2004; 351:2170–2178.

56. Frank JI. Large hemispheric infarction, deterioration, and intracranial pressure. Neurology 1995; 45:1286–1290.

57. D'Ambrosio AL, Hoh DJ, Mack WJ, et al. Interhemispheric intracranial pressure gradients in nonhuman primate stroke. Surg Neurol 2002; 58:295–301.

58. Schwab S, Aschoff A, Spranger M, et al. The value of intracranial pressure monitoring in acute hemispheric stroke. Neurology 1996; 47:393–398.

59. Schwarz S, Schwab S, Bertram M, et al. Effects of hypertonic saline hydroxyethyl starch solution and mannitol in patients with increased intracranial pressure after stroke. Stroke 1998; 29:1550–1555.

60. Schwarz S, Georgiadis D, Aschoff A, et al. Effects of hypertonic (10%) saline in patients with raised intracranial pressure after stroke. Stroke 2002; 33:136–140.

61. Keller E, Steiner T, Fandino J, et al. Jugular venous oxygen saturation thresholds in trauma patients may not extrapolate to ischemic stroke patients: lessons from a preliminary study. J Neurosurg Anesthesiol 2002; 14:130–136.

62. Keller E, Wietasch G, Ringleb P, et al. Bedside monitoring of cerebral blood flow in patients with acute hemispheric stroke. Crit Care Med 2000; 28:511–516.

63. Steiner T, Pilz J, Schellinger P, et al. Multimodal online monitoring in middle cerebral artery territory stroke. Stroke 2001; 32:2500–2506.

64. Dohmen C, Bosche B, Graf R, et al. Identification and clinical impact of impaired cerebrovascular autoregulation in patients with malignant middle cerebral artery infarction. Stroke 2007; 38:56–61.

65. Persson L, Valtysson J, Enblad P, et al. Neurochemical monitoring using intra-cerebral microdialysis in patients with subarachnoid hemorrhage. J Neurosurg 1996; 84:606–16.

66. Bullock R, Zauner A, Woodward J, et al. Massive persistent release of excitatory amino acids following human occlusive stroke. Stroke 1995; 26:2187–2189.

67. Berger C, Annecke A, Aschoff A, et al. Neurochemical monitoring of fatal middle cerebral artery infarction. Stroke 1999; 30:460–463.

68. Schneweis S, Grond M, Staub F, et al. Predictive value of neurochemical monitoring in large middle cerebral artery infarction. Stroke 2001;32:1863–1867.

69. Cillessen JP, van Huffelen AC, Kappelle LJ, et al. Electroencephalography improves the prediction of functional outcome in the acute stage of cerebral ischemia. Stroke 1994; 25:1968–1972.

70. Finnigan SP, Rose SE, Walsh M, et al. Correlation of quantitative EEG in acute ischemic stroke with 30-day NIHSS score: comparison with diffusion and perfusion MRI. Stroke 2004; 35:899–903.

71. Jordan KG. Emergency EEG and continuous EEG monitoring in acute ischemic stroke. J Clin Neurophysiol 2004; 21:341–352.

72. Arboix A, Comes E, García-Eroles L, et al. Prognostic value of very early seizures for in-hospital mortality in atherothrombotic infarction. Eur Neurol 2003;50:78–84.

73. Hargadine JR, Branston NM, Symon L. Central conduction time in primate brain ischemia—a study in baboons. Stroke 1980;11:637–642.

74. Symon L. The relationship between CBF, evoked potentials and the clinical features in cerebral ischaemia. Acta Neurol Scand Suppl 1980;78:175–190.
75. Schweiger H, Kamp HD, Dinkel M. Somatosensory-evoked potentials during carotid artery surgery: experience in 400 operations. Surgery 1991; 109:602–609.
76. Haupt WF, Pawlik G, Thiel A. Initial and serial evoked potentials in cerebrovascular critical care patients. J Clin Neurophysiol 2006; 23:389–394.
77. Tzvetanov P, Rousseff RT, Atanassova P. Prognostic value of median and tibial somatosensory evoked potentials in acute stroke. Neurosci Lett 2005; 380:99–104.
78. Minahan RE, Bhardwaj A, Williams MA. Critical care monitoring for cerebrovascular disease. New Horiz 1997; 5:406–421.

11

Surgical Management of Intracerebral Hemorrhage

Patrick C. Hsieh, MD, Resident
Patrick Sugrue, MD, Resident
H. Hunt Batjer, MD, Professor and Chairman
Issam Awad, MD, Professor

Department of Neurological Surgery, Northwestern University Feinberg School of Medicine, Chicago, Illinois, U.S.A.

INTRODUCTION

Over the past several years, major gains have been made in the diagnosis and management of cerebral vascular events, with most of those advances centered on the management of ischemic stroke and hemorrhagic stroke that result from aneurysms, arteriovenous malformations (AVMs), and cavernous malformations. However, spontaneous intracerebral hemorrhage (ICH), which accounts for as many as 10% to 30% of all strokes (1), has until recently received comparatively little attention and seen little impact in therapeutic advances. Rupture of small blood vessels that penetrate and perfuse brain tissue leads to ICH, and prognosis for patients remains poor. Compounding the issue is the fact that patients with hemorrhagic stroke are on average 10 years younger than those who suffer ischemic strokes, magnifying the socioeconomic impact of such an event.

A great deal of controversy surrounds the appropriate management of ICH, some of which concerns the role of surgical intervention and other aspects of acute resuscitation and critical care. The debate of medical-versus-surgical management of ICH dates back several decades to an early prospective randomized trial (2).

Regardless of whether a medical or surgical approach is taken, ICH continues to be a devastating event with high rates of mortality and disability. The 30-day mortality rate for patients with ICH is reported to be 35% to 44%, and the 60-day mortality rate is nearly 50% (3–5). Moreover, for those fortunate enough to survive an initial ICH, only 20% are able to function independently at six months (6). As a result, the annual cost per patient following ICH is approximately $125,000, totaling nearly $6 billion in annual costs (7,8). From this data, it has been extrapolated that ICH, while accounting for a small fraction of all strokes, accounts for nearly half of all stroke-related disabilities, deaths, and costs. Therefore, to optimally treat patients and to attempt to change the paradigm for patients and their families, a better understanding of ICH is imperative.

EPIDEMIOLOGY AND PATHOETIOLOGY

Approximately 700,000 new strokes occur in the United States each year; of that number, approximately 15% are hemorrhagic strokes related to ICH (1,9,10), which equates to approximately 20 of 100,000 people afflicted annually. However, despite the relatively small number in comparison with ischemic strokes, patients who have an ICH suffer from some of the worst outcomes. As mentioned above, the mortality rate for an ICH patient approaches nearly 50%, and only a small percentage are able to ultimately achieve independent functional status (3–6).

Spontaneous ICH is typically considered distinct from traumatic cerebral bleeds and contusions, although overlap may exist in the pathophysiology and treatment. Furthermore, differences are often difficult to ascertain in elderly patients following a trivial fall, when the distinction is merely made by the presence or lack of external evidence of trauma. For the purpose of this chapter, ICH (including the so-called primary and secondary categories) will strictly refer to nontraumatic etiologies.

ICH can be separated into two categories: primary and secondary. Primary ICH is more common, accounts for 70% to 88% of ICH cases, and is the result of either chronic uncontrolled hypertension or cerebral amyloid angiopathy (1,11). On the other hand, the secondary form of ICH (15–30%) is associated with vascular malformations, tumors, substance abuse, coagulation disorders, and the use of anticoagulation or thrombolytic agents. Primary ICH is more common in the elderly, males, African-Americans, and Asians (12,13). The most common location for primary ICH is the deep subcortical area, with more than 50% of all spontaneous ICHs occuring in the basal ganglia (Fig. 1). Other locations include the lobar areas of the cerebral hemispheres and infratentorial locations, such as the cerebellum or the pons. Secondary etiology is typically sought, especially in younger patients, in whom vascular anomaly, tumor, or coagulopathy account for more than half of the bleeds. The term *primary* is not very useful, as these cases are caused by age and hypertension-related vasculopathy, as noted below, and are not truly idiopathic.

Developing an ICH is associated with several important risk factors (14,15). Aging inherently leads to increased degenerative changes in the cerebral

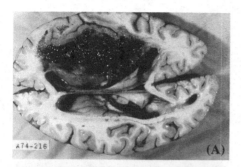

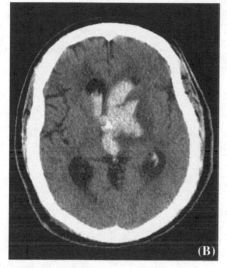

Figure 1 Intracerebral hemorrhage. (A) Gross specimen of basal ganglia ICH. (B) CT scan of left thalamic ICH with ventricular extension. The red arrow demonstrates the tip of external ventricular drain within IVH. *Abbreviations*: ICH, intracerebral hemorrhage; CT, computer tomography.

blood vessels and thus renders a greater risk of vessel rupture. Cerebral parenchyma in the elderly can also manifest progressive dilatation of the Virchow-Robin perivascular spaces and general rarefaction and demyelination of the brain parenchyma in association with chronic ischemia, i.e., leukoaraiosis. Such a process in this fragile state is thought to predispose an aged brain to hemorrhage, even in the face of minimal trauma. Moreover, it is believed that such parenchymal tissue is also at increased risk for hemorrhage expansion.

Another common etiology of primary ICH in the aged patient is cerebral amyloid angiopathy, which accounts for as many as 15% of all ICH cases (11,16–18). Hemorrhage from cerebral amyloid angiopathy is more common in the elderly and typically occurs in a more lobar distribution (Fig. 2). It is important to note that cerebral amyloid is not associated with systemic amyloidosis. The small-to-

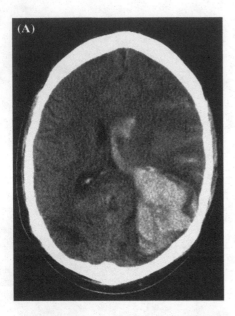

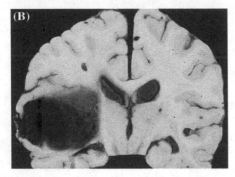

Figure 2 Lobar intracerebral hemorrhage. (**A**) CT scan demonstrating left parietal-occipital lobar ICH. (**B**) Gross specimen demonstrating lobar ICH. *Abbreviations*: ICH, intracerebral hemorrhage; CT, computer tomography.

medium-sized vessels of the brain and leptomeninges have been shown histologically to have amyloid β-peptide deposits in the vessel wall (17,19). The deposition of amyloid in the vessel wall contributes to vessel wall fragility, which ultimately leads to increased rupture susceptibility and, thus, lobar hemorrhage. Moreover, recurrent hemorrhage can occur in 5% to 15% of all cases of lobar hemorrhage, where cerebral amyloid angiopathy is thought to be the likely etiology, as well as in those patients who have evidence of numerous chronic hemorrhages, as demonstrated on gradient echo magnetic resonance imaging (MRI) (20,21) (Fig. 3). Likewise, it has been demonstrated that the ε2 and ε4 alleles of the apolipoprotein E gene are associated with increased risk of recurrent

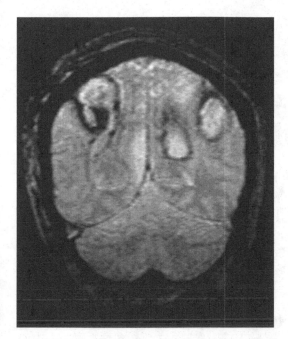

Figure 3 Gradient echo demonstrating multiple intracerebral hemorrhages.

hemorrhages in these patients (20–22). The above considerations and the overall increase in life expectancy of the general population contribute to a predicted doubling in the incidence of ICH in the next 50 years.

Hypertension is another major risk factor for ICH. It is one of the most common medical problems in the general population and considered a modifiable risk factor of ICH (23). However, because of poor compliance with medications, failure to make lifestyle modifications, or simply failure to treat, many individuals suffer the consequences of uncontrolled chronic hypertension. Chronically elevated blood pressure leads to lipohyalinosis, which includes degradation, fragmentation, and necrosis of small penetrating cerebral vessels (Fig. 4). Also, as a result of chronic hypertension, arteriolar microaneurysms, known as Charcot-Bouchard aneurysms, can develop. Rupture of these aneurysms or of the fragile vessel walls of small- and medium-sized arteries during pressure spikes may result in the extravasation of blood into the brain parenchyma. Hemorrhage as a result of hypertension has most commonly been associated with deep or brain stem hemorrhage, but uncontrolled hypertension can contribute to the risk of stroke in all cerebral locations. Lipohyalinosis leads to occlusive changes and microaneurysm formation on the same vessel, lending some explanation to the presence of lacunar infarcts in areas adjacent to an ICH. Hence, hypertension predisposes the possibility of ICH at an earlier age.

While chronic uncontrolled hypertension, cerebral amyloid, and age-related angiopathy are the most common etiologies for ICH, they are not the only

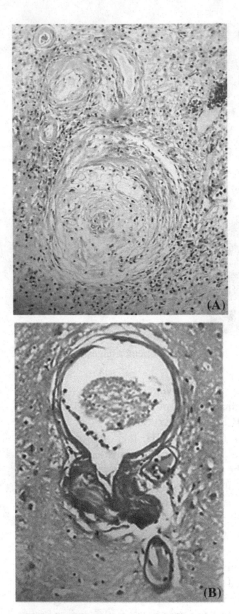

Figure 4   Vasculopathic changes associated with chronic hypertension. (**A**) Lipohyalinosis.
(**B**) Microaneurysm.

associated risk factors. Other etiologies include use of coumadin or other anticoagulation agents, alcohol consumption, use of cocaine and amphetamine,
antiplatelet therapy, and systemic or intra-arterial recombinant tissue plasminogen activator (rtPA) therapy. Heavy alcohol consumption, even during a

binge, can lead to decreased platelet function and induce hypertension (24–26). Additionally, snorting or smoking cocaine is associated with increased risk of ICH (27), as these activities cause an induced cerebral vasculopathy (28). Similar to cocaine, amphetamine use is associated with ICH, as it contributes to an induced transient hypertension by blocking norepinephrine uptake and causing a sympathetic surge. Many antiplatelet and anticoagulation agents have a tremendous therapeutic value but not without risk. Agents such as aspirin, coumadin, and rtPA all increase the risk for ICH (29–33). However, because these agents have been shown to help to decrease the morbidity and mortality associated with serious diseases such as coronary artery disease, peripheral vascular disease, and cerebrovascular ischemic disease, the use of such agents must be carefully evaluated in terms of risk versus reward.

PATHOPHYSIOLOGY

The morbidity and mortality associated with ICH is closely correlated with a few key variables, including patient age, volume of the hematoma, location of hemorrhage, and neurologic status at presentation, as measured by the Glasgow Coma Scale (GCS) (4,34,35). For example, patients with a supratentorial hemorrhage with a volume greater than 60 mL have a 71% to 93% mortality rate, while those with cerebellar hemorrhages with volumes of 30 to 60 mL have a 75% mortality rate (10,11). In addition, nearly all pontine hemorrhages greater than 5 mL are considered lethal. An ICH score has been devised that takes into account GCS score, ICH volume, intraventricular hemorrhage (IVH), location of hemorrhage (supratentorial vs. infratentorial), and age (36) (Table 1 and Fig. 5). This score was correlated with a corresponding 30-day mortality rate. A higher ICH score corresponded with a higher 30-day mortality rate, with the GCS score at presentation being the most powerful independent predictor of mortality.

Likewise, IVH can be associated with ICH in as many 40% of all cases (Fig. 1). Blood within the ventricular system can lead to hydrocephalus and to increased intracranial pressure (ICP). Therefore, IVH is an additional negative predictor of overall clinical outcome in ICH, especially when associated with ventricular obstruction (37). An ICH score like the one developed by Hemphill and colleagues not only helps the physician guide clinical management, but certainly aids the treating physician when discussing the patient's prognosis with family.

Overall, the poor outcomes associated with ICH are related to the extent of brain damage. Of the above-mentioned factors that influence outcome following ICH, the most important is hemorrhage volume (4,10,11). Large clots both exert mass effect, thus elevating ICP, and cause direct compression and destruction of surrounding brain tissue. The clot and its mass effect can lead to poor perfusion and poor venous drainage of the surrounding brain tissue, leading to ischemia. Likewise, the penumbra, which of all the brain regions most requires the appropriate perfusion, cannot receive the required blood supply,

Table 1 Determination of the ICH score

Component	ICH score points
GCS score	
3–4	2
5–12	1
13–15	0
ICH volume, mL	
≥30	1
<30	0
IVH	
Yes	1
No	0
Infratentorial origin of ICH	
Yes	1
No	0
Age, years	
≥80	1
<80	0

Abbreviations: ICH, intracerebral hemorrhage; GCS, Glasgow coma score; IVH, intraventricular hemorrhage. *Source*: From Ref. 36.

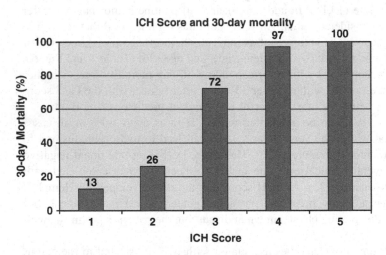

Figure 5 ICH score and 30-day mortality. *Abbreviation*: ICH, intracerebral hemorrhage. *Source*: From Ref. 36.

leading to greater ischemic damage. Furthermore, the extravasated blood and the ischemic brain tissue release vasoactive and toxic substances that compound the cerebral insult and ultimately contribute to the morbidity and mortality associated with ICH (38–44).

Hematoma growth, a critical risk factor known to occur in one-third or one-half of all cases in the first few hours after ICH symptom onset, is associated with neurologic deterioration and, independently, with worsened outcome (45). Hematoma growth is also associated with new or worsened IVH, which may also be a factor that contributes to worsened outcome (46). With earlier referral of patients with ICH to tertiary institutions, hematoma growth becomes a critical and potentially modifiable factor impacting on outcome (47–49). Risk factors of hematoma growth include anticoagulation and, possibly, uncontrolled hypertension. Other factors that underlie hematoma growth are not well understood.

ESTABLISHING THE DIAGNOSIS AND ICH ETIOLOGY

The diagnosis of ICH is largely based on clinical history and radiographic findings. The most common presenting symptoms from ICH are the result of mass effect from the hematoma itself. For example, those with smaller hemorrhages may complain only of headache, nausea, or vomiting, while those who have sustained a larger hemorrhage often present with depressed mental status, low GCS score, and even focal neurologic deficits related to the site of the hemorrhage and its mass effect.

Therefore, a clinical history with acute onset and focal neurologic deficit in the context of intracranial hypertension is highly suspicious for ICH, especially when confirmed on noncontrast head computed tomography (CT). Therefore, patients with acute onset of severe headache, nausea, vomiting, or depressed mental status should immediately be evaluated for ICH or other hemorrhagic event with a noncontrast head CT (Fig. 6). A CT of the head is an extremely valuable tool in the evaluation of intracranial pathology and has a sensitivity and specificity that approaches nearly 100% in the face of ICH. In addition, the pattern of hyperdensity on CT can be helpful in determining the etiology of the hemorrhage. The location of the hemorrhage, the characteristics of the clinical history, the patient's risk factors, and the onset of symptoms together help to determine the need for further diagnostic studies and reveal the etiology of the hemorrhage. For example, an elderly patient with a history of chronic hypertension and a CT revealing a hyperdensity or hemorrhage in the putamen, thalamus, cerebellum, or pons most likely suffered from spontaneous ICH as a result of uncontrolled hypertension. By contrast, the presence of a temporal lobe ICH associated with sylvian fissure subarachnoid blood or frontal hemorrhage associated with interhemispheric fissure blood (Fig. 6) is highly suggestive of a ruptured aneurysm that leads to both parenchymal hemorrhage and subarachnoid hemorrhage. An ICH associated with intralesional or perilesional large blood vessels is suggestive of an AVM (Fig. 6), while evidence of calcification within the ICH suggests either tumor or cavernous malformation as the underlying cause.

One of the most important predictors of ultimate outcome following ICH is hematoma volume, which can be easily approximated using the CT. Volume is

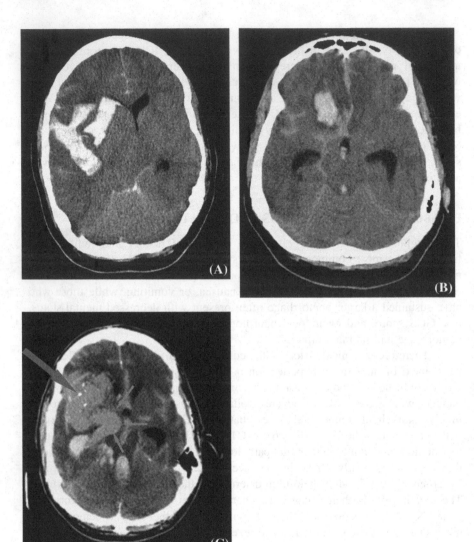

Figure 6 Intracerebral hemorrhages associated with ruptured aneurysms or AVM. (**A**) Right ICH associated with sylvian fissure hematoma. (**B**) Right frontal ICH associated with interhemispheric fissure and sylvian fissure subarachnoid hemorrhage. (**C**) ICH resulting from AVM hemorrhage. The small arrows indicate the large draining varix and the large arrowhead points to the intranidal calcification. *Abbreviations*: AVM, arteriovenous malformation; ICH, intracerebral hemorrhage.

an essential prognostic indicator and criterion for therapeutic intervention. More importantly, its expansion can be associated with continued neurologic deterioration. Volume can be easily calculated using a simple formula, $(A \times B \times C)/2$, where A is the largest diameter (cm) of the hemorrhage as measured on an axial

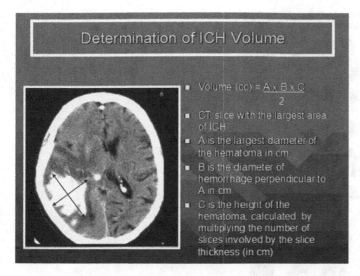

Figure 7 The ABC method for determining ICH volume. *Abbreviation*: ICH, intracerebral hemorrhage.

CT slice, B is the largest diameter (cm) perpendicular to A as measured on the same slice, and C is the thickness of the hematoma (cm) as measured by the number of slices on which the hematoma can be seen (excluding the most superior and most inferior slices on which the hematoma is visualized) multiplied by the thickness in centimeters of each slice. The product of this equation is then divided in half to produce the volume of the hematoma (Fig. 7). This formula is based on the geometric volume of an ellipse of the same dimensions that has been correlated with true volume measurements and has been shown to have excellent interobserver agreement (4,50).

The use of contrast-enhanced CT and CT angiography (CTA), which can be obtained very quickly with modern CT scanners, rapidly excludes most gross vascular and tumor etiologies of hemorrhage. Thus, it can play a tremendous role in formulating an appropriate treatment plan. Aneurysms and AVMs can be invisible on noncontrast CT but are often revealed easily on CTA (Fig. 8), which can significantly impact the treatment plan in determining the need for emergent surgical evacuation of the hematoma. MRI is less commonly used in the acute setting for establishing a diagnosis of ICH. While a highly sensitive method for evaluating ICH, MRI is typically reserved for use as a supplementary evaluation method. When an evaluation with CT and a clinical exam are insufficient to determine an etiology of ICH, MRI can be used. For instance, MRI is highly sensitive for the detection of flow voids or gliosis associated with an AVM. Likewise, detection of heme degradation products associated with cavernous malformations or diffusion abnormalities is suggestive of underlying ischemic infarct. MRI evidence of an underlying contrast-enhancing mass associated with

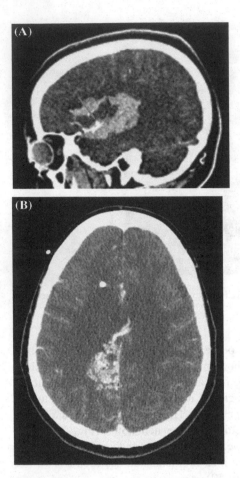

Figure 8 CT angiogram demonstrating aneurysms and arteriovenous malformation. (**A**) Sagittal CTA image demonstrating a right middle cerebral artery aneurysm within the hematoma. (**B**) Axial CTA image demonstrating right frontal-parietal arteriovenous malformation with a draining vein anteriorly. *Abbreviations*: CT, computer tomography; CTA; CT angiography.

ICH is highly suggestive of a hemorrhagic tumor (Fig. 9). In evaluating ICH, the MRI sequences obtained should include fluid-attenuated inversion recovery (FLAIR), T2-weighted images, gradient echo (T2*), diffusion-weighted images with apparent diffusion coefficient mapping, and T1-weighted images before and after contrast enhancement. Conversely, it should be noted that the acute and subacute paramagnetic effects of hemorrhage on MRI may obscure subtle underlying pathologies. Delayed use of MRI after clinical stabilization of the patient and acute resolution of ICH is an important tool to utilize in attempts to exclude such etiologies. However, it should not be postponed too long, given the possible presence of some malignant etiology such as a primary or metastatic

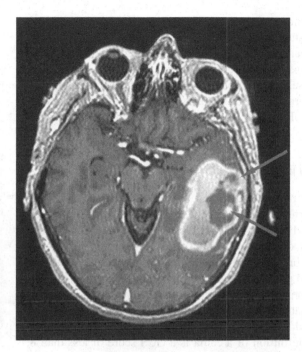

Figure 9 Contrast-enhanced, T1-weighted image demonstrating enhancing nodule associated with an ICII. *Abbreviation*. ICH, intracerebral hemorrhage.

tumor with rapid growth potential that could lead to further neurologic decline or even hasten death if untreated. Follow-up MRI scans are recommended at six to eight weeks, if an underlying neoplastic process is suspected, or at three to four months, for evaluation to rule out occult vascular abnormality. MR angiography (MRA) is not likely to provide additional information to the work up. MRA is best utilized for the evaluation of aneurysms, large vessel occlusive disease, and AVMs. However, CTA is often employed in the acute setting and provides the same information. However, it should be noted that MRI does not contain the radiation risk or iodine contrast dye complications that are associated with the CT modality. Conventional catheter-based cerebral angiogram with digital subtraction views remain the study of choice for demonstrating or at least helping to exclude small AVMs (dural or parenchymal) and small aneurysms and elucidating their anatomy as well as various arteriopathies, including Moya Moya disease and vasculitis. An angiogram is considered necessary in younger patients and in cases in which such etiologies are suspected or when an aneurysm is suspected but not fully clarified on CTA or MRA.

It is important to note that the majority of spontaneous ICH is found in the elderly population, in those who have a history of chronic hypertension, and in those who are far less likely to harbor any underlying cerebrovascular anomaly. However, in young and nonhypertensive patients whose ICH is in an atypical location, cerebral angiogram should still be considered even if CTA and/or MRA are negative. In a prospective study of 206 cases, it was found that 48% of patients who were younger than 45 years and were without preexisting hypertension and who had evidence of putamenal, thalamic, or posterior fossa ICH had positive angiographic findings. Likewise, in those young and nonhypertensive patients who suffered lobar ICH, the angiographic yield was 65% (51). For those patients with a suspected cocaine abuse etiology of ICH, an underlying vasculopathy is often discovered (52,53).

RESUSCITATION AND ACUTE MANAGEMENT

Like any trauma patient or rapidly deteriorating patient, the primary consideration in evaluating ICH patients in the acute phase is to follow the Advanced Cardiac Life Support or Advanced Trauma Life Support guidelines. The "ABCs" in the management of an acute patient include securing the airway, ensuring that the patient can breathe, and maintaining appropriate cerebral and systemic circulation and blood pressure. After completion of the primary survey, evaluation should begin of the symptoms at presentation that will guide management. Depressed mental status is a symptom found in 30% of all patients who have suffered a supratentorial ICH and in almost all patients following brain stem ICH (54). The clinical definition of a coma is a GCS score of less than 8, and all patients with a GCS score of less than 8 should be considered unable to protect their airway. They should be intubated to avoid aspiration, hypoxemia, and hypercapnia. Hypoxemia and hypercapnia in this setting will lead to further cerebral ischemia and can worsen intracranial hypertension.

Over 90% of ICH patients have acute hypertension, typically greater than 160/90 mmHg (18), and an elevated blood pressure has been associated with the expansion of the hematoma, intraventricular extension, and worse overall outcome (55–58). With that in mind, blood pressure should be aggressively controlled to achieve normotension without compromising cerebral perfusion in the face of elevated ICP (Table 2). Moreover, studies have shown that a reduction in blood pressure by 20% has no adverse side effects with regard to cerebral perfusion (59,60), and the American Heart Association recommends that blood pressure be maintained so that the mean arterial pressure (MAP) is less than 130 mmHg in patients with a history of hypertension (59). To appropriately monitor these parameters and administer IV antihypertensive medications, an arterial catheter and often a central venous catheter are typically required in these patients.

For those patients who present with a GCS score of less than 8 or in those whose neurologic status cannot be reliably measured by serial clinical neurologic exam, an ICP monitor should be placed, unless the hematoma is promptly evacuated (see below). Both fiberoptic intraparenchymal monitors and intraventricular catheters with extraventricular drainage (EVD) are commonly utilized in patients who have suffered ICH. The intraparenchymal ICP bolt is more accurate and less vulnerable to obstruction. On the other hand, the EVD catheter allows for the

Table 2 Blood Pressure Management in Hemorrhagic Stroke

Elevated blood pressure (some suggested medications)

Labetalol	5–100 mg/hr by intermittent bolus doses of 10–40 mg or continuous drip (2–8 mg/min)
Esmolol	500 µg/kg as a load; maintenance use, 50–200 $\mu g \cdot kg^{-1} \cdot min^{-1}$
Nitroprusside	0.5–10 $\mu g \cdot kg^{-1} \cdot min^{-1}$
Hydralazine	10–20 mg every 4–6 hr
Enalapril	0.625–1.2 mg every 6 hr as needed
Nicardipine	5–15 mg/hr infusion

The following algorithm, adapted from guidelines for antihypertensive therapy in patients with acute stroke, may be used in the first few hours of ICH (level of evidence V, grade C recommendation)

1. If *systolic* BP is > 230 mmHg or *diastolic* BP is > 140 mmHg on two readings 5 min apart, nitroprusside should be instituted.
2. If *systolic* BP is 180–230 mmHg, *diastolic* BP is 105–140 mmHg, or mean arterial BP is ≥ 130 mmHg on two readings 20 min apart, IV labetalol, esmolol, enalapril, or other smaller doses of easily titratable IV medications, such as diltiazem, lisinopril, or verapamil, should be instituted.
3. If *systolic* BP is < 180 mmHg and *diastolic* BP is < 105 mmHg, antihypertensive therapy should be deferred. Choice of medication depends on other medical contraindications (e.g., labetalol should be avoided in patients with asthma).
   If ICP monitoring is available, cerebral perfusion pressure should be kept at > 70 mmHg.

Low blood pressure

Volume replenishment is the first line of approach. Isotonic saline or colloids can be used and monitored with central venous pressure or pulmonary artery wedge pressure. If hypotension persists after correction of volume deficit, continuous infusions of vasopressors should be considered, particularly for low systolic BP, such as < 90 mmHg.

Phenylephrine	2–10 $\mu g \cdot kg^{-1} \cdot min^{-1}$
Dopamine	2–20 $\mu g \cdot kg^{-1} \cdot min^{-1}$
Norepinephrine	Titrate from 0.05–0.2 $\mu g \cdot kg^{-1} \cdot min^{-1}$

Abbreviations: ICH, intracerebral hemorrhage; ICP, intracranial pressure; BP, blood pressure.
Source: From Ref. 8.

simultaneous monitoring of ICP and the ability to drain cerebrospinal fluid if the ICP rises. An EVD catheter is considered a necessity in cases of demonstrated or suspected ventricular obstruction from associated IVH (Fig. 1).

Elevated ICP is defined by an ICP measurement greater than 20 mmHg for more than five minutes, and the goal of treatment is to keep the ICP less than 20 mmHg and cerebral perfusion pressure to greater than 60 to 70 mmHg. The cerebral perfusion pressure is determined by the measurement of MAP minus ICP (MAP − ICP), and it represents the pressure gradient that drives cerebral blood flow. The inability to maintain appropriate cerebral perfusion pressure will result in additional cerebral ischemia.

Elevations in ICP can be managed in numerous ways, including drainage of cerebrospinal fluid, decreasing brain tissue bulk, or decreasing cerebral blood volume. In extreme cases, other methods include sedation and pharmacologic paralysis to reduce brain metabolic demand and lower ICP. EVD allows for the diversion of cerebrospinal fluid in cases of hydrocephalus and whenever ICP exceeds a certain level. Maintaining a certain ICP can be performed continuously by titrating the level of the drip chamber or intermittently by adjusting the level of the drip chamber when needed. However, EVD is ineffective in managing ICP elevation when the ventricles are compressed or slit from brain edema and over drainage or if the catheter is obstructed by clotted blood. It may be possible to restore EVD patency and enhance ventricular drainage of IVH with the use of intraventricular rtPA administered through the EVD catheter in doses of 0.3 to 2 mg every 8 to 12 hours (61–63) (Fig. 10). If the benefit of intraventricular thrombolysis is proven in currently ongoing studies, it may significantly impact the outcome of ICH. For now, while the use of intraventricular rtPA remains under investigation in clinical trials, this treatment may only be used as an off-label compassionate application, after due consideration of all options and risks, when the patient is deteriorating from an obstructed EVD and when AVM and unsecured aneurysm have been excluded.

Brain bulk may be decreased to lower ICP with osmotic agents such as mannitol (0.25–0.5 g/kg every 4 hours) and furosemide (10 mg every 2–8 hours). Alternating the use of these two agents is routine in the management of ICP spikes. With the use of these agents, it is important to measure serum osmolarity and serum sodium concentrations serially every six hours for a goal serum osmolarity of less than 310 mOsm/L. Likewise, fluid management should aim to maintain overall euvolemia and normonatremia; thus, osmotherapy cannot be utilized to treat ICP if extremes of hypovolemia or hyponatremia are allowed to develop. Corticosteroids should not be used in the treatment of ICH, as randomized trials have shown a lack of efficacy (64–66).

Hyperventilation is also utilized in the treatment of ICP to achieve hypocarbia (25–35 mmHg), which decreases ICP by causing cerebral vasoconstriction in response to a reduction in the intravascular hydrogen ion concentration. This method has been shown to be very effective in treating acute crises with waves of elevated ICP. However, it is important to note that extreme hyperventilation ($PCO_2 < 20$ mmHg) can exacerbate cerebral ischemia by decreasing cerebral blood flow and cerebral perfusion pressure. Hyperventilation and hypocarbia can only be used in the acute setting because of the metabolic compensation achieved in response to respiratory alkalosis. Further response to life-threatening ICP elevations becomes ineffective after chronic hypertension, and the patient becomes at risk for rebound increased ICP when normocapnia is restored.

Sedation from neuromuscular paralysis can reduce elevated ICP by preventing agitation and straining, while at the same time reducing brain metabolic

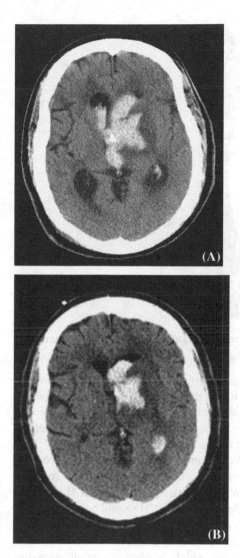

Figure 10 CT axial images demonstrating decreased IVH and improved EVD drainage with intrathecal rtPA without any evidence of rehemorrhage. (**A**) Preintrathecal rtPA infusion with dense IVH in bilateral frontal horns and third ventricle. (**B**) Postintrathecal rtPA infusion with decreased IVH with complete resolution of right frontal horn and third ventricular IVH. *Abbreviations*: CT, computer tomography; IVH, intraventricular hemorrhage; EVD, extraventricular drainage, rtPA, recombinant tissue plasminogen activator.

demand. If the ICP remains high despite maximal medical/pharmacologic intervention as discussed above, induced barbiturate coma may be employed with continuous electroencephalographic monitoring. A central line and an arterial line are necessary for appropriate hemodynamic monitoring, and a Swan-Ganz

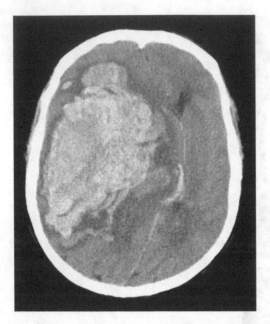

Figure 11 Large ICH resulting from uncorrected coagulopathy from use of coumadin. *Abbreviation*: ICH, intracerebral hemorrhage.

catheter should be placed when vasopressors are employed during barbiturate-induced coma. Barbiturates can decrease ICP in proportion to the level of sedation, including burst suppression as shown on electroencephalography. The use of barbiturates beyond burst suppression likely does not offer any additional benefits with respect to ICP management, while it increases toxic side effects.

The highest risk of neurologic deterioration and cardiovascular decompensation is within the first 24 hours after hemorrhage. In fact, early neurologic decline within the first 24 hours occurs in approximately 25% of all ICH patients (34,67). With that in mind, patients who have suffered ICH should be admitted to an intensive care unit, preferably one with expertise in cerebrovascular disease. As alluded to earlier, the most common cause of early neurologic deterioration following ICH is expansion of the hematoma, which is often a complication in patients with uncorrected coagulation profiles (Fig. 11). A study of 103 patients reported that 26% of ICH patients experienced hematoma expansion within one hour following initial CT scan and that 38% of ICH patients experienced hematoma expansion by greater than 33% within the first three hours after onset (68).

Hematoma expansion may be related to coagulopathy but is more often thought to be related to active bleeding from the primary source and due to mechanical disruption and shearing of surrounding vasculature. In addition, breakdown of the blood-brain barrier, reduction of venous outflow, and transient creation of local coagulopathy are other possible etiologies for hematoma expansion. Recombinant activated factor VII (rVIIa) is a hemostatic agent that has been approved for use in treating active bleeding in hemophilia for those patients who have proven to be refractory to factor VIII replacement therapy. rVIIa initiates the coagulation cascade and enhances thrombin formation on the surface of activated platelets, which leads to the formation of stable lysis-resistant clot at the site of vascular injury. In a randomized double-blinded, placebo-controlled trial of 399 ICH patients, the use of rVIIa within four hours of hemorrhage onset limited hematoma expansion by approximately 50% (69). In this study, rVIIa was administered in doses of 40 µg/kg, 80 µg/kg, and 160 µg/kg. The placebo group displayed a mean increase of 29% in hematoma volume. By contrast, the mean increase in hematoma volume in the three treatment groups was 16% at 40 µg/kg, 14% at 80 µg/kg, and 11% at 160 µg/kg. Overall, the study determined that rVIIa reduced the mortality rate at three months from 29% in the placebo group to 18% in the three treatment groups. Moreover, significant improvements in functional outcome at 90 days were observed in the treatment groups. However, a 7% rate of thromboembolic adverse events was seen in comparison to 2% in the placebo group. Many of the thromboembolic events were seen at higher doses, and, overall, it was determined that the benefits far outweighed the risks. At this time, rVIIa is still awaiting approval for use in noncoagulopathic ICH patients in an ongoing clinical trial (the FAST trial), which is investigating the use of rVIIa in ICH by comparing 20 µg/kg and 80 µg/kg doses with placebo.

Warfarin is used in approximately 15% of ICH cases and has been shown to increase the risk of ICH fivefold (33), while anticoagulation is associated with progressive bleeding, clinical deterioration, and overall increased mortality (31). The delayed reversal of coagulopathy has been associated with worsened outcome (70). While it is recommended that any patient who suffers an ICH and who is on warfarin receive both vitamin K and fresh frozen plasma in attempts to reverse the anticoagulation, such treatment is not without consequence. For example, the anticoagulation reversal by vitamin K and fresh frozen plasma is typically delayed and accompanies a significant fluid load. The reversal may be required to stop further deterioration or to take the patient to the operating room. Likewise, some patients may be unable to tolerate the associated fluid load because of other medical comorbidities. rVIIa has been shown to expedite the reversal of warfarin anticoagulation without significant fluid load. In fact, rVIIa when given intravenously can normalize the prothrombin time and international normalized ratio within minutes. More importantly, rVIIa has been used to reverse warfarin anticoagulation in acute ICH and expedite the effect of neurosurgical intervention with favorable clinical results (71). Thus, rVIIa should be considered as an adjunct to vitamin K and fresh frozen plasma in anticoagulation reversal. While higher doses of rVIIa can produce a longer duration of affect, the reversal affects of rVIIa only last several hours. The use of rVIIa is likely contraindicated in patients with known arterial or venous occlusive disease, acute thromboembolic sources, or metal prostheses, and should only be used in clinical trials or in compassionate use when further clot expansion or delayed surgery would likely be fatal or severely disabling.

HEMATOMA EVACUATION

On average, 7000 patients/yr will require surgical evacuation of a hematoma following ICH (10). The goals of surgical evacuation are to remove the hematoma, reduce the mass effect, and remove potential neurotoxic elements and prevent their interaction with healthy brain tissue. However, the surgical approach for deep hematomas requires dissection through otherwise healthy brain tissue, which may cause damage in the process.

In the first reported prospective randomized trial of surgical evacuation of hematoma following ICH, it was found that surgical intervention was associated with worse clinical outcomes and resulted in an increased mortality rate when compared with conservative medical management (2). One caveat regarding this study is that it was conducted in 1961, prior to routine CT use, and factors such as undetermined hematoma volume and delayed treatment may have confounded the study results. Many studies have been conducted with more modern technologies and practices and confirmed the findings of the first study. In a 1989 randomized study of 52 patients comparing craniotomy evacuation within 48 hours of presentation to conservative medical management, increased mortality was found in the surgical group (72). In 1990, a randomized trial was begun to compare surgical evacuation versus medical management or medical management with EVD and ICP monitoring. However, it was terminated prematurely because of poor outcomes in all treatment groups and poor recruitment (73).

One study since the 1961 study showed improved neurologic and overall outcomes with a reduced mortality rate in the surgical study population when stereotactic navigation was utilized (74). In this study, investigators evaluated ultrasound-guided endoscopic hematoma evacuation versus medical therapy alone in a group of 100 patients. They reported mortality rates of 42% in the surgical group and 70% in the medical group. Moreover, they found an improvement in overall functional outcome in the surgical population in comparison with the medical population. It is important to point out, however, that the surgical patients were younger and that subsequent subgroup analysis revealed that on the whole the younger patients did better in both treatment groups.

The most recent study to address this issue is the International Surgical Trials in Intracerebral Hemorrhage (STICH), which included 1033 patients (75). This landmark study compared early surgical evacuation of the hematoma and initial medical management. Inclusion criteria for patients on this study were spontaneous supratentorial ICH and presentation to the health delivery system within 72 hours of onset of symptoms. Moreover, each patient had to meet the additional criterion of uncertainty between the need for surgical evacuation and best medical therapy before randomization. Hence, the study excluded from randomization most young patients with ongoing neurologic deterioration in whom surgeons considered operation helpful. In randomized patients with such equipoise, no difference in mortality was observed between the two groups.

Moreover, the only difference between the two groups was in regard to favorable outcome at six months, which was slight, with 26% for the surgical group and 24% in the medical group. The overall conclusion of this comprehensive study was that no clear advantage was associated with early surgical intervention when compared with initial conservative medical management in patients who suffered from spontaneous supratentorial ICH. Furthermore, it is important to reiterate that the results of this study cannot be generalized to those patients who were thought by the surgeon to be able to benefit from surgical evacuation, including many young patients and those who were rapidly deteriorating from lobar hemorrhages (Fig. 2). In more than two-thirds of the patients screened for this study, the treating neurosurgeon expressed certainty about the appropriate treatment plan, and surgery was performed in approximately one-third. Most of these patients were younger with lower GCS scores, and their neurologic decline was likely because of the mass effect caused by the hematoma. Furthermore, the best timing of surgery in these patients remains unclear. The average time from ictus to surgical intervention was nearly 30 hours. Therefore, it is yet unclear if such patients would benefit further from surgery within the first 12 to 24 hours after the onset of symptoms. Future phases of STICH will attempt to resolve some of these uncertainties about the role of surgical intervention.

A Phase II multicentered randomized prospective analysis of the role of minimally invasive surgery and rtPA versus the best medical therapy for treatment of ICH, known as the "MISTIE" trial and sponsored by the National Institutes of Health (NIH), is ongoing at the time of this writing. The procedure involves drilling a burr hole and placing a catheter using stereotactic or other image guidance (CT or MR) into the hematoma, which is followed by hematoma aspiration and administration of rtPA over the following 72 hours (Fig. 12). Patients included in this study are aged between 18 and 80 years; they have GCS scores of less than 15 or NIH Stroke Scale scores of greater than 6 and ICH greater than or equal to 25 mL that is diagnosed within 12 hours of the onset of symptoms. A repeat CT six hours later must confirm a stable volume of the lesion within 5 mL of that on the initial CT. Those who are excluded from the study include, but are not limited to, patients who have an infratentorial hemorrhage, irreversible coagulopathy, uncorrected thrombocytopenia less than 100,000, are older than 80 years, are pregnant, have an IVH that requires EVD drainage, have significant comorbidities or multisystem organ failure, or have an ICH secondary to aneurysm or vascular malformation. Patients are randomized in a 1–3 scheme to protocol-driven best medical therapy or to this therapy in association with a catheter procedure and escalating doses of rtPA administered through the ICH catheter every eight hours for 72 hours or until the ICH reaches a volume of less than or equal to 15 mL or less than 80% of baseline ICH volume (Fig. 13). The primary outcome measurements are the 30-day mortality rate for the two groups and surgery or procedure-related morbidities. Secondary outcome assessments include clot size reduction rate at days 4 to 5 and the 90-day and 180-day clinical outcomes measured by Glasgow Outcome Score, Rankin Scale,

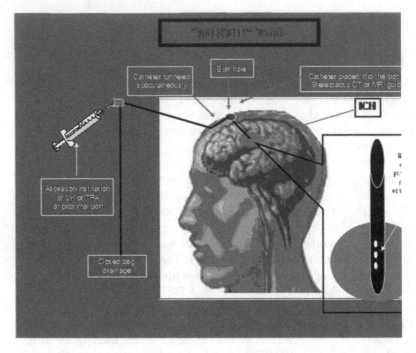

Figure 12 Schematic diagram demonstrating the operative technique involved in the MISTIE (Minimally Invasive Surgery Plus rtPA for Intracerebral Hemorrhage Evacuation) trial.

and Stoke Impact Scale. The hypothesis of the investigators is that this minimally invasive intervention would reduce the hematoma volume, thereby facilitating more rapid recovery of neurologic function and decreasing mortality from ICH in comparison with conventional medical management.

CONCLUSION

Despite many studies evaluating the efficacy of various treatment modals, the best treatment for ICH remains controversial, perhaps due in large part to the fact that ICH continues to be a formidable disease that is associated with high rates of morbidity and mortality. Nevertheless, as the population continues to age and as hypertension continues to be undertreated, the incidence of ICH will likely continue to rise, resulting in significant socioeconomic impact.

A promising trend is the range of ongoing research efforts investigating the most optimal treatment algorithms and a number of novel interventions to improve outcomes for ICH patients. The task of finding the solutions so desperately needed must be shared by neurosurgeons, stroke neurologists, critical care physicians, and other health care providers. It is hoped that the combination

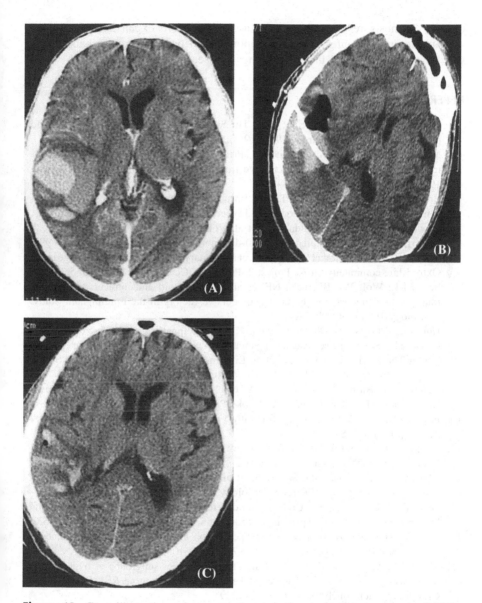

Figure 13 Case illustration of stereotactic aspiration and rtPA treatment of ICH. (A) Preoperative CT showing right parietotemporal ICH. (B) CT showing insertion of catheter and reduction of ICH volume following immediate aspiration. (C) Postcatheter removal CT illustrating dramatic reduction of ICH volume. *Abbreviations*: rtPA, recombinant tissue plasminogen activator; CT, computer tomography; ICH, intracerebral hemorrhage.

of early diagnosis, resuscitation, prevention of hematoma expansion, selection of appropriate surgical intervention, and judicious critical care and rehabilitation will lessen the burden of this devastating disease.

REFERENCES

1. Foulkes MA, Wolf PA, Price TR, et al. The Stroke Data Bank: design, methods, and baseline characteristics. Stroke 1988; 19(5):547–554.
2. McKissock WA, Richardson, Taylot J. Primary intracerebral haemorrhage: a controlled trial of surgical and conservative treatment in 180 unselected cases. Lancet 1961; 2:221–226.
3. Broderick JP, Brott T, Tomsick T, et al. Intracerebral hemorrhage more than twice as common as subarachnoid hemorrhage. J Neurosurg 1993; 78(2):188–191.
4. Broderick JP, Brott TG, Duldner JE, et al. Volume of intracerebral hemorrhage. A powerful and easy-to-use predictor of 30-day mortality. Stroke 1993; 24(7):987–993.
5. Counsell C, Boonyakarnkul S, Dennis M, et al. Primary intracerebral haemorrhage in the Oxfordshire community Stroke Project 2. Prognosis. Cerebrovasc Dis 1995; 5:26–34.
6. Sacco RL, Wolf PA, Bharucha NE, et al. Subarachnoid and intracerebral hemorrhage: natural history, prognosis, and precursive factors in the Framingham Study. Neurology 1984; 34(7):847–854.
7. Holloway RG, Witter DM Jr., Lawton KB, et al. Inpatient costs of specific cerebrovascular events at five academic medical centers. Neurology 1996; 46(3):854–860.
8. Taylor TN, Davis PH, Torner JC, et al. Lifetime cost of stroke in the United States. Stroke 1996; 27(9):1459–1466.
9. Dennis MS, Burn JP, Sandercock PA, et al. Long-term survival after first-ever stroke: the Oxfordshire Community Stroke Project. Stroke 1993; 24(6):796–800.
10. Fayad PB, Awad IA. Surgery for intracerebral hemorrhage. Neurology 1998; 51(3 suppl 3):S69–S73.
11. Qureshi AI, Tuhrim S, Broderick JP, et al. Spontaneous intracerebral hemorrhage. N Engl J Med 2001; 344(19):1450–1460.
12. Klatsky AL, Friedman GD, Sidney S, et al. Risk of hemorrhagic stroke in Asian American ethnic groups. Neuroepidemiology 2005; 25(1):26–31.
13. Qureshi AI, Giles WH, J.B. Croft. Racial differences in the incidence of intracerebral hemorrhage: effects of blood pressure and education. Neurology 1999; 52(8): 1617–1621.
14. Brott T, Thalinger K, Hertzberg V. Hypertension as a risk factor for spontaneous intracerebral hemorrhage. Stroke 1986; 17(6):1078–1083.
15. Thrift AG, McNeil JJ, Forbes A, et al. Three important subgroups of hypertensive persons at greater risk of intracerebral hemorrhage. Melbourne Risk Factor Study Group. Hypertension 1998; 31(6):1223–1229.
16. Ishihara T, Takahashi M, Yokota T, et al. The significance of cerebrovascular amyloid in the aetiology of superficial (lobar) cerebral haemorrhage and its incidence in the elderly population. J Pathol 1991; 165(3):229–234.
17. Iwamoto N, Ishihara T, Ito H, et al. Morphological evaluation of amyloid-laden arteries in leptomeninges, cortices and subcortices in cerebral amyloid angiopathy with subcortical hemorrhage. Acta Neuropathol (Berl) 1993; 86(5):418–421.
18. Mayer SA, Rincon F. Treatment of intracerebral haemorrhage. Lancet Neurol 2005; 4(10):662–672.

19. Vonsattel JP, Myers RH, Hedley-Whyte ET, et al. Cerebral amyloid angiopathy without and with cerebral hemorrhages: a comparative histological study. Ann Neurol 1991; 30(5):637–649.
20. Greenberg SM, Eng JA, Ning M, et al. Hemorrhage burden predicts recurrent intracerebral hemorrhage after lobar hemorrhage. Stroke 2004; 35(6):1415–1420.
21. O'Donnell HC, Rosand J, Knudsen KA, et al. Apolipoprotein E genotype and the risk of recurrent lobar intracerebral hemorrhage. N Engl J Med 2000; 342(4):240–245.
22. Greenberg SM, Rebeck GW, Vonsattel JP, et al. Apolipoprotein E epsilon 4 and cerebral hemorrhage associated with amyloid angiopathy. Ann Neurol 1995; 38(2): 254–259.
23. Feldmann E, Broderick JP, Kernan WN, et al. Major risk factors for intracerebral hemorrhage in the young are modifiable. Stroke 2005; 36(9):1881–1885.
24. Gorelick PB. Alcohol and stroke. Stroke 1987; 18(1):268–271.
25. Klatsky AL, Armstrong MA, Friedman GD. Alcohol use and subsequent cerebrovascular disease hospitalizations. Stroke 1989; 20(6):741–746.
26. Klatsky AL, Armstrong MA, Friedman GD, et al. Alcohol drinking and risk of hemorrhagic stroke. Neuroepidemiology, 2002; 21(3):115–122.
27. MacKenzie JM. Intracerebral haemorrhage. J Clin Pathol 1996; 49(5):360–364.
28. Fredericks RK, Lefkowitz DS, Challa VR, et al. Cerebral vasculitis associated with cocaine abuse. Stroke 1991; 22(11):1437–1439.
29. Berrouschot J, Rother J, Glahn J, et al. Outcome and severe hemorrhagic complications of intravenous thrombolysis with tissue plasminogen activator in very old (> or = 80 years) stroke patients. Stroke 2005; 36(11):2421–2425.
30. Hart RG, Benavente O, Pearce LA. Increased risk of intracranial hemorrhage when aspirin is combined with warfarin: a meta-analysis and hypothesis. Cerebrovasc Dis 1999; 9(4):215–217.
31. Hart RG, Boop BS, Anderson DC. Oral anticoagulants and intracranial hemorrhage. Facts and hypotheses. Stroke 1995; 26(8):1471–1477.
32. Kidwell CS, Saver JL, Carneado J, et al. Predictors of hemorrhagic transformation in patients receiving intra-arterial thrombolysis. Stroke 2002; 33(3):717–724.
33. Wintzen AR, de Jonge H, Loeliger EA, et al. The risk of intracerebral hemorrhage during oral anticoagulant treatment: a population study. Ann Neurol 1984; 16(5): 553–558.
34. Qureshi AI, Safdar K, Weil J, et al. Predictors of early deterioration and mortality in black Americans with spontaneous intracerebral hemorrhage. Stroke 1995; 26(10): 1764–1767.
35. Tuhrim S, Horowitz DR, Sacher M, et al. Validation and comparison of models predicting survival following intracerebral hemorrhage. Crit Care Med 1995; 23(5): 950–954.
36. Hemphill JC III, Bonovich DC, Besmertis L, et al. The ICH Score : a Simple, Reliable Grading Scale for Intracerebral Hemorrhage. Editorial Comment: a Simple, Reliable Grading Scale for Intracerebral Hemorrhage. Stroke 2001; 32(4):891–897.
37. Tuhrim S, Horowitz DR, Sacher M, et al. Volume of ventricular blood is an important determinant of outcome in supratentorial intracerebral hemorrhage. Crit Care Med 1999; 27(3):617–621.
38. Lee KR, Betz AL, Kim S, et al. The role of the coagulation cascade in brain edema formation after intracerebral hemorrhage. Acta Neurochir (Wien) 1996; 138(4): 396–400 (discussion 400–401).

39. Lee KR, Colon GP, Betz AL, et al. Edema from intracerebral hemorrhage: the role of thrombin. J Neurosurg 1996; 84(1):91–96.

40. Lee KR, Kawai N, Kim S, et al. Mechanisms of edema formation after intracerebral hemorrhage: effects of thrombin on cerebral blood flow, blood-brain barrier permeability, and cell survival in a rat model. J Neurosurg 1997; 86(2):272–278.

41. Xi G, Fewel ME, Hua Y, et al. Intracerebral hemorrhage: pathophysiology and therapy. Neurocrit Care 2004; 1(1):5–18.

42. Xi G, Hua Y, Bhasin RR, et al., Mechanisms of edema formation after intracerebral hemorrhage: effects of extravasated red blood cells on blood flow and blood-brain barrier integrity. Stroke 2001; 32(12):2932–2938.

43. Xi G, Keep RF, Hoff JT. Mechanisms of brain injury after intracerebral haemorrhage. Lancet Neurol 2006; 5(1):53–63.

44. Xi G, Wagner KR, Keep RF, et al. Role of blood clot formation on early edema development after experimental intracerebral hemorrhage. Stroke 1998; 29(12):2580–2586.

45. Davis SM, Broderick J, Hennerici M, et al. Hematoma growth is a determinant of mortality and poor outcome after intracerebral hemorrhage. Neurology 2006; 66(8): 1175–1181.

46. Steiner T, Diringer MN, Schneider D, et al. Dynamics of intraventricular hemorrhage in patients with spontaneous intracerebral hemorrhage: risk factors, clinical impact, and effect of hemostatic therapy with recombinant activated factor VII. Neurosurgery 2006; 59(4):767–773 (discussion 773–774).

47. Mayer SA. Ultra-Early Hemostatic Therapy for Intracerebral Hemorrhage. Stroke 2003; 34(1):224–229.

48. Mayer SA, Brun NC, Begtrup K, et al., Recombinant activated factor VII for acute intracerebral hemorrhage. N Engl J Med 2005; 352(8):777–785.

49. Mayer SA, Brun NC, Broderick J, et al. Safety and feasibility of recombinant factor VIIa for acute intracerebral hemorrhage. Stroke 2005; 36(1):74–79.

50. Kothari RU, Brott T, Broderick JP, et al. The ABCs of measuring intracerebral hemorrhage volumes. Stroke 1996; 27(8):1304–1305.

51. Zhu XL, Chan MS, Poon WS. Spontaneous intracranial hemorrhage: which patients need diagnostic cerebral angiography? A prospective study of 206 cases and review of the literature. Stroke, 1997; 28(7):1406–1409.

52. Levine SR, Brust JC, Futrell N, et al., A comparative study of the cerebrovascular complications of cocaine: alkaloidal versus hydrochloride—-a review. Neurology 1991; 41(8):1173–1177.

53. Levine SR, Brust JC, Futrell N, et al. Cerebrovascular complications of the use of the "crack" form of alkaloidal cocaine. N Engl J Med 1990; 323(11):699–704.

54. Gujjar AR, Deibert E, Manno EM, et al. Mechanical ventilation for ischemic stroke and intracerebral hemorrhage: indications, timing, and outcome. Neurology 1998; 51(2):447–451.

55. Dandapani BK, Suzuki S, Kelley RE, et al. Relation between blood pressure and outcome in intracerebral hemorrhage. Stroke 1995; 26(1):21–24.

56. Fogelholm R, Avikainen S, Murros K. Prognostic value and determinants of first-day mean arterial pressure in spontaneous supratentorial intracerebral hemorrhage. Stroke 1997; 28(7):1396–1400.

57. Terayama Y, Tanahashi N, Fukuuchi Y, et al. Prognostic value of admission blood pressure in patients with intracerebral hemorrhage. Keio Cooperative Stroke Study. Stroke, 1997. 28(6):1185–1188.

58. Willmot M, Leonardi-Bee J, Bath PM. High blood pressure in acute stroke and subsequent outcome: a systematic review. Hypertension 2004; 43(1):18–24.
59. Broderick JP, Adams HP Jr., Barsan W, et al. Guidelines for the management of spontaneous intracerebral hemorrhage: a statement for healthcare professionals from a special writing group of the Stroke Council, American Heart Association. Stroke 1999; 30(4):905–915.
60. Qureshi AI, Wilson DA, Hanley DF, et al. Pharmacologic reduction of mean arterial pressure does not adversely affect regional cerebral blood flow and intracranial pressure in experimental intracerebral hemorrhage. Crit Care Med 1999; 27(5):965–971.
61. Mayfrank L, Kim Y, Kissler J, et al. Morphological changes following experimental intraventricular haemorrhage and intraventricular fibrinolytic treatment with recombinant tissue plasminogen activator. Acta Neuropathol (Berl) 2000; 100(5): 561–567.
62. Mayfrank L, Rohde V, Gilsbach JM. Fibrinolytic treatment of intraventricular haemorrhage preceding surgical repair of ruptured aneurysms and arteriovenous malformations. Br J Neurosurg 1999; 13(2):128–131.
63. Wang YC, Lin CW, Shen CC, et al. Tissue plasminogen activator for the treatment of intraventricular hematoma: the dose-effect relationship. J Neurol Sci 2002; 202(1–2): 35–41.
64. Poungvarin N. Steroids have no role in stroke therapy. Stroke 2004; 35(1):229–30.
65. Poungvarin N. Bhoopat W, Viriyavejakul A, et al. Effects of dexamethasone in primary supratentorial intracerebral hemorrhage. N Engl J Med 1987; 316(20): 1229–1233.
66. Tellez H, Bauer RB. Dexamethasone as treatment in cerebrovascular disease. 1. A controlled study in intracerebral hemorrhage. Stroke 1973; 4(4):541–546.
67. Mayer SA, Sacco RL, Shi T, et al. Neurologic deterioration in noncomatose patients with supratentorial intracerebral hemorrhage. Neurology 1994; 44(8):1379–1384.
68. Brott T, Broderick J, Kothari R, et al. Early hemorrhage growth in patients with intracerebral hemorrhage. Stroke 1997; 28(1):1–5.
69. Mayer SA, Brun NC, Begtrup K, et al. Recombinant activated factor VII for acute intracerebral hemorrhage. N Engl J Med 2005; 352(8):777–785.
70. Goldstein JN, Thomas SH, Frontiero V, et al. Timing of fresh frozen plasma administration and rapid correction of coagulopathy in warfarin-related intracerebral hemorrhage. Stroke 2006; 37(1):151–155.
71. Park P, Fewel ME, Garton HJ, et al. Recombinant activated factor VII for the rapid correction of coagulopathy in nonhemophilic neurosurgical patients. Neurosurgery 2003; 53(1):34–38 (discussion 38–39).
72. Juvela S, Heiskanen O, Poranen A, et al. The treatment of spontaneous intracerebral hemorrhage. A prospective randomized trial of surgical and conservative treatment. J Neurosurg 1989; 70(5):755–758.
73. Batjer HH, Reisch JS, Allen BC, et al. Failure of surgery to improve outcome in hypertensive putaminal hemorrhage. A prospective randomized trial. Arch Neurol 1990; 47(10):1103–1106.
74. Auer LM, Deinsberger W, Niederkorn K, et al. Endoscopic surgery versus medical treatment for spontaneous intracerebral hematoma: a randomized study. J Neurosurg 1989; 70(4):530–535.
75. Mendelow AD, Gregson BA, Fernandes HM, et al. Early surgery versus initial conservative treatment in patients with spontaneous supratentorial intracerebral haematomas in the International Surgical Trial in Intracerebral Haemorrhage (STICH): a randomised trial. Lancet 2005; 365(9457):387–397.

12

Management of Blood Pressure and Intracranial Hypertension in Intracerebral Hemorrhage

Gustavo J. Rodríguez, MD, Fellow[a]
Qaisar A. Shah, MD, Fellow[a]
Adnan I. Qureshi, MD, Professor and Vice Chair of Neurology

[a]Endovascular Surgical Neuroradiology,
Zeenat Qureshi Stroke Research Center, University of Minnesota,
Minneapolis, Minnesota, U.S.A.

INTRODUCTION

Management of arterial hypertension and increased intracranial pressure (ICP) in patients with spontaneous intracerebral hemorrhage (ICH) is performed with the principal intent to decrease the morbidity and mortality associated with this condition. However, strong evidence-based guidelines are lacking.

Hypertension is the most common risk factor associated with spontaneous ICH, and it is frequently found at presentation. It is also considered a trigger and has been implicated in early hematoma growth. Long-term hypertension control has already shown to be of benefit, but whether acute hypertensive treatment is favorable in ICH is yet to be proven. Monitoring of increased ICP is useful when suspected; elevated pressures can potentially impair adequate cerebral blood flow (CBF), especially in patients with chronic hypertension. In severe cases, it may lead to herniation and death. Medical management and external ventricular drainage are often used to control raised ICP, but decompressive surgery may sometimes be required to stop the process.

The current understanding of limitations to and the ongoing research in the management of arterial hypertension and increased ICP in spontaneous ICH are reviewed in this chapter.

Spontaneous ICH accounts for approximately 10% to 15% of all strokes, which represents approximately 37,000 to 52,000 people every year in the United States (1). It is a devastating disease; mortality may affect up to half of patients in the first month, and as few as 20% will be independent at six months (2,3).

Primary ICH, when no obvious structural abnormality exists, generally results from chronic hypertension, accounting for 65% of cases (4). Acute hypertension is considered a responsible trigger and is often found at presentation (5–7). Elevated blood pressure among patients with spontaneous ICH is a predictor of hematoma expansion and poor outcome (8–10).

The presence of increased ICP requires close vigilance. Frequent neurological evaluation is advisable to detect herniation syndromes that require prompt treatment. In suspected cases, monitoring of ICP becomes useful. Appropriate treatment response can be assessed, and adequate cerebral perfusion pressure can be ensured when arterial hypertension is being lowered.

Ischemia in the perihematoma region was thought to contribute to brain injury and edema in the past (11). Global cerebral ischemia is still a concern if blood pressure is lowered in patients with chronic hypertension because of a shifted autoregulation response. Nonetheless, reductions in the mean arterial pressure of up to 15% in small- or medium-sized hematomas did not change the global CBF (12). Investigations are currently underway to study the safety of aggressive blood pressure control in spontaneous ICH and to further assess the efficacy of this intervention in lowering the rates of hematoma expansion (13).

One of the priorities in spontaneous ICH research is acute blood pressure management (14), especially its relationship with ICP. The establishment of evidence-based guidelines is desperately needed.

PATHOPHYSIOLOGY OF ICH

Implications of Chronic Hypertension in Spontaneous ICH

Elevated blood pressure was reported in two-thirds of patients with acute stroke and spontaneous reduction within 10 days without antihypertensive treatment (15,16). In a large cross-sectional study, a high prevalence (75%) of elevated systolic blood pressure ($\geq$ 140 mmHg) in patients with ICH was also found (17). Arterial hypertension at the time of admission may in some cases simply reflect chronically untreated hypertension (18). Other possibilities include a protective response to maintain cerebral perfusion when the brainstem is compressed, also known as the Cushing–Kocher response (1,19), or a stress secondary to abnormal sympathetic activity, altered parasympathetic activity, raised levels of circulating catecholamines, or brain natriuretic peptide that may also induce acute hypertension (20,21).

Chronic hypertension causes histologic changes in penetrating blood vessels, with degeneration of the media and smooth muscle, mainly in the bifurcations that make them susceptible to rupture (22). It also produces thickening of the vascular wall, increasing the resistance and providing tissue protection if cerebral perfusion pressure is high but diminishing the ability to dilate when cerebral perfusion pressure is reduced (23,24).

Cerebral autoregulation is the homeostatic mechanism that maintains CBF by modifying the cerebrovascular resistance when cerebral perfusion pressure fluctuates. The lumen of arterioles dilates or constricts if cerebral perfusion pressure lowers or rises, respectively. This mechanism keeps CBF constant in normal subjects when the cerebral perfusion pressure ranges between 50 and 150 mmHg. In patients with chronic hypertension, cerebral autoregulation is shifted to higher levels and the degree correlates with the severity of hypertension (23,24).

Initial Mass Effect

Spontaneous ICH results from the rupture of small penetrating arteries that originate from the main intracranial circulation. Common sites in the brain parenchyma are the basal ganglia, thalamus, pons, cerebellum, and cerebral lobes. The mass effect in the adjacent structures is responsible for the initial symptoms (25). Because of the common deep location in the ventricular system proximity, hematomas, especially if large, may extend to the ventricles, worsening outcome (26). Intracerebral hematomas are not monophasic events, and up to one-third may expand in the first 24 hours, mainly within the first six hours. It is not yet clear why this expansion happens, but it has been attributed to continuing bleeding from the source, to the disruption of surrounding vessels, hypertension, and coagulation deficits (27,28). Hematoma expansion causes additional mass effect and neuronal injury and is the main cause of clinical deterioration and death during the hyperacute phase (9,29–31).

Perihematoma Edema Without Ischemia: Additional Mass Effect

In survivors of the initial event, edema around the hematoma soon develops and may persist for as long as two weeks (32,33). Edema in the surrounding parenchyma that develops within eight hours of onset is interstitial in nature and results from the accumulation of osmotically active serum proteins from the clot and movement of water across an intact blood-brain barrier into the extracellular space (34,35). Between 24 and 48 hours after the onset, cell death and inflammation that result from direct cellular toxicity and blood-brain barrier disruption are the main processes (32,36–41). Cytotoxic edema and breakdown of the blood-brain barrier, from blood and blood products are most likely the explanation for the late edema formation (42–43).

Cerebral ischemia was initially thought to contribute to neuronal injury and edema (44–48). More recent studies refute this hypothesis and suggest that three phases of CBF and metabolism changes follow ICH (11). In an initial hibernation

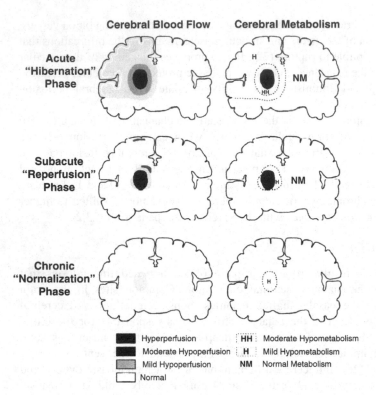

Cerebral Blood Flow   Cerebral Metabolism

Acute "Hibernation" Phase

Subacute "Reperfusion" Phase

Chronic "Normalization" Phase

	Hyperperfusion	HH	Moderate Hypometabolism
	Moderate Hypoperfusion	H	Mild Hypometabolism
	Mild Hypoperfusion	NM	Normal Metabolism
	Normal		

Figure 1 Diagrammatic representation of the three phases of cerebral blood flow and metabolism changes in spontaneous intracerebral hemorrhage: hibernation, reperfusion, and normalization. *Source*: From Ref. 11.

phase, concomitant hypoperfusion and hypometabolism that involve the peri-hematoma region are identified within 48 hours of hemorrhage onset. Reductions in CBF and cerebral oxygen consumption can be observed using positron emission tomography scanning (49–51). A reperfusion phase is seen between days 2 and 14 with a mixed pattern of CBF, consisting of areas of relatively normal flow, hypoperfusion, and hyperperfusion. Finally, a normalization phase is observed after day 14, with normal CBF reestablished in all regions except those with nonviable tissue. Despite low CBF in the perihematoma region during the acute phase, complementary low metabolism prevents ischemia (Fig. 1).

MANAGEMENT OF ACUTE HYPERTENSION IN ICH

American Heart Association Guidelines

Evidence-based guidelines in the management of blood pressure in patients with spontaneous ICH are lacking. The stroke council for the American Heart Association (52), in their guidelines for management of spontaneous ICH, encourages tight blood pressure control in an attempt to stop the ongoing bleeding but also considers that aggressive treatment may decrease cerebral perfusion and worsen brain damage, especially if increased ICP is present. On the basis of these two rationales, the recommendation is for the systemic arterial pressure to be maintained around 160/90 mmHg (mean of 110 mmHg). However, in patients with suspected increased ICP, the goal is to ensure a cerebral perfusion pressure >60 to 80 mmHg (Class IIb, Level of Evidence C). Continuous intravenous infusions (Labetalol, Nicardipine, Esmolol, Hydralazine, Nitroprusside, Nitroglycerin) or intermittent (Labetalol, Esmolol, Enalapril, Hydralazine) intravenous medications are recommended. Nitroprusside may be associated with further increases in ICP, thus accentuating any Cushing–Kocher response that may be occurring.

Clinical Trials and Experimental Studies

Elevated blood pressure is associated with hematoma expansion and poor neurologic outcome. Ischemia in the perihematoma region is no longer a concern. Thus, on the basis of the above-mentioned evidence, it is reasonable to treat hypertension in patients who present with spontaneous ICH. The ideal blood pressure goals to improve the clinical outcome with adequate maintenance of cerebral perfusion pressure are unknown. Several small clinical trials have addressed this issue. A nonrandomized, prospective trial in 1962 was the first to demonstrate an improvement in mortality with the use of antihypertensive medication in patients with ICH (53). Limitations included the fact that less severe symptoms were present in the treatment group. In a 1995 retrospective study of blood pressure control at presentation, blood pressure control in the initial two to six hours improved mortality and morbidity (54). However, the study did not consider variables such as hematoma volume, ventricular blood, and initial Glasgow Coma Scale, all of which confounded the results. In 1999, an animal study showed that pharmacologic reduction of the mean arterial pressure had no adverse effects on ICP or CBF in regions around and distant to the hematoma (55). The study was limited by the fact that all of the experimental animals were normotensive, as opposed to patients who often suffer from long-standing hypertension and changes in cerebral flow dynamics. In a 2001 study of 14 patients within 6 to 22 hours with small- to medium-sized hematomas, the patients were randomized to receive either nicardipine or labetalol for blood pressure control (12). CBF was measured using positron emission tomography before and after treatment. No significant changes in CBF, either globally or around the hematoma, were seen with a 15% reduction in the mean arterial pressure. In 2004, a prospective multicentered study on the safety and feasibility of early antihypertensive treatment in 27 patients showed low rates of neurologic deterioration and hematoma expansion (56). Patients who were treated within six hours were more likely to be independent at one month compared to those who were treated between 6 and 24 hours. Limitations to the study included

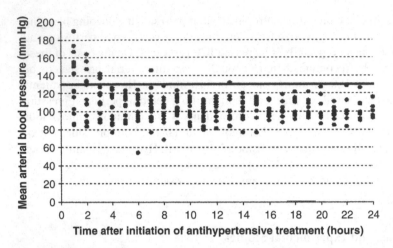

Figure 2 Systolic blood pressure control with intravenous nicardipine. Hourly mean arterial blood pressure changes for the initial 24-hr period after initiation of anti-hypertensive treatment with IV infusion of nicardipine in 28 patients with intracerebral hemorrhage. Mean arterial blood pressure goal <130 mmHg. *Source*: From Ref. 57.

unmatched controls with variable characteristics. Also, 24-hour follow-up CT of the head was not obtained for every patient, and thus asymptomatic hematoma expansion could have been missed. In a single- centered prospective registry in 2006, 29 patients were treated with nicardipine to achieve a mean arterial pressure goal of below 130 mmHg within the first 24 hours (following American Heart Association guidelines) (57). The study was unique, as it was the first study that utilized the guidelines, and nicardipine was used to maintain an even and more effective reduction in blood pressure, versus boluses of labetalol and hydralazine, which resulted in uneven reduction in blood pressure (Figs. 2 and 3). Nicardipine was well tolerated in 86% of the patients, and rates of neurologic deterioration and hematoma expansion were lower than previously reported (13% and 18% of the patients, respectively).

Ongoing Clinical Trials

The Antihypertensive Treatment of Acute Cerebral Hemorrhage (ATACH) trial (13) is designed to determine the tolerability of blood pressure control with IV infusion of nicardipine for 18 to 24 hours after ICH. Three different systolic blood pressure targets have to be achieved and maintained. The presence of neurologic deterioration and any serious adverse event during the treatment are being studied. Inclusion criteria require a presentation within six hours of symptom onset and an initial systolic blood pressure above 200 mmHg. Three treatment tiers are being studied: systolic blood pressure between 170 and 200 mmHg, between 140 and 170 mmHg, and between 110 and 140 mmHg.

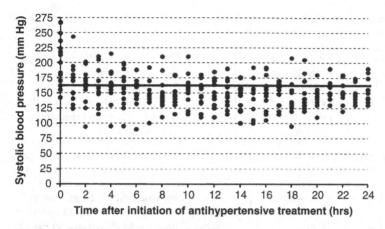

Figure 3 Systolic blood pressure control with IV labetolol and hydralazine. Hourly systolic blood pressure changes for the initial 24-hr period after initiating antihypertensive treatment with IV boluses of labetalol and hydralazine in 13 patients with intracerebral hemorrhage. Systolic arterial blood pressure goal <180 mmHg. *Source*: From Ref. 56.

The current study will be the largest of its kind and will help to increase our understanding about the principles of blood pressure control in acute ICH. A sample protocol for IV nicardipine infusion that is currently being used is detailed in Table 1.

ORAL INITIATION OF ANTIHYPERTENSIVE AGENTS IN PATIENTS WITH ICH

Long-term blood pressure control has been shown to reduce the incidence of stroke by 35% to 40%, myocardial infarction by 20% to 25%, and heart failure by more than 50% (58). The latest report of the Joint National Committee on Prevention, Detection, Evaluation, and Treatment of High Blood Pressure highlights a number of issues: (*i*) In individuals older than 50, an elevated systolic blood pressure is of more concern than an elevated diastolic blood pressure. (*ii*) The risk of cardio-vascular disease, beginning at 115/75 mmHg, doubles with each increment of 20/10 mmHg. If normotensive at 55 years of age, the lifetime risk for developing hypertension is 90%. (*iii*) A new term, *prehypertension*, has been introduced for individuals with a systolic blood pressure between 120 and 139 mmHg or a dia-stolic between 80 and 89 mmHg. Individuals with prehypertension are recom-mended to make lifestyle modifications to prevent cardiovascular disease. (*iv*) Thiazide-type diuretics, either alone or in combination with other classes, should be considered as the initial treatment of choice for most patients with uncomplicated hypertension. Certain high-risk conditions are compelling indications for the initial

Table 1 Nicardipine Infusion Protocol

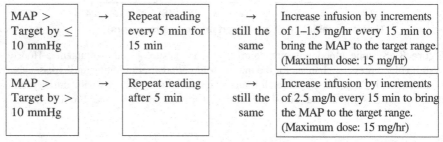

| Start infusion at 5 mg/hr | → | Titrate by 2.5 mg/hr every 15 min to bring the MAP to the target range. (Maximum dose: 15 mg/hr) | → | Once [a]target MAP is reached, decrease nicardipine by 2.5 mg/hr every 15 min until the target MAP is maintained in the target range or the medication is discontinued |

- If after stabilization in the target range, the MAP becomes more than the target range:

| MAP > Target by ≤ 10 mmHg | → | Repeat reading every 5 min for 15 min | → still the same | Increase infusion by increments of 1–1.5 mg/hr every 15 min to bring the MAP to the target range. (Maximum dose: 15 mg/hr) |
| MAP > Target by > 10 mmHg | → | Repeat reading after 5 min | → still the same | Increase infusion by increments of 2.5 mg/h every 15 min to bring the MAP to the target range. (Maximum dose: 15 mg/hr) |

- If after stabilization in the target range, the MAP becomes less than the target range:

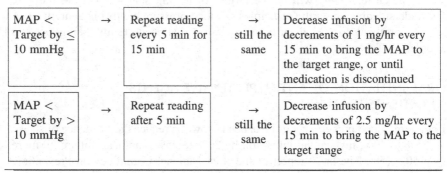

| MAP < Target by ≤ 10 mmHg | → | Repeat reading every 5 min for 15 min | → still the same | Decrease infusion by decrements of 1 mg/hr every 15 min to bring the MAP to the target range, or until medication is discontinued |
| MAP < Target by > 10 mmHg | → | Repeat reading after 5 min | → still the same | Decrease infusion by decrements of 2.5 mg/hr every 15 min to bring the MAP to the target range |

[a]target MAP: 90–130 mmHg. *Abbreviation*: MAP, mean arterial pressure.

use of other antihypertensive drug classes (e.g., angiotensin-converting enzyme inhibitors, angiotensin-receptor blockers, β blockers, calcium channel blockers). (*v*) Blood pressures that are 20/10 mmHg above the desired goal will require two agents, one of which should be a thiazide-type diuretic. (*vi*) Most patients with hypertension will require two or more antihypertensive medications to achieve the goal (<140/90 mmHg, or lower for patients with diabetes or chronic kidney disease) (59). For patients with spontaneous ICH and persistent hypertension, oral anti-hypertensives can be initiated after 72 hours of onset to gradually achieve the preferred blood pressure (60).

INTRACRANIAL HYPERTENSION IN SPONTANEOUS ICH

Intracranial hypertension is defined as ICP above 19 mmHg for more than five minutes. It may result initially if hematomas are large or if there is associated hydrocephalus, but it can also develop later when edema begins to collect in the region immediately around the hematoma. Intracranial hypertension contributes to morbidity and mortality in ICH and should be suspected in patients with sudden decrease in the level of consciousness, headache, or vomiting. Increased pressure due to progressive mass effect may lead to herniation because of restricted intracranial space (61,62), and it should be addressed quickly since treatment may be life saving (19).

MEDICAL MANAGEMENT OF INTRACRANIAL HYPERTENSION

Patients with ICH should be admitted to a monitored unit for at least the initial 24 hours (63). Standard critical care measures in the management of intracranial hypertension include frequent neurologic examinations, elevation of the head of the bed by 30° to 40°, treatment of fever, tachycardia, extreme hypertension, and adequate sedation (preferably short-acting agents that can be easily reversed) when patients are stimulated or mobilized. No evidence supports the use of prophylactic agents to prevent herniation.

In the presence of increased ICP or herniation syndromes, treatment should be instituted without delay; the following protocol can be followed (18,64,65):

1. Emergent intubation (medications and stimuli that increase ICP should be prevented), and hyperventilation or manual hyperventilation with a ventilation bag should be performed initially. The goal is to maintain $PaCO_2$ between 25 and 30 mmHg by ventilating at a rate between 30 and 40 breaths/min.
2. Hypertonic saline (a bolus of 30 mL of 23.4% NaCl or 5 mL/kg of 3% NaCl given in 30–60 minutes) through a central venous catheter or an osmotic agent, such as IV mannitol (0.5–1 gm/kg, bolus), can then be administered. If an adequate response is not observed with one agent in the first 10 minutes of initiating treatment, the other agent may be added. Thiopental can be used in case of a pronounced hypertensive response (defined as mean arterial pressure > 150 mmHg) accompanying the herniation episode. Vasopressors and fluid boluses may be required to keep a systolic arterial pressure above 90 mmHg.
3. Once the first round of treatment is completed, an emergent CT scan of the head can be obtained to determine a possible requirement for surgical decompression.
4. Either a maintenance infusion of hypertonic saline to achieve a serum sodium between 145 and 155 mmol/L or boluses of mannitol (0.5 g/kg q6 hr) to achieve a serum osmolality between 310 and 315 mOsm/L, or a combination of both, may then be started.

5. Barbiturate coma can also be considered if other medical and surgical options are not feasible or the patient's signs and symptoms are refractory to initial treatment efforts.

Controlled hyperventilation causes cerebral vasoconstriction, which quickly decreases ICP. Its benefit lasts for a few hours, and it is typically used as a bridging therapy. Slow normalization of the $PaCO_2$ over 24 hours is recommended to avoid a rebound effect (66,67).

Mannitol is an osmotic and rheologic agent that produces an osmotic gradient from the interstitium to the intravascular compartment. In the kidneys, mannitol prevents resorption of water and is eliminated unmetabolized. Mannitol also reduces blood viscosity, producing a transient increase in CBF and volume, with a compensating vasoconstriction and a net reduction in cerebral blood volume (68). Side effects include reversed osmolality and renal failure. Reversed osmolality refers to the accumulation of mannitol in the brain after multiple doses, causing a reversed osmotic shift.

Hypertonic saline has shown a favorable effect in the treatment of intracranial hypertension in laboratory and clinical settings. It has a better reflection coefficient than mannitol (1 as compared to 0.9), meaning the blood-brain barrier is virtually impermeable to hypertonic saline. Hypertonic saline should be used with caution in patients with heart failure (69). Studies to compare both hyperosmolar agents are needed to define which is superior in the treatment of intracranial hypertension.

Barbiturates decrease ICP by reducing metabolic activity and secondarily reducing the CBF and volume. Their maximum effect is obtained when a burst-suppression pattern is seen on the electroencephalogram, with no further benefit seen with higher doses. Barbiturate coma successfully reduces intracranial hypertension but is not exempt from side effects, and it is unclear whether these patients gain long-term benefits from this intervention (70,71). Hypothermia (temperatures in the range of 32–33°C) lowers ICP, although its long-term benefit is not clear. Ongoing research may reveal its advantage in the future (72–74).

SURGICAL MANAGEMENT OF INTRACRANIAL HYPERTENSION

Patients with a Glasgow Coma Scale score of less than 9 or those who are clinically deteriorating because of suspected mass effect should have an intracranial monitoring device placed (level of evidence V, grade C recommendation) (75). External ventricular drainage devices are more invasive, increasing the risk of infection (unlike fiberoptic bolt systems), but they help to control the increased ICP by draining cerebrospinal fluid. In cases of acute hydrocephalus, ICP may quickly increase, making the rapid placement of an external ventricular drain of extreme importance (76). The stroke council for the American Heart Association recommends monitoring ICP in patients with elevated ICP to maintain a cerebral perfusion pressure above 70 mmHg (Class IIa, level of evidence B) (52).

Although it is known that intracerebral hematomas may lead to progressive mass effect and brain herniation, a pertinent question arises as to whether early clot removal would be an appropriate preventive therapy. Randomized trials that compared best medical treatment with early surgical clot removal failed to demonstrate differences in outcome (77). It is becoming clearer that draining hematomas that are deep and do not involve posterior fossa may lead to worse outcomes, and that some superficial hemorrhages in clinically deteriorating patients could benefit from urgent surgical intervention (77–81). Hematomas larger than 3 cm located in the cerebellum and causing hydrocephalus or brain stem compression are also likely to benefit from surgery (82).

Recently, minimally invasive methods have become an investigational procedure of choice. In a recent study, 72 patients with supratentorial ICH were randomized to either conservative treatment or to treatment with urokinase and subsequent drainage every 6 hours for 48 hours. Although no difference was found in mortality, this therapy was proven to be safe (83).

CONCLUSION

Spontaneous ICH carries great morbidity and mortality. Hematoma expansion, one of the major causes of neurologic deterioration, is a delayed process amenable of intervention. Measures to decrease the rate and extent of hematoma growth are urgently needed. Tight blood pressure control may be of benefit in this regard. Ongoing research may help to determine the blood pressure target at which cerebral perfusion pressure is not compromised in patients with increased ICP and a shifted autoregulation. Increased ICP often predisposes patients with spontaneous ICH to worsening outcomes. Its management may be life saving. More research is necessary to develop evidence-based protocols of intervention.

REFERENCES

1. Qureshi AI, Tuhrim S, Broderick JP, et al. Spontaneous intracerebral hemorrhage. N Engl J Med 2001; 344:1450–1460.
2. Counsell C, Boonyakamkul S, Dennis M, et al. Primary intracerebral haemorrhage in the Oxfordshire Community Stroke Project, 2: prognosis. Cerebrovasc Dis 1995; 5:26–34.
3. Kojima S, Omura T, Wakamatsu W, et al. Prognosis and disability of stroke patients after 5 years in Akita, Japan. Stroke 1990; 21:72–77.
4. Foulkes MA, Wolf PA, Price TR, et al. The Stroke Data Bank: design, methods, and baseline characteristics. Stroke 1988; 19(5):547–554.
5. Simoons ML, Maggioni AP, Knatterud G, et al. Individual risk assessment for intracranial hemorrhage during thrombolytics therapy. Lancet 1993; 342:1523–1528.
6. Brott T, Thalinger K, Hertzberg V. Hypertension as a risk factor for spontaneous intracerebral hemorrhage. Stroke 1986; 17:1078–1083.

7. Thrift AG, McNeil JJ, Forbes A, et al. Three important subgroups of hypertensive persons at greater risk of intracerebral hemorrhage. Hypertension 1998; 31:1223–1229.

8. Fogelholm R, Avikainen S, Murros K. Prognostic value and determinants of first-day mean arterial pressure in spontaneous supratentorial intracerebral hemorrhage. Stroke 1997; 28:1396–1400.

9. Kazui S, Minematsu K, Yamamoto H, et al. Predisposing factors to enlargement of spontaneous intracerebral hematoma. Stroke 1997; 28(12):2370–2375.

10. Ohwaki K, Yano E, Nagashima H, et al. Blood pressure management in acute intracerebral hemorrhage: relationship between elevated blood pressure and hematoma enlargement. Stroke 2004; 35(6):1364–1367.

11. Qureshi AI, Hanel RA, Kirmani JF, et al. Cerebral blood flow changes associated with intracerebral hemorrhage. Neurosurg Clin N Am 2002; 13(3):355–370.

12. Powers WJ, Zazulia AR, Videen TO, et al. Autoregulation of cerebral blood flow surrounding acute (6 to 22 hours) intracerebral hemorrhage. Neurology 2001; 57(1):18–24.

13. Qureshi AI. Antihypertensive Treatment of Acute Cerebral Hemorrhage (ATACH): rationale and design. Neurocrit Care 2007; 6(1):56–66.

14. NINDS ICH Workshop Participants. Priorities for clinical research in intracerebral hemorrhage: report from a National Institute of Neurological Disorders and Stroke workshop. Stroke 2005; 36(3):E23–E41.

15. Wallace JD, Levy LL. Blood pressure after stroke. JAMA 1981; 246(19):2177–2180.

16. Britton M, Carlsson A, de Faire U. Blood pressure course in patients with acute stroke and matched controls. Stroke 1986; 17(5):861–864.

17. Qureshi AI, Ezzeddine MA, Nasar A, et al. Prevalence of elevated blood pressure in 563,704 adult patients with stroke presenting to the ED in the United States. Am J Emerg Med 2007; 25(1):32–38.

18. Arboix A, Roig H, Rossich R, et al. Differences between hypertensive and non-hypertensive ischemic stroke. Eur J Neurol 2004; 11(10):687–692.

19. Qureshi AI, Geocadin RG, Suarez JI, et al. Long-term outcome after medical reversal of transtentorial herniation in patients with supratentorial mass lesions. Crit Care Med. 2000; 28(5):1556–1564.

20. Cheung RT, Hachinski V, et al. Cardiac effects of stroke. Curr Treat Options Cardiovasc Med 2004; 6(3):199–207.

21. Nakagawa K, Yamaguchi T, Seida M, et al. Plasma concentrations of brain natriuretic peptide in patients with acute ischemic stroke. Cerebrovasc Dis 2005; 19(3):157–164.

22. Olson JD. Mechanisms of homeostasis: effect on intracerebral hemorrhage. Stroke 1993; 24:Suppl:I109–I114.

23. Baumback GL, Heistad DD. Cerebral circulation in chronic arterial hypertension. Hypertension 1988; 12:89–95.

24. Agnoli A, Fieschi C, Bozzao L, et al. Autoregulation of cerebral blood flow. Studies during drug-induced hypertension in normal subjects and in patients with cerebral vascular diseases. Circulation 1968; 38:800–812.

25. Mutlu N, Berry RG, Alpers BJ. Massive cerebral hemorrhage: clinical and pathological correlations. Arch Neurol 1963; 8:644–661.

26. Young WB, Lee KP, Pessin MS, et al. Prognostic significance of ventricular blood in supratentorial hemorrhage: a volumetric study. Neurology 1990; 40(4):616–619.

27. Olson JD. Mechanisms of homeostasis. Effect on intracerebral hemorrhage. Stroke 1993; 24(12 suppl):I109–I114.

28. Brott T, Broderick J, Kothari R, et al. Early hemorrhage growth in patients with intracerebral hemorrhage. Stroke 1997; 28:1–5.
29. Kazui S, Naritomi H, Yamamoto H, et al. Enlargement of spontaneous intracerebral hemorrhage: incidence and time course. Stroke 1996; 27:1783–1787.
30. Fujii Y, Tanaka R, Takeuchi S, et al. Hematoma enlargement in spontaneous intracerebral hemorrhage. J Neurosurg 1994; 80:51–57.
31. Fehr MA, Anderson DC. Incidence of progression or rebleeding in hypertensive intracerebral hemorrhage. J Stroke Cerebrovasc Dis 1991; 1:111–116.
32. Zazulia AR, Diringer MN, Derdeyn CP, et al. Progression of mass effect after intracerebral hemorrhage. Stroke 1999; 30:1167–173.
33. Yang GY, Betz AL, Chenevert TL, et al. Experimental intracerebral hemorrhage: relationship between brain edema, blood flow, and blood-brain barrier permeability in rats. J Neurosurg 1994; 81:93–102.
34. Wagner KR, Xi G, Hua Y, et al. Lobar intracerebral hemorrhage model in pigs: rapid edema development in perihematomal white matter. Stroke 1996; 27:490–497.
35. Wagner KR, Xi G, Hau Y, et al. Early metabolic alterations in edematous peri-hematomal brain regions following experimental intracerebral hemorrhage. J Neurosurg 1998; 88:1058–1065.
36. Qureshi AI, Suri MF, Ostrow PT, et al. Apoptosis as a form of cell death in intra-cerebral hemorrhage. Neurosurgery 2003; 52:1041–1048.
37. Rosenberg GA, Navratil M. Metalloproteinase inhibition blocks edema in intracerebral hemorrhage in the rat. Neurology 1997; 48:921–926.
38. Nath FP, Kelly PT, Jenkins A, et al. Effects of experimental intracerebral hemor-rhage on blood flow, capillary permiability, and histochemistry. J Neurosurg 1987; 66:555–562.
39. Lee KR, Colon GP, Betz AL, et al. Edema from intracerebral hemorrhage: the role of thrombin. J Neurosurg 1996; 84:91–96.
40. Xi G, Keep RF, Hoff JT. Erythrocytes and delayed brain edema formation following intracerebral hemorrhage in rats. J Neurosurg 1998; 89:991–996.
41. Suzuki J, Ebina T. Sequential changes in tissue surrounding ICH. In: Pia HW, Longmaid C, Zierski J, eds. Spontaneous Intracerebral Hematomas. Berlin: Springer-Verlag 1980:121–128.
42. Jenkins A, Mendelow AD, Graham DI, ét al. Experimental intracranial hematoma: the role of blood constituents in early ischemia. Br J Neurosurg 1990; 4:45–51.
43. Lee KR, Betz AL, Keep RF, et al. Intracerebral infusion of thrombin as a cause of brain edema. J Neurosurg 1995; 83:1045–1050.
44. Kobari M, Gotoh F, Tomita M, et al. Bilateral hemispheric reduction of cerebral blood volume and blood flow immediately after experimental cerebral hemorrhage in cats. Stroke 1988; 19:991–996.
45. Bullock R, Brock-Utne J, van Dellen J, et al. Intracerebral hemorrhage in a primate model: effect on regional blood flow. Surg Neurol 1988; 29:101–107.
46. Nehls DG, Mendelow AD, Graham DI, et al. Experimental intracerebral hemorrhage: progression of hemodynamic changes after production of a spontaneous mass lesion. Neurosurgery 1988; 23:439–444.
47. Nehls DG, Mendelow AD, Graham DI, et al. Experimental intracerebral hemorrhage: early removal of a spontaneous mass lesion improves late outcome. Neurosurgery 1990; 27:674–682.

48. Hirano T, Read SJ, Abbott DF, et al. No evidence of hypoxic tissue on 18F-fluoromisonidazole PET after intracerebral hemorrhage. Neurology 1999; 53:2179–2182.

49. Uemura K, Shishido F, Higano S, et al. Positron emission tomography in patients with a primary intracerebral hematoma. Acta Radiol Suppl 1986; 369:426–428.

50. Videen TO, Dunford-Shore JE, Diringer MN, et al. Correction for partial volume effects in regional blood flow measurements adjacent to hematomas in humans with intracerebral hemorrhage: implementation and validation. J Comput Assist Tomogr 1999; 23:248–256.

51. Zazulia AR, Diringer MN, Videen TO, et al. Hypoperfusion without ischemia surrounding acute intracerebral hemorrhage. J Cereb Blood Flow Metab 2001; 21:804–810.

52. Broderick J, Connolly S, Feldmann E, et al. Guidelines for the management of spontaneous intracerebral hemorrhage in adults: 2007 update: a guideline from the American Heart Association/American Stroke Association Stroke Council, High Blood Pressure Research Council, and the Quality of Care and Outcomes in Research Interdisciplinary Working Group. Stroke 2007; 38(6):2001–2023.

53. Meyer JS, Bauer RB. Medical treatment of spontaneous intracranial hemorrhage by the use of hypotensive drugs. Neurology 1962; 12:36–47.

54. Dandapani BK, Suzuki S, Kelley RE, et al. Relation between blood pressure and outcome in intracerebral hemorrhage. Stroke 1995; 26(1):21–24.

55. Qureshi AI, Wilson DA, Hanley DF, et al. Pharmacologic reduction of mean arterial pressure does not adversely affect regional cerebral blood flow and intracranial pressure in experimental intracerebral hemorrhage. Crit Care Med 1999; 27(5):965–971.

56. Qureshi AI, Mohammad YM, Yahia AM, et al. A prospective multicenter study to evaluate the feasibility and safety of aggressive antihypertensive treatment in patients with acute intracerebral hemorrhage. J Intensive Care Med 2005; 20(1):34–42.

57. Qureshi AI, Harris-Lane P, Kirmani JF, et al. Treatment of acute hypertension in patients with intracerebral hemorrhage using American Heart Association guidelines. Crit Care Med 2006; 34(7):1975–1980.

58. Neal B, MacMahon S, Chapman N. Effects of ACE inhibitors, calcium antagonists, and other blood-pressure-lowering drugs: results of prospectively designed overviews of randomised trials. Blood Pressure Lowering Treatment Trialists' Collaboration. Lancet 2000; 356(9246):1955–1964.

59. Chobanian AV, Bakris GL, Black HR, et al. National Heart, Lung, and Blood Institute Joint National Committee on Prevention, Detection, Evaluation, and Treatment of High Blood Pressure; National High Blood Pressure Education Program Coordinating Committee. The Seventh Report of the Joint National Committee on Prevention, Detection, Evaluation, and Treatment of High Blood Pressure: the JNC 7 report. JAMA 2003; 289(19):2560–2572.

60. Qureshi AI, Bliwise DL, Bliwise NG, et al. Rate of 24-hour blood pressure decline and mortality after spontaneous intracerebral hemorrhage: a retrospective analysis with a random effects regression model. Crit Care Med 1999; 27:480–485.

61. Janny P, Papo I, Chazal J, et al. Intracranial hypertension and prognosis of spontaneous intracerebral haematomas: a correlative study of 60 patients. Acta Neurochir (Wien) 1982; 61:181–186.

62. Papo I, Janny P, Caruselli G, et al. Intracranial pressure time course in primary intracerebral hemorrhage. Neurosurgery 1979; 4:504–511.

63. Diringer MN, Edwards DF. Admission to a neurologic/neurosurgical intensive care unit is associated with reduced mortality rate after intracerebral hemorrhage. Crit Care Med 2001; 29:635–640.

64. Bhardwaj A, Ulatowski JA. Cerebral edema: hypertonic saline solutions. Curr Treat Options Neurol 1999; 1:179–188.

65. Suarez JI, Qureshi AI, Bhardwaj A, et al. Treatment of refractory intracranial hypertension with 23.4% saline. Crit Care Med 1998; 26(6):1118–1122.

66. Bendo AA, Luba K. Recent changes in the management of intracranial hypertension. Int Anesthesiol Clin 2000; 38(4):69–85.

67. Schneider GH, Sarrafzadeh AS, Kiening KL, et al. Influence of hyperventilation on brain tissue-PO_2, PCO_2, and pH in patients with intracranial hypertension. Acta Neurochir Suppl 1998; 71:62–65.

68. Mendelow AD, Teasdale GM, Russell T, et al. Effect of mannitol on cerebral blood flow and cerebral perfusion pressure in human head injury. J Neurosurg 1985; 63(1):43–48.

69. Qureshi AI, Suarez JI. Use of hypertonic saline solutions in treatment of cerebral edema and intracranial hypertension. Crit Care Med 2000; 28(9):3301–3313.

70. Rockoff MA, Marshall LF, Shapiro HM. High-dose barbiturate therapy in humans: a clinical review of 60 patients. Ann Neurol 1979; 6(3):194–199.

71. Piatt JH Jr., Schiff SJ. High-dose barbiturate therapy in neurosurgery and intensive care. Neurosurgery 1984; 15(3):427–444.

72. Jiang J, Yu M, Zhu C. Effect of long-term mild hypothermia therapy in patients with severe traumatic brain injury: 1-year follow-up review of 87 cases. J Neurosurg 2000; 93:546–549.

73. Clifton GL, Miller ER, Choi SG, et al. Lack of effect of induction of hypothermia after acute brain injury. N Engl J Med 2001; 344:556–563.

74. Schwab S, Georgiadis D, Berrouschot J, et al. Feasibility and safety of moderate hypothermia after massive hemispheric infarction. Stroke 2001; 32:2033–2035.

75. Diringer MN. Intracerebral hemorrhage. Pathophysiology and management. Crit Car Med 1993; 21:1591–1603.

76. Liliang PC, Liang CL, Lu CH, et al. Hypertensive caudate hemorrhage prognostic predictor, outcome, and role of external ventricular drainage. Stroke 2001:32(5):1195–1200.

77. Mendelow AD, Gregson BA, Fernandes HM, et al. Early surgery versus initial conservative treatment in patients with spontaneous supratentorial intracerebral haematomas in the International Surgical Trial in Intracerebral Haemorrhage (STICH): a randomised trial. Lancet 2005; 365(9457):387–397.

78. Batjer HH, Reisch JS, Allen BC, et al. Failure of surgery to improve outcome in hypertensive putaminal hemorrhage: a prospective randomized trial. Arch Neurol 1990; 47:1103–1106.

79. Juvela S, Heiskanen O, Poranen A, et al. The treatment of spontaneous intracerebral hemorrhage: a prospective randomized trial of surgical and conservative treatment. J Neurosurg 1989; 70:755–758.

80. Auer LM, Deinsberger W, Niederkorn K, et al. Endoscopic surgery versus medical treatment for spontaneous intracerebral hematoma: a randomized study. J Neurosurg 1989; 70:530–535.

81. Morgenstern LB, Frankowski RF, Shedden P, et al. Surgical treatment for intracerebral hemorrhage (STICH): a single-center, randomized clinical trial. Neurology 1998; 51:1359–1363.

82. Chen HJ, Lee TC, Wei CP. Treatment of cerebellar infarction by decompressive suboccipital craniectomy. Stroke 1992; 23:957–961.
83. Teernstra OP, Evers SM, Lodder J, et al. Multicenter randomized controlled trial (SICHPA). Stereotactic treatment of intracerebral hematoma by means of a plasminogen activator: a multicenter randomized controlled trial (SICHPA). Stroke 2003; 34(4):968–974.

13

Diagnostic Evaluation of Aneurysmal Subarachnoid Hemorrhage

Jonathan A. Edlow, MD, FACEP, Vice Chairman[a] and Associate Professor[b]

[a]Department of Emergency Medicine, Beth Israel Deaconess Medical Center,
and [b]Department of Medicine, Harvard Medical School,
Boston, Massachusetts, U.S.A.

INTRODUCTION

In treating patients with aneurysmal subarachnoid hemorrhage (aSAH) the best outcomes are predicated on the early, correct diagnosis of patients who are in good clinical condition. Delay in treatment often results in early complications and worse outcomes (1,2); therefore, early diagnosis is the key. The foundations of the diagnosis of aSAH will be outlined in this chapter.

Nearly all awake patients with aSAH present with headache (3). The ability of the frontline physician to recognize that the patient has suffered an aSAH is hampered by the fact that headache is an extremely common chief complaint in an emergency department (ED) (4). Because most patients who present to the ED with the complaint of a headache have primary headache disorders (e.g., migraine or tension), extensive, urgent evaluation of the entire group for aSAH is inappropriate (5,6). On the other hand, a small percentage of these patients have far more serious pathology (4,7) (Table 1). In these cases, failure to diagnosis or a delay in diagnosis can lead to significant morbidity and mortality (8). aSAH is most commonly caused by trauma; of nontraumatic cases, 80% are due to ruptured intracranial aneurysms, which is the focus of this chapter (3).

Table 1 Life, Limb, Vision, or Brain-threatening Causes of Headache

Subarachnoid hemorrhage
Meningitis and encephalitis
Cervicocranial artery dissections
Temporal arteritis
Acute narrow angle closure glaucoma
Hypertensive emergencies
Carbon monoxide poisoning
Idiopathic intracranial hypertension (pseudotumor cerebri)
Cerebral venous and dural sinus thrombosis
Spontaneous intracranial hypotension
Acute strokes: hemorrhagic or ischemic
Pituitary apoplexy
Mass lesions
   Tumor
   Abscess
   Intracranial hematomas (parenchymal, subdural, epidural)
   Parameningeal infections
   Colloid cyst of third ventricle

Slightly less than 1% of all patients who present to the ED with headache have aSAH (4,7,9,10). Furthermore, several studies have shown that of neurologically normal patients with severe and acute-onset headaches, roughly 12% have aSAH (11–13). In a Canadian study of ED patients with lower acuity of headache (not abrupt onset and not necessarily "worst of life" in severity), 6.7% of headache patients had an aSAH (14).

Despite the widespread availability of neuroimaging equipment, misdiagnosis of aSAH has been surprisingly common, occurring in 25% to 50% of patients with aSAH on their first physician consultation. Misdiagnosis has been documented in many different settings over the past three decades (15–19). However, more recent studies suggest that this misdiagnosis rate may be falling. In 2004, a report of the largest single-institution data found a misdiagnosis rate of 12% (20), and in 2007, a population-based study found a misdiagnosis rate of 5.4% in patients seen in an ED in Ontario, Canada (21). These data suggest the possibility that increased scrutiny of the misdiagnosis phenomenon in emergency medicine has resulted in an improved rate of diagnosis (22). Another study in Japan found that doctor-related misdiagnosis is decreasing but that patient-related delays have increased, highlighting the need for better public education regarding stroke symptoms (23).

As with most conditions, aSAH is associated with a bell-shaped curve of presentations. The classic presentation (abrupt onset of a severe, unique, and distinctive headache that begins during exertion and is associated with neck pain, vomiting, and transient loss of consciousness) or a severe presentation (severe headache followed by overt neurologic deficits) poses few diagnostic problems (3).

Table 2 Reasons for Misdiagnosis of aSAH

Failure to know the spectrum of presentations of subarachnoid hemorrhage
  Not evaluating patients with unusual (for the patient) headaches
    Is the onset abrupt?
    Is the quality different from prior headaches?
    Is the severity greater than prior headaches?
    Are there associated symptoms that have been absent with prior headaches (such as
      vomiting, diplopia, syncope, or seizure)?
  Failure to appreciate that the headache can improve spontaneously or with nonnarcotic
    analgesics
  Overreliance on the classic presentation with misdiagnosis of
  Viral syndrome, viral meningitis, and gastroenteritis
  Migraine and tension-type headache
  Sinus-related headache
  Neck pain (rarely, back pain)
  Psychiatric diagnoses
  Focus on the secondary head injury (resulting from syncope and fall or car crash)
  Focus on the electrocardiographic abnormalities
  Focus on the elevated blood pressure
  Lack of knowledge of presentations of the unruptured aneurysm
Failure to understand the limitations of CT scans
  CT scans are less sensitive with increasing time from onset of headache.
  CT scans can be falsely negative with small volume bleeds (spectrum bias).
  Interpretation factors (expertise of physician reading the scan).
  Technical factors (Have thin cuts been taken at the base of the brain? Is motion artifact
    observed?)
  CT scans be falsely negative for blood at hematocrit level of <30%.
Failure to perform LP and correctly interpret cerebrospinal fluid findings
  Failure to do LP in patients with negative, equivocal, or suboptimal CT scans
  Failure to recognize that xanthochromia may be absent very early (<12 hr) and very late
    (>2 wks)
  Failure to realize that visual inspection for xanthochromia is less sensitive than
    measurement by spectrophotometry
  Failure to properly distinguish traumatic tap from true aSAH

The problem arises in those mildly affected patients, who account for nearly half of the total and who present on the left side of the curve. These awake, alert, and neurologically normal patients are simultaneously the most likely to be misdiagnosed and the most likely to benefit from early identification and definitive treatment (3). Three generic causes lead to misdiagnosis: failure to appreciate the spectrum of clinical presentation, failure to understand the limitations of computed tomography (CT), and failure to perform and correctly interpret the results of lumbar puncture (LP) (3,5,6) (Table 2). Improvements in identifying which patients should be evaluated for aSAH and how the workup should proceed would likely reduce the frequency of misdiagnoses.

WHO SHOULD BE EVALUATED?

Physicians must pay careful attention to four aspects of the patient history to best identify which patients with headache should be further evaluated for aSAH. While the severity of the headache is often reported as "worst ever," variability exists. Headaches from aSAH may improve spontaneously (24) or after administration of narcotic or nonnarcotic analgesics sumatriptan or prochlorperazine (25,26). Because the pathophysiologic mechanisms that mediate pain in the head are limited (27,28), interventions that relieve pain do not necessarily distinguish benign from serious causes. Therefore, pain relief alone should not be used as a criterion to exclude aSAH (or other serious neurologic problems) if the history is otherwise worrisome.

Most but not all patients with aSAH describe an abrupt onset of pain that often reaches maximal intensity within seconds. Onset frequently occurs during exercise or Valsalva maneuver, but it may begin at any time, including during quiet activity or even sleep (29). Perhaps the most useful historic element is the quality of the pain. Even when patients have frequent headaches from another cause, during careful evaluation, they describe the pain from aSAH as unique and distinct—somehow "different" from prior headaches (5). Headaches that are associated with vomiting, which may occur in primary headache disorders, should suggest the possibility of intracranial bleeding, especially if vomiting did not accompany prior episodes. Other associated symptoms, such as syncope, diplopia, and seizure make aSAH more likely (30).

Epidemiologic context is important. Alcohol (especially a recent binge), cigarette smoking, hypertension, and use of cocaine and other sympathomimetic drugs are risk factors for aSAH (31). Another strong risk factor is past or family history of aSAH. Various connective tissue disorders have also been associated with aSAH (8). Physical examination may disclose meningismus, cranial neuropathy, retinal or vitreous bleeding, or any other focal or generalized neurologic finding (5,6). Caused by meningeal irritation from blood, meningismus (nuchal rigidity) occurs in approximately 70% to 85% cases of aSAH, but may take hours to days to develop. In a series of 312 cases of aSAH, 50 (16%) had no stiffness on admission, while another 56 (18%) had slight or moderate stiffness (32). Third cranial nerve palsy may lead to limited ipsilateral eye movements and a dilated pupil. The pupil is dilated in the classic aneurysmal third cranial nerve palsy (also referred to as a "surgical third nerve") because the peripherally located pupillary constrictor fibers are more vulnerable to external compression (33). This third cranial nerve palsy is usually from a posterior communicating artery aneurysm; therefore, the finding is only present in 10% to 15% cases of aSAH (32,34). Funduscopy may disclose retinal hemorrhage (which may be the only clue of aSAH in comatose patients) and papilledema (which may suggest idiopathic intracranial hypertension or intracranial mass) (5,6). Importantly, physical examination may be entirely normal, and it is in this scenario that the diagnosis is most often missed.

After the history and physical examination, the physician must decide if further evaluation is necessary. If no plausible alternative hypothesis is indicated, the physician should proceed with further testing (5,6). Of particular note is that a first-ever severe headache cannot be confidently diagnosed as tension or migraine, both of which require multiple episodes before they can be definitively diagnosed (35). While it is true that all patients with these primary headache disorders must have their first episode at some point in time, they usually do not seek medical attention for them; if they do, these diagnoses cannot be definitively made on the first episode by history and physical examination alone.

EVALUATION FOR aSAH—CT SCANNING

Once the decision to pursue the diagnosis of aSAH is made, the current standard evaluation is straightforward (Fig. 1). The first test to be performed is the noncontrast cranial CT scan (3,5,6,36,37). While this test has revolutionized the diagnosis of aSAH, it has limitations (38). Spectrum bias occurs in patients with smaller bleeds, who are more likely to be conscious, well appearing, and to have normal scans (17). Also, errors in interpretation inevitably occur, especially in this mildly affected group (3). The sensitivity of CT decays rapidly with time (39). Even in the first 12 hour-posticctus, when CT displays excellent sensitivity (40–42), the confidence intervals are sufficiently wide for further testing to be recommended in patients with normal CT scans despite clinical suspicion of aSAH (38,43). Early studies demonstrated that by day 3, only 85% of patients with aSAH have abnormal CT scans and by one week, this figures drops to 50% (39). While evidence suggests that newer scanners have higher sensitivity (44), until this is confirmed, a negative CT should be followed by an LP in patients with clinical suspicion of aSAH. It is noteworthy that anemia (hematocrit <30), motion artifact, or other technical factors may cause falsely normal scans (3). In patients who have mild symptoms that present early, it should be realized that the factors that influence the CT sensitivity are conflicting. Early presenting patients are much more likely to have positive scans, while patients with mild symptoms are more likely to have normal scans. Therefore, the decision to solidify the diagnosis by performing an LP is appropriate in patients with a history that is consistent with aSAH but with a negative (or nondiagnostic) CT scan (38,40,43,45).

In patients with head injury, subarachnoid blood on the CT scan may be traumatic in origin; however, the possibility that a ruptured aneurysm caused the trauma must be considered (46,47). Location of the blood high on the cerebral convexities suggests a traumatic origin, whereas blood from a ruptured aneurysm is more likely to be in the basal cisterns. Because the literature contains several reports of nonaneurysmal aSAH cases with blood in atypical locations, clinicians must be careful in making decisions about which patients to further evaluate with vascular imaging, even when the blood is in the higher cortical areas (48,49). False-positive CTs are distinctly unusual but may occur in the setting of

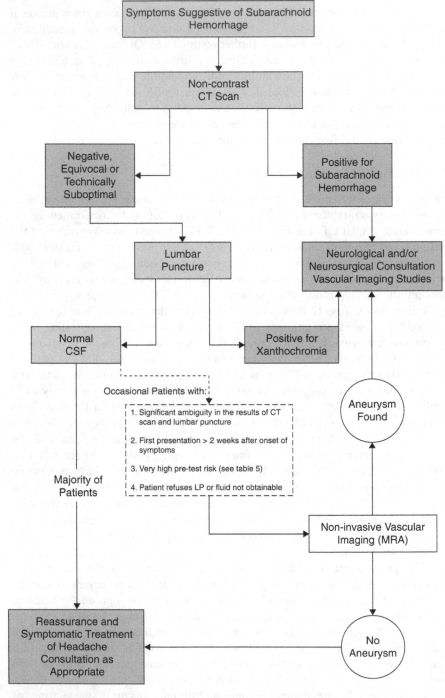

Figure 1 Flowchart showing symptoms of suggestive subarachnoid hemorrhage (courtesy Jonathan Edlow, copyright owner).

intravenous (IV) contrast neurotoxicity (50,51), purulent meningitis (52,53), spontaneous intracranial hypotension (54), bilateral subdural hematomas (55,56), and increased density of dural structures (57). In each of these settings, the next diagnostic steps—LP and/or specialist consultation—should lead to the correct diagnosis. Therefore, for patients with positive CT scans, immediate consultation with a cerebrovascular specialist is indicated. Whenever meningitis is a serious consideration, IV antibiotics should be administered promptly and should not be delayed by diagnostic testing (6). For patients with negative, equivocal, or suboptimal scans, LP is indicated (3,5,6).

EVALUATION FOR aSAH—LP

LP also has limitations, the most significant of which is the physician failing to perform one in the first place (11). Performing an LP will also diagnose the occasional patient with an atypical presentation of meningitis and other intracranial conditions. Careful attention to the technique may reduce the likelihood of traumatic puncture, which occurs in approximately 15% of cases (58). Measuring the opening pressure is helpful in distinguishing traumatic puncture from true aSAH, as two-thirds of patients with aSAH will demonstrate elevated pressure (32). Furthermore, elevated pressure may provide clues to other potential diagnoses, such as idiopathic intracranial hypertension and cerebral venous sinus thrombosis (1), and low pressure suggests the diagnosis of spontaneous intracranial hypotension (59). The cerebrospinal fluid (CSF) may contain erythrocytes [or red blood cells (RBCs)] and/or show xanthochromia, the yellow discoloration caused by hemoglobin breakdown products—primarily oxyhemoglobin and bilirubin.

Again, details are important. The results must also be interpreted in the context of time: how many hours have elapsed since the onset of headache? Just as time from ictus affects the sensitivity of CT, timing also affects the interpretation of the results of the CSF findings. RBCs are absent in LP samples done in the first minutes after aSAH but should be abundant in the ensuing hours. In Walton's classic work, all 21 of the 21 patients assessed by LP in the first four hours after the ictus were positive for blood (including 4 patients inside of 2 hours) (32) (Table 3). Rare case reports from the pre-CT era documented patients with aSAH without blood in the lumbar theca (60,61). The mechanisms in these cases were (*i*) aneurysmal rupture directly into the intraparenchymal or subdural compartments, and (*ii*) tonsillar herniation with CSF block. In each of these rare instances, modern CT scanning would be expected to be diagnostic. On average, RBCs gradually disappear over the course of 7 to 14 days (32,62), although exceptions exist on either end, and the disappearance of blood in the CSF has been reported as early as 24 hours after the ictus (32).

A specific threshold number of RBCs in the CSF below which aSAH is excluded has not been determined, and smaller bleeds obviously result in fewer cells. Anecdotally, aSAH has been reported in a patient with "a couple of

Table 3 Findings from CSF Analysis (from Walton's study)

Time from ictus (hours)	# of cases	Blood present	Xanthochromia present (not present; not recorded)
0–2	4	4	0
2–4	17	17	1(15 not; 1 NR)
4–6	28	28	16(9 not; 3 NR)
6–12	40	40	26(4 not; 10 NR)
12–24	35	32	31(0 not; 4 NR)
25–72	57	51	53(0 not; 4 NR)

hundred'' red cells in the CSF, but this low number is probably very unusual (63). Most patients will have many thousands of cells, but the time interval between the LP and the onset of the headache must be factored into this analysis.

Oxyhemoglobin can develop within hours, whereas bilirubin formation is an enzyme-dependent, in vivo process that requires time to develop (64,65). Xanthochromia can be assessed visually or by spectrophotometry (66). Some authorities recommend a delay of 12 hours before performing LP because xanthochromia, as measured by spectrophotometry, may not be present until this time (67,68). However, the particular study on which this recommendation is based was flawed (69): First, entry into the study required a positive CT scan. The patients in whom the significance of xanthochromia must be understood are those with negative CT scans, and they were not studied. Second, the study did not perform any LPs prior to 12 hours after the ictus; therefore, it was not designed to evaluate the utility of the earlier LP.

More recently, investigators have evaluated CSF spectrophotometry in the clinically relevant population of patients with negative CT scans (and normal physical examinations). They found that spectrophotometry resulted in the diagnosis of an aneurysm in 2% of 463 such patients; however, they did not compare spectrophotometry with visual inspection (70). In a survey of approximately 2500 North American hospital laboratories, 99.4% used the method of visual inspection (71). Therefore, waiting for 12 hours makes no sense if the clinical laboratory in the particular hospital uses visual inspection rather than spectrophotometry to measure xanthochromia. Furthermore, even when measured visually, many patients do have early xanthochromia. In Walton's series, which used visual inspection, one patient had xanthochromia within 4 hours of the ictus and of patients seen within four to six hours, 57% (16 of 28) had xanthochromia (32) (Table 3). In patients who presented between 6 and 12 hours after the ictus, this figure rose to 65% (26/40), which does not include 10 (of the 40) additional patients for whom the presence or absence of xanthochromia was not recorded. Thus, xanthochromia can occur very early, possibly from oxyhemoglobin. After 12 hours, nearly all had xanthochromia, suggesting that the kinetics of visually apparent versus spectrophotometrically apparent xanthochromia are quite similar. For all these reasons, some authors do not recommend the 12- hour delay (3,72).

Despite the fact that some claim that the human eye cannot reliably detect xanthochromia (73), recent data suggest that visual inspection is quite useful if a clinician sees the CSF as colorless (74). Furthermore, while spectrophotometry of CSF may be very sensitive, its specificity is quite low (11,75). If spectrophotometry were routinely used, it could lead to a significant increase in unnecessary cerebrovascular imaging and diagnoses of asymptomatic aneurysms (75). Practically speaking, in almost all patients with query aSAH, at least several hours will have passed from the onset of their headache until their LP, even if they rapidly seek medical attention. Time elapses as they are transported to an ED, triaged and registered, evaluated by a physician, and undergo a CT scan, which must then be interpreted. Bloody CSF will be present in all CT-negative early cases, and xanthochromia will be observed in many such cases (32). Physicians who decide to wait for 12 hours must weigh the risks of waiting, such as ultra-early rebleeding, against the benefit of improving diagnostic sensitivity of xanthochromia (76,77).

DISTINGUISHING TRAUMATIC LP FROM TRUE aSAH

Traumatic LP occurs when RBCs enter the CSF via needle trauma, and not from a preexisting aSAH. The visual threshold for seeing bloody fluid is approximately 400 RBCs/mm^3, and an arbitrary level frequently used to define a traumatic tap is 1000 cells (58,65,78). At this latter threshold, traumatic LP occurs approximately 10% of the time (58,78). At the threshold of 400 cells, the rate is 15% (58). Distinguishing traumatic LP from true aSAH is essential (65,79). Patients with traumatic LPs ideally should not be evaluated with expensive and potentially risky diagnostic tests, and patients with true aSAH should not be sent home with the diagnosis of traumatic LP. Traumatic LP can be distinguished from true aSAH via many potential methods (79). Many of these methods, such as analysis for crenated RBCs, or erythrophages, are without value, and others, such as D-dimer measurement, are of unproven value. Another method—repeating the LP at another interspace—is poorly studied and rarely done in practice but may be useful. An abnormal opening pressure suggests aSAH or other central nervous system pathology (see above).

The three-tube test, in which the RBC counts in successive tubes of CSF are compared, is commonly used. In a traumatic LP, the numbers will fall substantially from the first to the last tube. Ideally, for this test to be meaningful, the number of RBCs in the last tube should be close to or trend toward zero. One practical way to maximize the likelihood of this happening is to allow extra CSF to drain out between the first and last tubes (79). While the three-tube test has some value, it is clearly imperfect (65,80–82). If the number of RBCs in the final tube is not close to zero, it does not exclude the possibility of a simultaneous traumatic tap and an aSAH. Using the arbitrary reduction of 25% from the first to the last tube is not sufficiently sensitive (82).

Clearly, xanthochromia (when present) is the best way of distinguishing traumatic LP from true aSAH. Although many articles mention that visual inspection is only 50% sensitive (using spectrophotometry as the criterion standard) (3,66,83), these data are primarily based on one study that included only eight patients with aSAH (84) and one experimental study (85). It is logical that a machine is more accurate than the human eye, but the price of high sensitivity is markedly decreased specificity (11,75). Specific causes of false-positive xanthochromia are transported to the lab via a pneumatic tube, very high numbers of RBCs (from an LP), longer time from LP to CSF analysis, elevated serum bilirubin or CSF protein, hypercarotinemia, and rifampin use (65,86,87). Therefore, CSF samples should be rapidly taken to the lab, centrifuged, and analyzed, no matter how one measures for xanthochromia.

In the Walton study, all patients who presented in the first 12 hour (both with and without xanthochromia) had bloody CSF, although the specific numbers of RBCs were not reported (32). Therefore, patients presented within 12 hour of onset of headache will have bloody CSF and some will have xanthochromia (no matter how it is measured). Of patients who presented from 12 hour to 2 weeks after onset of headache, many will have RBCs and nearly all will have xanthochromia. After 2 weeks, almost none will show RBCs and the frequency of xanthochromia will begin to decline.

OTHER DIAGNOSTIC ISSUES

Can the Workup be Stopped in the Setting of Normal CT and CSF?

With the increasing availability of noninvasive cerebrovascular imaging, some investigators recommend angiography even when the CT scan and LP are both normal (88). Does this strategy make sense? In part, this sequence of tests stems from a 1986 report of a patient with a thunderclap headache who, despite a normal CT and LP, was diagnosed with a cerebral aneurysm and vasospasm (89). The aneurysm was treated, and the patient did not suffer further headaches. Since then at least five studies have examined groups of patients with thunderclap headaches and normal CTs and LPs (12,13,90–92). The results of all these studies are concordant; none of the approximately 300 patients pooled from these studies was found to have an aSAH or die suddenly during the months of follow-up. Therefore, although unruptured aneurysms can and do sometimes cause symptoms (93), stopping the workup in patients with negative test results is borne out by the literature. The patient in the 1986 study likely had an asymptomatic aneurysm and benign thunderclap headache, which has been associated with reversible cerebral vasospasm (94,95).

Other Imaging Options to Primarily Diagnose aSAH

Because of greater availability, lower cost, greater experience with its interpretation, and generally easier use in sick patients, CT remains the imaging study of choice for the diagnosis of aSAH (3,5,6). In many parts of the world, including many parts of North America, it is the de facto only choice. Furthermore, information, such as presence of a hematoma or hydrocephalus drives therapy. Nonetheless, MRI and MR angiography (MRA) (see below) are increasingly used. Several points are relevant when using MRI. First, it is important that the radiologist understands exactly what the clinician is looking for. Various acquisition sequences have differing abilities to detect acute blood. In both experimental and clinical studies, some have suggested that MRI, especially using fluid-attenuated inversion recovery (FLAIR) sequences, can reliably diagnose acute aSAH (96–100). As with CT, however, false positives (100) and false negatives can still occur (98), often in low-volume bleeds. At present, this tool is not the standard of care; however, in medical centers where both the equipment and expertise exist, it is possible that these modalities are clinically useful.

Other authors have suggested that CT angiography (CTA) can be used to diagnose aSAH (as opposed to being performed for surgical planning after establishing the diagnosis of aSAH) (88). Because asymptomatic aneurysms have prevalence in the general population of 2% to 6% (8), this practice could increase the amount of testing done on patients who harbor asymptomatic aneurysms without necessarily improving diagnosis of aSAH. Furthermore, the occasional patient whose diagnosis is made by CSF analysis would be missed if LP were not part of the diagnostic algorithm.

LP—FIRST STRATEGY

Some have advocated an LP-first strategy in carefully selected patients who have severe and acute-onset headaches and completely normal physical examinations (including vital signs and no stiff neck), whose LP is delayed by 12 hours from onset of headache, and in whom xanthochromia is measured by spectrophotometry (101). They argue that this strategy speeds ED throughput, decreases total resource utilization, and forces physicians to do the LP, which otherwise is frequently omitted in practice (11). Most of the studies that address this issue were conducted 20 years ago, when access to CT scanning was more restricted.

Some investigators have found performing LP first to be safe, even in patients who are Hunt and Hess grades 2 and 3, have meningismus, and may be drowsy (102,103). These investigators contend that early detection of bacterial meningitis is another reason to perform LP. Others suggest that this practice is unsafe because collecting CSF in those patients who have a ruptured aneurysm may precipitate rebleeding or herniation from an unrecognized intracranial hematoma (104,105), which can occur in the absence of localizing neurologic findings. Most of the patients who deteriorated in these two latter studies had neck stiffness and were Hunt and Hess grades 1–3 (mostly 2); however, one patient was documented to have no neck stiffness (104).

It is important to note that the justification for an LP-first strategy comes from mathematic modeling, not from clinical trials (101). At present, while this practice may well be safe in carefully selected patients, data are insufficient to broadly recommend a routine LP-first strategy. Physicians who use this strategy should be compulsive in patient selection, documentation of their medical decision making, and their discussions with the patient. They should pay meticulous attention to LP technique and understand the limitations of whatever tests are being used.

ANGIOGRAPHY

Once aSAH is diagnosed, the last diagnostic steps are vascular imaging (MRI, CT, or conventional cerebral angiography) to define the vascular lesion and consultation with a cerebrovascular specialist. All patients with positive CT scans or persistently bloody or xanthochromic CSF should undergo vascular imaging (3,5,6). In addition, vascular imaging should be performed in patients whose other tests are ambiguous, such as these early-presenting patients with bloody CSF but no xanthochromia, and patients who present more than two weeks beyond the original ictus whose CT scans and CSF findings may have normalized (3,5,6). Finding hemosiderin deposition by T2-weighted MRI may be useful in this latter group of patients (106). In addition (Fig. 1), clinicians should consider vascular imaging in patients with an extremely high likelihood of aSAH and in those from whom CSF cannot be obtained (6).

The criterion standard for vascular imaging remains digital subtraction angiography (DSA). Because of the decreased morbidity with, and major improvements in, hardware and software of noninvasive imaging (MRA and CTA), these modalities are being increasingly employed. Nevertheless, the neurologic and systemic morbidity of DSA in contemporary series is quite low (107,108). In one prospective series of nearly 3000 procedures, morbidity was reported in only 1.3% of cases, more than half of which were transient or reversible (108).

Regardless of the type of cerebrovascular imaging study, neuroradiologists may be more accurate than other physicians in interpreting the images (109). Some studies have cautioned about lower sensitivity for small aneurysms in the noninvasive studies (110–114); however, more germane are investigations that study the actual use of these modalities in series of patients with aSAH. Controversy exists regarding whether MRA or CTA should be used in place of DSA for surgical planning. Two recent studies suggest that MRA can replace DSA in the preoperative planning for aSAH patients (115,116). Importantly, some patients in both of those studies required DSA to resolve ambiguity based on the MRA alone, and these patients were identified on a case-by-case basis.

More data exist for CTA than for MRA. Again, some caution that CTA has much lower sensitivity for aneurysms that are less than 4 mm in size (113), while others have found that CTA has excellent sensitivity even for smaller aneurysms (117). Because of this issue of sensitivity at the lower size range, some authors argue that if the CTA shows a clinically appropriate lesion, it is sufficient, but if not, DSA ought to be performed (114,118). Four studies have evaluated a strategy

Table 4 Management Issues to be Addressed when aSAH is Diagnosed

1. Airway management, if relevant
2. Arranging an angiogram
3. Arranging for transfer to a neurovascular center, if appropriate
4. Treatment of hypertension
5. Volume status and IV fluids
6. Seizure prophylaxis
7. Acute treatment of hydrocephalus, extra-axial or intracerebral hematomas
8. Nimodipine administration for vasospasm prophylaxis
9. Discuss short-term antifibrinolytics to prevent rebleeding
10. Cardiac telemetry
11. Analgesia and anxiolytics
12. Intracranial pressure monitoring, if appropriate

of CTA-only for planning the surgical approach in large numbers of patients with aSAH (118–121). These studies demonstrate the feasibility of going directly to surgery with CTA as the only preoperative imaging data. As of 2007, this practice is in evolution and will depend on local resources, philosophy, and experience.

DISPOSITION AND TRANSITION TO IN-PATIENT CARE

If a patient's condition deteriorates after initial evaluation, repeat CT scans may show the reason; common findings include early hydrocephalus, rebleeding, intracranial hematoma, and brain infarction. Each of these has a different treatment strategy. Newer data strongly suggest that aSAH patients have substantially better outcomes when treated at medical centers that offer comprehensive cerebrovascular care, where surgical, endovascular, and neurocritical care specialists work in concert (122–124). Therefore, practitioners who diagnose patients with aSAH at hospitals that do not offer comprehensive cerebrovascular care should routinely transfer them to centers that do. Furthermore, once the diagnosis of aSAH is established, the treating physician should follow the guidance of the accepting cerebrovascular specialist regarding initial management issues, such as blood pressure and airway control, seizure and vasospasm prophylaxis, treatment of pain and anxiety, and possibly short-term agents to prevent early rebleeding, even if they are only used over a period of hours (125) (Table 4).

SUMMARY

Physicians should focus on specific elements of the patient history—onset, severity, quality of the headache, and associated symptoms—to decide which patients with headache ought to be evaluated for aSAH. The physical examination should be compulsive with regard to vital signs, head, retinal, neck, and neurologic examinations. At this juncture, the physician should form an explicit differential diagnosis and have specific reasons for diagnosing migraine, tension, or sinus headache and other benign causes.

If no alternative hypothesis is clear, the patient should be evaluated by CT and LP (if the CT is negative, equivocal, or technically inadequate). Physicians should understand the limitations of this diagnostic algorithm. The CSF should be carefully analyzed, including measuring the opening pressure. In patients whose CT scans and CSF analysis are normal, further testing is rarely indicated. Once aSAH has been diagnosed, vascular imaging to define the cause of the hemorrhage and specialty consultation are indicated.

REFERENCES

1. Broderick J, Brott T, Duldner J, et al. Initial and recurrent bleeding are the major causes of death following subarachnoid hemorrhage. Stroke 1994; 25:1342–1347.
2. Naidech AM, Janjua N, Kreiter KT, et al. Predictors and impact of aneurysm rebleeding after subarachnoid hemorrhage. Arch Neurol 2005; 62(3):410–416.
3. Edlow JA, Caplan LR. Avoiding pitfalls in the diagnosis of subarachnoid hemorrhage [comments]. N Engl J Med 2000; 342(1):29–36.
4. Goldstein JN, Camargo CA Jr., Pelletier AJ, et al. Headache in United States Emergency Departments: demographics, work-up and frequency of pathological diagnoses. Cephalalgia 2006; 26(6):684–690.
5. Edlow JA. Diagnosis of subarachnoid hemorrhage. Neurocrit Care 2005; 2(2):99–109.
6. Edlow JA. Diagnosis of subarachnoid hemorrhage in the emergency department. Emerg Med Clin North Am 2003; 21(1):73–87.
7. Ramirez-Lassepas M, Espinosa CE, Cicero JJ, et al. Predictors of intracranial pathologic findings in patients who seek emergency care because of headache. Arch Neurol 1997; 54(12):1506–1509.
8. Schievink WI. Intracranial aneurysms. N Engl J Med 1997; 336(1):28–40.
9. Dhopesh V, Anwar R, Herring C. A retrospective assessment of emergency department patients with complaints of headache. Headache 1979; 19:37–42.
10. Leicht M. Non-traumatic headache in the emergency department. Ann Emerg Med 1980; 9(8):404–409.
11. Morgenstern LB, Luna-Gonzales H, Huber JC Jr., et al. Worst headache and subarachnoid hemorrhage: prospective, modern computed tomography and spinal fluid analysis. Ann Emerg Med 1998; 32(3 pt 1):297–304.
12. Linn FH, Wijdicks EF, van der Graaf Y, et al. Prospective study of sentinel headache in aneurysmal subarachnoid haemorrhage. Lancet 1994; 344(8922):590–593.
13. Landtblom AM, Fridriksson S, Boivie J, et al. Sudden onset headache: a prospective study of features, incidence and causes. Cephalalgia 2002; 22(5):354–360.
14. Perry JJ, Stiell IG, Wells GA, et al. Attitudes and judgment of emergency physicians in the management of patients with acute headache. Acad Emerg Med 2005; 12(1):33–37.
15. Adams HP Jr., Jergenson DD, Kassell NF, et al. Pitfalls in the recognition of subarachnoid hemorrhage. Jama 1980; 244(8):794–796.

16. Kassell N, Kongable G, Torner J, Adams H, Mazuz H. Delay in referral of patients with ruptured aneurysms to neurosurgical attention. Stroke 1985; 16(4):587–590.

17. Kassell NF, Torner JC, Haley EC Jr., et al. The International Cooperative Study on the Timing of Aneurysm Surgery. Part 1: Overall management results. J Neurosurg 1990; 73(1):18–36.

18. Mayer PL, Awad IA, Todor R, et al. Misdiagnosis of symptomatic cerebral aneurysm: prevalence and correlation with outcome at four institutions. Stroke 1996; 27(9):1558–63.

19. Neil-Dwyer G, Lang D. 'Brain attack'—aneurysmal subarachnoid haemorrhage: death due to delayed diagnosis. J R Coll Physicians (London) 1997; 31(1):49–52.

20. Kowalski RG, Claassen J, Kreiter KT, et al. Initial misdiagnosis and outcome after subarachnoid hemorrhage. JAMA 2004; 291(7):866–869.

21. Vermeulen M, Schull MJ. Missed diagnosis of subarachnoid hemorrhage in the emergency department. Stroke 2007; 38(4):1216–1221.

22. Edlow JA. Diagnosis of subarachnoid hemorrhage—are we doing better? Stroke 2007; 8(4):1129–1131.

23. Miyazaki T, Ohta F, Moritake K, et al. The key to improving prognosis for aneurysmal subarachnoid hemorrhage remains in the pre-hospitalization period. Surg Neurol 2006; 65(4):360–365 (discussion 5–6).

24. Liedo A, Calandre L, Martinez-Menendez B, et al. Acute headache of recent onset and subarachnoid hemorrhage: a prospective study. Headache 1994; 34(4):172–74.

25. Pfadenhauer K, Schönsteiner T, Keller H. The risks of sumatriptan administration in patients with unrecognized subarachnoid haemorrhage (SAH). Cephalalgia 2006; 26(3):320–323.

26. Seymour JJ, Moscati RM, Jehle DV. Response of headaches to nonnarcotic analgesics resulting in missed intracranial hemorrhage. Am J Emerg Med 1995; 13(1):43–45.

27. Moskowitz MA, Henrikson BM, Markowitz S. Experimental studies on the sensory innervation of the cerebral blood vessels. Cephalalgia 1986; 6 (suppl 4):63–66.

28. Limmroth V, Cutrer FM, Moskowitz MA. Neurotransmitters and neuropeptides in headache. Curr Opin Neurol 1996; 9(3):206–210.

29. Schievink WI, Karemaker JM, Hageman LM, et al. Circumstances surrounding aneurysmal subarachnoid hemorrhage. Surg Neurol 1989; 32(4):266–272.

30. Linn F, Rinkel G, Algra A, et al. Headache characteristics in subarachnoid hemorrhage and benign thunderclap headache. J Neurol, Neurosurg Psychiatry 1998; 65:791–793.

31. Feigin VL, Rinkel GJ, Lawes CM, et al. Risk factors for subarachnoid hemorrhage: an updated systematic review of epidemiological studies. Stroke 2005; 36(12):2773–2780.

32. Walton J. Subarachnoid hemorrhage. Edinburgh: E & S Livingstone Ltd 1956.

33. Woodruff M, Edlow JA. Evaluation of third nerve palsy in the emergency department. J Emerg Med 2007 (in press).

34. Sarner M, Rose F. Clinical presentation of ruptured intracranial aneurysm. J Neurol Neurosurg Pschiat 1967; 30:67–70.

35. Anonymous. Classification and diagnostic criteria for headache disorders, cranial neuralgias and facial pain. Cephlalgia 1988; 8(suppl.7):1–73.

36. Findlay JM. Current management of aneurysmal subarachnoid hemorrhage guidelines from the Canadian Neurosurgical Society. Can J Neurol Sci 1997; 24(2):161–170.

37. Mayberg MR, Batjer HH, Dacey R, et al. Guidelines for the management of aneurysmal subarachnoid hemorrhage. Stroke 1994; 25(11):2315–2328.

38. Edlow JA, Wyer PC. How good is a negative cranial computed tomographic scan result in excluding subarachnoid hemorrhage? Ann Emerg Med 2000; 36(5):507–516.

39. van Gijn J, van Dongen K. The time course of aneurysmal haemorrhage on computed tomograms. Neuroradiology 1982; 23:153–156.

40. van der Wee N, Rinkel GJ, Hasan D, et al. Detection of subarachnoid haemorrhage on early CT: is lumbar puncture still needed after a negative scan? J Neurol Neurosurg Psychiatry 1995; 58(3):357–359.

41. Sames TA, Storrow AB, Finkelstein JA, Magoon MR. Sensitivity of new-generation computed tomography in subarachnoid hemorrhage. Acad Emerg Med 1996; 3(1): 16–20.

42. Sidman R, Connolly E, Lemke T. Subarachnoid hemorrhage diagnosis: lumbar puncture is still needed when the computed tomography scan is normal. Acad Emerg Med 1996; 3(9):827–831.

43. Prosser RL Jr., Feedback: computed tomography for subarachnoid hemorrhage. Which review should we believe regarding the diagnostic power of computed tomography for ruling out subarachnoid hemorrhage? Ann Emerg Med 2001; 37(6): 679–680 (discussion 680–685).

44. Boesiger BM, Shiber JR. Subarachnoid hemorrhage diagnosis by computed tomography and lumbar puncture: are fifth generation CT scanners better at identifying subarachnoid hemorrhage? J Emerg Med 2005; 29(1):23–27.

45. Hoffman JR. Computed tomography for subarachnoid hemorrhage: what should we make of the "evidence"? Ann Emerg Med 2001; 37(3):345–349.

46. Sakas DE, Dias LS, Beale D. Subarachnoid haemorrhage presenting as head injury. BMJ 1995; 310(6988):1186–1187.

47. Vos PE, Zwienenberg M, O'Hannian KL, et al. Subarachnoid haemorrhage following rupture of an ophthalmic artery aneurysm presenting as traumatic brain injury. Clin Neurol Neurosurg 2000; 102(1):29–32.

48. Spitzer C, Mull M, Rohde V, et al. Non-traumatic cortical subarachnoid haemorrhage: diagnostic work-up and aetiological background. Neuroradiology 2005; 47(7):525–531.

49. Patel KC, Finelli PF. Nonaneurysmal convexity subarachnoid hemorrhage. Neurocrit Care 2006; 4(3):229–233.

50. Sharp S, Stone J, Beach R. Contrast agent neurotoxicity presenting as subarachnoid hemorrhage [comments]. Neurology 1999; 52(7):1503–1505.

51. Velden J, Milz P, Winkler F, et al. Nonionic contrast neurotoxicity after coronary angiography mimicking subarachnoid hemorrhage. Eur Neurol 2003; 49(4):249–251.

52. Mendelsohn DB, Moss ML, Chason DP, et al. Acute purulent leptomeningitis mimicking subarachnoid hemorrhage on CT. J Comput Assist Tomogr 1994; 18(1): 126–128.

53. Chatterjee T, Gowardman JR, Goh TD. Pneumococcal meningitis masquerading as subarachnoid haemorrhage. Med J Aust 2003; 178(10):505–507.

54. Schievink WI, Maya MM, Tourje J, et al. Pseudo-subarachnoid hemorrhage: a CT-finding in spontaneous intracranial hypotension. Neurology 2005; 65(1):135–137.

55. Huang D, Abe T, Ochiai S, et al. False positive appearance of subarachnoid hemorrhage on CT with bilateral subdural hematomas. Radiat Med 1999; 17(6): 439–442.

56. Rabinstein AA, Pittock SJ, Miller GM, et al. Pseudosubarachnoid haemorrhage in subdural haematoma. J Neurol Neurosurg Psychiatry 2003; 74(8):1131–1132.
57. Spiegel SM, Fox AJ, Vinuela F, et al. Increased density of tentorium and falx: a false positive CT sign of subarachnoid hemorrhage. Can Assoc Radiol J 1986; 37(4):243–247.
58. Shah KH, Richard KM, Nicholas S, Edlow JA. Incidence of traumatic lumbar puncture. Acad Emerg Med 2003; 10(2):151–154.
59. Schievink WI. Spontaneous spinal cerebrospinal fluid leaks and intracranial hypotension. JAMA 2006; 295(19):2286–2296.
60. Voris H. Subarachnoid hemorrhage. Illinois Medical Journal 1949; 95:160–167.
61. Wolfe H. Spontaneous subarachnoid hemorrhage. British Journal of Surgery 1955; 50:319–325.
62. Richardson J, Hyland H. Intracranial aneurysms. Medicine (Baltimore) 1941; 20:1–83.
63. Weir B. Diagnostic aspects of subarachnoid hemorrhage. In: Weir B, ed. Subarachnoid Hemorrhage: causes and cures. New York: Oxford University Press, 1998:144–176.
64. Roost KT, Pimstone NR, Diamond I, et al. The formation of cerebrospinal fluid xanthochromia after subarachnoid hemorrhage. Neurology 1972; 22:973–977.
65. Fishman R. Chapter 8: Composition of the Cerebrospinal Fluid. 2nd ed. Philadelphia: WB Saunders, 1992.
66. Beetham R, Fahie-Wilson MN, Park D. What is the role of CSF spectrophotometry in the diagnosis of subarachnoid haemorrhage? Ann Clin Biochem 1998; 35 (pt 1): 1–4.
67. van Gijn J. Slip-ups in diagnosis of subarachnoid haemorrhage. Lancet 1997; 349(9064):1492.
68. Vermeulen M. Subarachnoid haemorrhage: diagnosis and treatment. J Neurol 1996; 243(7):496–501.
69. Vermeulen M, Hasan D, Blijenberg BG, et al. Xanthochromia after subarachnoid haemorrhage needs no revisitation. J Neurol Neurosurg Psychiatry 1989; 52(7): 826–828.
70. Gunawardena H, Beetham R, Scolding N, et al. Is cerebrospinal fluid spectrophotometry useful in CT scan-negative suspected subarachnoid haemorrage? Eur Neurol 2004; 52(4):226–229.
71. Edlow JA, Bruner KS, Horowitz GL. Xanthochromia. Arch Pathol Lab Med 2002; 126(4):413–415.
72. Gerber CJ, Crawford P, Mendelow AD, et al. Lumbar puncture should not be delayed in subarachnoid haemorrhage [letter; comment]. BMJ 1998; 317(7151): 148.
73. Petzold A, Keir G, Sharpe TL. Why human color vision cannot reliably detect cerebrospinal fluid xanthochromia. Stroke 2005; 36(6):1295–1297.
74. Linn FH, Voorbij HA, Rinkel GJ, et al. Visual inspection versus spectrophotometry in detecting bilirubin in cerebrospinal fluid. J Neurol Neurosurg Psychiatry 2005; 76(10):1452–1454.
75. Perry JJ, Sivilotti ML, Stiell IG, et al. Should spectrophotometry be used to identify xanthochromia in the cerebrospinal fluid of alert patients suspected of having subarachnoid hemorrhage? Stroke 2006; 37(10):2467–2472.
76. Inagawa T. Effect of ultra-early referral on management outcome in subarachnoid haemorrhage. Acta Neurochir (Wien) 1995; 136(1–2):51–61.

77. Ohkuma H, Tsurutani H, Suzuki S. Incidence and significance of early aneurysmal rebleeding before neurosurgical or neurological management. Stroke 2001; 32(5): 1176–1180.

78. Eskey CJ, Ogilvy CS. Fluoroscopy-guided lumbar puncture: decreased frequency of traumatic tap and implications for the assessment of CT-negative acute subarachnoid hemorrhage. AJNR Am J Neuroradiol 2001; 22(3):571–576.

79. Shah KH, Edlow JA. Distinguishing traumatic lumbar puncture from true subarachnoid hemorrhage. J Emerg Med 2002; 23(1):67–74.

80. Buruma OJS, Janson HLF, den Bergh FAJTM, et al. Blood-stained cerebrospinal fluid: traumatic puncture or haemorrhage. J Neurol Neurosurg Psychiatry 1981; 44: 144–147.

81. Tourtellotte W, Somers J, Parker J, et al. A study of traumatic lumbar punctures. Neurology 1958; 8:129–134.

82. Heasley DC, Mohamed MA, Yousem DM. Clearing of red blood cells in lumbar puncture does not rule out ruptured aneurysm in patients with suspected subarachnoid hemorrhage but negative head CT findings. AJNR Am J Neuroradiol 2005; 26(4):820–824.

83. Beetham R, Fahie-Wilson MN, Holbrook I, et al. CSF spectrophotometry in the diagnosis of subarachnoid haemorrhage. J Clin Pathol 2002; 55(6):479–480 (author reply 80).

84. Soderstrom CE. Diagnostic significance of CSF spectrophotometry and computer tomography in cerebrovascular disease. A comparative study in 231 cases. Stroke 1977; 8(5):606–612.

85. Sidman R, Spitalnic S, Demelis M, et al. Xanthrochromia? By what method? A comparison of visual and spectrophotometric xanthrochromia. Ann Emerg Med 2005; 46(1):51–55.

86. Wenham PR, Hanson T, Ashby JP. Interference in spectrophotometric analysis of cerebrospinal fluid by haemolysis induced by transport through a pneumatic tube system. Ann Clin Biochem 2001; 38(pt 4):371–375.

87. Graves P, Sidman R. Xanthochromia is not pathognomonic for subarachnoid hemorrhage. Acad Emerg Med 2004; 11(2):131–135.

88. Carstairs SD, Tanen DA, Duncan TD, et al. Computed tomographic angiography for the evaluation of aneurysmal subarachnoid hemorrhage. Acad Emerg Med 2006; 13(5):486–492.

89. Day JW, Raskin NH. Thunderclap headache: symptom of unruptured cerebral aneurysm. Lancet 1986; 2(8518):1247–1248.

90. Harling DW, Peatfield RC, van Hille PT, et al. Thunderclap headache: is it migraine? Cephalgia 1989; 9:87–90.

91. Markus HS. A prospective follow-up of thunderclap headache mimicking subarachnoid hemorrhage. J Neurol Neurosurg Psychiatry 1991; 54:1117–1125.

92. Wijdicks EFM, Kerkhoff H, van Gijn J. Long-term follow-up of 71 patients with thunderclap headache mimicking subarachnoid hemorrhage. Lancet 1988; 2(8602): 68–69.

93. Raps EC, Rogers JD, Galetta SL, et al. The clinical spectrum of unruptured intracranial aneurysm. Arch Neurol 1993; 50:265–268.

94. Calabrese LH, Dodick DW, Schwedt TJ, et al. Narrative review: reversible cerebral vasoconstriction syndromes. Ann Intern Med 2007; 146(1):34–44.

95. Slivka A, Philbrook B. Clinical and angiographic features of thunderclap headache. Headache 1995; 35(1):1–6.
96. Mitchell P, Wilkinson ID, Hoggard N, et al. Detection of subarachnoid haemorrhage with magnetic resonance imaging. J Neurol Neurosurg Psychiatry 2001; 70(2): 205–211.
97. Rumboldt Z, Kalousek M, Castillo M. Hyperacute subarachnoid hemorrhage on T2-weighted MR images. AJNR Am J Neuroradiol 2003; 24(3):472–475.
98. Woodcock RJ Jr., Short J, Do HM, et al. Imaging of acute subarachnoid hemorrhage with a fluid-attenuated inversion recovery sequence in an animal model: comparison with non-contrast-enhanced CT. AJNR Am J Neuroradiol 2001; 22(9):1698–1703.
99. Wiesmann M, Mayer TE, Yousry I, et al. Detection of hyperacute subarachnoid hemorrhage of the brain by using magnetic resonance imaging. J Neurosurg 2002; 96(4):684–689.
100. Dechambre SD, Duprez T, Grandin CB, et al. High signal in cerebrospinal fluid mimicking subarachnoid haemorrhage on FLAIR following acute stroke and intravenous contrast medium. Neuroradiology 2000; 42(8):608–611.
101. Schull MJ. Lumbar puncture first: an alternative model for the investigation of lone acute sudden headache. Acad Emerg Med 1999; 6(2):131–136.
102. French JK, Glasgow GL. Lumbar puncture in subarachnoid haemorrhage: yes or no? N Z Med J 1985; 98(779):383–384.
103. Patel MK, Clarke MA. Lumbar puncture and subarachnoid haemorrhage. Postgrad Med J 1986; 62(733):1021–1024.
104. Hillman J. Should computered tomography scanning replace lumbar puncture in the diagostic process in suspected subarachnoid hemorrhage? Surg Neurol 1986; 26:547–550.
105. Duffy GP. The warning leak in spontaneous subarachnoid haemorrhage. Med J Aust 1983; 1:514–516.
106. Imaizumi T, Chiba M, Honma T, et al. Detection of hemosiderin deposition by T2*-weighted MRI after subarachnoid hemorrhage. Stroke 2003; 34(7):1693–1698.
107. Cloft HJ, Joseph GJ, Dion JE. Risk of cerebral angiography in patients with subarachnoid hemorrhage, cerebral aneurysm, and arteriovenous malformation: a meta-analysis. Stroke 1999; 30(2):317–320.
108. Willinsky RA, Taylor SM, TerBrugge K, et al. Neurologic complications of cerebral angiography: prospective analysis of 2,899 procedures and review of the literature. Radiology 2003; 227(2):522–528.
109. White PM, Wardlaw JM, Lindsay KW, et al. The non-invasive detection of intracranial aneurysms: are neuroradiologists any better than other observers? Eur Radiol 2003; 13(2):389–396.
110. White PM, Teasdale EM, Wardlaw JM, Easton V. Intracranial aneurysms: CT angiography and MR angiography for detection prospective blinded comparison in a large patient cohort. Radiology 2001; 219(3):739–749.
111. White PM, Wardlaw JM, Easton V. Can noninvasive imaging accurately depict intracranial aneurysms? A systematic review. Radiology 2000; 217(2):361–370.
112. Johnson MR, Good CD, Penny WD, et al. Lesson of the week: playing the odds in clinical decision making: lessons from berry aneurysms undetected by magnetic resonance angiography. BMJ 2001; 322(7298):1347–1349.
113. Teksam M, McKinney A, Casey S, et al. Multi-section CT angiography for detection of cerebral aneurysms. AJNR Am J Neuroradiol 2004; 25(9):1485–1492.

114. Dammert S, Krings T, Moller-Hartmann W, et al. Detection of intracranial aneurysms with multislice CT: comparison with conventional angiography. Neuroradiology 2004; 46(6):427–434.

115. Westerlaan HE, van der Vliet AM, Hew JM, et al. Magnetic resonance angiography in the selection of patients suitable for neurosurgical intervention of ruptured intracranial aneurysms. Neuroradiology 2004; 46(11):867–875.

116. Sato M, Nakano M, Sasanuma J, et al. Preoperative cerebral aneurysm assessment by three-dimensional magnetic resonance angiography: feasibility of surgery without conventional catheter angiography. Neurosurgery 2005; 56(5):903–912 (discussion 12).

117. Jayaraman MV, Mayo-Smith WW, Tung GA, et al. Detection of intracranial aneurysms: multi-detector row CT angiography compared with DSA. Radiology 2004; 230(2):510–518.

118. Caruso R, Colonnese C, Elefante A, et al. Use of spiral computerized tomography angiography in patients with cerebral aneurysm. Our experience. J Neurosurg Sci 2002; 46(1):4–9 (discussion 9)

119. Boet R, Poon WS, Lam JM, et al. The surgical treatment of intracranial aneurysms based on computer tomographic angiography alone—streamlining the acute mananagement of symptomatic aneurysms. Acta Neurochir (Wien) 2003; 145(2): 101–105 (discussion 5).

120. Hoh BL, Cheung AC, Rabinov JD, et al. Results of a prospective protocol of computed tomographic angiography in place of catheter angiography as the only diagnostic and pretreatment planning study for cerebral aneurysms by a combined neurovascular team. Neurosurgery 2004; 54(6):1329–1340 (discussion 40–2).

121. Pechlivanis I, Schmieder K, Scholz M, et al. 3-Dimensional computed tomographic angiography for use of surgery planning in patients with intracranial aneurysms. Acta Neurochir (Wien) 2005; 147(10):1045–1053 (discussion 53).

122. Berman MF, Solomon RA, Mayer SA, et al. Impact of hospital-related factors on outcome after treatment of cerebral aneurysms. Stroke 2003; 34(9):2200–2207.

123. Bardach NS, Zhao S, Gress DR, et al. Association between subarachnoid hemorrhage outcomes and number of cases treated at California hospitals. Stroke 2002; 33(7):1851–1856.

124. Johnston SC. Effect of endovascular services and hospital volume on cerebral aneurysm treatment outcomes. Stroke 2000; 31(1):111–117.

125. Hillman J, Fridriksson S, Nilsson O, et al. Immediate administration of tranexamic acid and reduced incidence of early rebleeding after aneurysmal subarachnoid hemorrhage: a prospective randomized study. J Neurosurg 2002; 97(4):771–778.

14

Surgical Versus Endovascular Aneurysm Exclusion

Aaron W. Grossman, PhD, Medical Student
University of Illinois College of Medicine at Urbana-Champaign, Urbana, Illinois, U.S.A.

Anil V. Yallapragada, MD, Resident
Department of Internal Medicine, SUNY Downstate Medical Center, Brooklyn, New York, U.S.A.

Giuseppe Lanzino, MD, Professor
Department of Neurological Surgery, Mayo Clinic College of Medicine, Rochester, Minnesota, U.S.A.

INTRODUCTION

Surgical clipping is considered the "gold standard" in the treatment of intracranial aneurysms, ruptured and unruptured, and it has been proven to be effective in preventing aneurysmal growth and rupture. Despite technical advances, however, aneurysm surgery remains quite challenging, even in the most experienced hands. Moreover, in the setting of subarachnoid hemorrhage (SAH), the swollen brain poorly tolerates even the most gentle surgical manipulation. These challenges have stimulated a constant search for "less-invasive" therapeutic modalities.

Pioneering efforts to treat aneurysms from an endovascular route have been attempted for many years (1–4). It was not until the early 1990s that, with the introduction of the Guglielmi detachable coil, intracranial aneurysms could be safely and effectively treated from the endovascular route. Following the introduction of detachable coils, numerous technical advances have occurred. Newer coils of various sizes and shapes and with different coating materials have been introduced in an attempt to increase the likelihood of aneurysm obliteration. In addition, the availability of adjuvant techniques to coiling such as "balloon-assisted" or "stent-assisted" techniques has broadened the indications for endovascular treatment to include large and wide-necked aneurysms not optimally obliterated with coils alone (5,6).

In the setting of an SAH, endovascular embolization allows obliteration of the aneurysm without any external brain or vessel manipulation. These characteristics have made endovascular treatment particularly appealing in elderly patients, patients with poor neurologic baseline, patients with significant systemic comorbidities, and patients with aneurysms posing particular surgical challenges such as those located at the basilar bifurcation (7). However, a major limitation of endovascular treatment is the risk of aneurysmal recanalization and recurrence, which requires mid- and long-term neuroimaging surveillance and possibly retreatment. In the past decade, a heated debate has arisen regarding the best treatment for ruptured and unruptured intracranial aneurysms: surgical or endovascular? In this chapter, we discuss the indications for either treatment modality, with particular emphasis on the treatment of ruptured aneurysms.

CURRENT STATUS OF NEUROSURGICAL TREATMENT

Since Walter Dandy's first surgical occlusion of an intracranial aneurysm (8), significant advances have been made in the surgical treatment of this condition. The introduction of the surgical microscope, advances in neuroanesthesia and perioperative management, and more recently, the introduction of skull-base approaches to minimize the degree of brain retraction during clipping of complex aneurysms have allowed many centers to achieve good outcome in most patients who undergo surgical repair of an intracranial aneurysm. Yet, the surgical procedure remains invasive and, especially in the setting of SAH, poorly tolerated. Although excellent outcomes have been reported at several highly specialized centers, a more realistic snapshot of the current status of surgery for ruptured intracranial aneurysms can be extrapolated from the Intraoperative Hypothermia for Aneurysm Surgery Trial (IHAST), a multicentered study that was designed to test whether mild hypothermia can be neuroprotective in the setting of surgical treatment of aneurysmal SAH (aSAH) (9). Since the study did not show any difference between the two experimental groups, the results can be considered together to obtain a view of the current status of surgical treatment across a wide spectrum of academic medical centers in North America, Europe, and Australia.

Between February 2000 and April 2003, 1001 nonobese patients (body mass index < 35) considered to have a good neurologic grade were enrolled.

Good neurologic grade was defined as a modified Rankin Score (mRS) of 0 or 1 before hemorrhage and World Federation of Neurosurgical Societies (WFNS) grades I–III on admission. All patients experienced SAH no more than 14 days before treatment (although 90% of patients were treated within 7 days of SAH) and received surgical clipping of the ruptured aneurysm. Just prior to treatment, patients were randomized to receive either intraoperative hypothermia (33°C) or no change in temperature during the procedure.

The average patient age was 51.5 years, and twice as many women as men participated in the study. Of all aneurysms, 35.5% were anterior communicating artery (ACom) aneurysms, 23.5% were posterior communicating artery (PCom) aneurysms, 21% were middle cerebral artery (MCA) aneurysms, 5.5% were vertebrobasilar aneurysms, and 14.5% were associated with other vessels. During surgery, a temporary clip was applied to the parent vessel 44.5% of the time, occluding the vessel for an average of 10.5 minutes. Perioperatively, moderate brain swelling was observed on dural opening 37% of the time, and the aneurysm leaked or ruptured in 31.5% of cases.

A neurologic exam performed 24 hours after surgery revealed a postoperative deterioration from baseline ($\geq$ 4 points on the NIH Stroke Scale) in 28% of patients. Study participants stayed an average of 6 ± 5 days in the intensive care unit and 16 ± 10 days in the hospital; 60% of patients were discharged home. Out of 1001 patients, 47 died in the hospital (in-hospital mortality rate of 4.7%). Perioperative and postoperative complications included delayed ischemic neurologic deficits in 22.5% of patients, cerebral infarction in 28%, brain swelling in 25%, and congestive heart failure or pulmonary edema in 11%. Overall, 6.5% of patients experienced severe hemorrhage during or soon after surgery, and 32.5% of patients required red blood cell transfusions at some point during surgery or recovery. Infectious complications included urinary tract infections (16.5% of patients), pneumonia (7%), meningitis or ventriculitis (5%), and incision or bone-flap infection (2%). Complication rates did not differ between the hypothermia and normothermia groups, except for the rate of bacteremia, which was higher in the hypothermic group (5% vs. 3%).

Approximately 90 days after surgery, patients were contacted and their condition was evaluated. Using the mRS, 65% of patients rated themselves as having mild or no neurologic disability (mRS = 0 or 1). On the Glasgow Outcome Scale, 64% of patients had a score of 1, indicating minor or no disability. Moderate disability was noted in 21% of patients, and severe disability was noted in 8%. Only one patient out of 1000 available for follow-up was in a persistent vegetative state (Glasgow Outcome Scale score = 4), and 61 patients had passed away since treatment, for an overall mortality of 10% (including patients who died during the first admission). No differences on outcome measures were noted between hypothermia and normothermia groups. Consistent with other studies of surgical treatment of aneurysms, increasing age, worse WFNS and Fisher grades on admission, and temporary clipping of the parent vessel were all associated with worse outcome (9).

STUDIES THAT COMPARE SURGERY TO ENDOVASCULAR TREATMENT

The first large-scale multicentered study of endovascular treatment in patients with intracranial aneurysms was published in 1997 and reported on data that were collected at eight participating centers as part of the multicentered study that eventually led to approval of the Guglielmi detachable coil system by the Food and Drug Administration (10).

Following that report, endovascular treatment became an accepted treatment modality as an alternative to surgery in patients who are considered to be high-risk surgical candidates. In the mid to late 1990s, numerous investigators began reporting their experiences in high-risk surgical patients, focusing on locations that were traditionally considered to be surgical challenges (particularly the basilar bifurcation), with excellent clinical and angiographic results (e.g., 11). As the techniques evolved and an increasing number of centers were obtaining adequate experience, it became clear that a study to compare endovascular treatment to surgical treatment "head-to-head" was required to address in a scientific manner some of the outstanding questions regarding efficacy.

Two prospective randomized clinical trials have compared surgical ligation with endovascular coiling of ruptured intracranial aneurysms. The first was conducted in Finland between February 1995 and August 1997 (12). The authors enrolled 109 patients with intracranial aneurysms that had ruptured less than 72 hours earlier. To be enrolled, patients had to have aneurysms that could be obliterated using either of the two treatment modalities, and patients were randomly assigned to surgery ($n = 57$) or coil embolization ($n = 52$). Seventy patients evaluated for treatment during the same period were not included in the study because their condition precluded one of the two modalities. Initial angiographic assessment revealed statistically significant benefits of surgery over embolization for anterior circulation aneurysms and benefits of embolization over surgery for posterior circulation aneurysms. Three months following treatment, patient outcome was assessed using the Glasgow Outcome Scale; good or moderate recovery was achieved in 79% of patients assigned to surgery and in 81% of patients assigned to embolization (12). Though not statistically significant, these results indicated that the newly emerging endovascular techniques could yield clinical outcome comparable to surgical ligation. At follow-up one year after treatment, patient survival was not significantly different between the two groups, and no group differences in neuropsychologic measures were noted in patients with good clinical recovery (13).

Following the Finnish study, the International Subarachnoid Aneurysm Trial (ISAT) was initiated (14). ISAT remains the largest prospective randomized clinical trial to compare neurosurgical clipping versus endovascular coiling in the treatment of ruptured intracranial aneurysms. The authors enrolled 2143 patients who presented with aSAH from a ruptured intracranial aneurysm that could have been treated with either modality. Most of the patients randomized into the trial were considered to have good neurologic grade (88% had WFNS

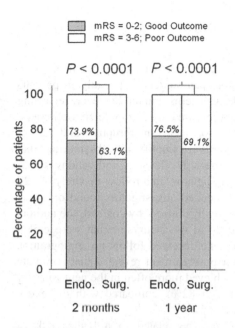

Figure 1 Two-month and one-year outcomes after surgical and endovascular treatment of ruptured intracranial aneurysms in ISAT. *Abbreviations*: mRS, modified Rankin Scale; ISAT, International Subarachnoid Aneurysm Trial. *Source*: From Ref. 15.

grades I and II), most patients had anterior circulation aneurysms (97.3%), and most aneurysms were small in size (93% were < 11 mm). Patients were randomly assigned to receive surgical ($n = 1070$) or endovascular ($n = 1073$) treatment and were assessed using the mRS at two months and again at one year (this was the primary outcome measure). Trial enrollment was stopped prematurely because it was revealed during interim analysis that the proportion of patients who were dependent or dead (mRS scores of 3–6) by two months or by one year was significantly higher in the neurosurgical group than in the endovascular group (14). When all the patients were followed to one year, the absolute risk reduction in those randomized to coiling was 7.4% compared with those randomized to neurosurgery (95% confidence interval, CI = 3.6–11.2; $p < 0.0001$) (Fig. 1) (15). This treatment advantage for survival and independence in the endovascular group was maintained for at least seven years (15).

Interestingly, subgroup analysis of the ISAT data reveals further group differences in the relative risk of death or dependency at one year. Patients in relatively good clinical condition at presentation (WFNS grades I–III) experienced better outcome with embolization (relative risk, RR, 0.71; 95% CI, 0.61–0.83), as did patients with smaller aneurysms (<11) and those whose aneurysms emerged from the internal carotid artery (RR, 0.56; 95% CI, 0.43–0.72). Additionally, patients treated with embolization were less likely to experience seizures after the procedure (RR, 0.52; 95% CI, 0.37–0.74) (15).

RATES OF RUPTURE AFTER ENDOVASCULAR
AND SURGICAL TREATMENT

On the basis of current evidence derived from ISAT and daily practice, endo-vascular treatment is better tolerated than open surgery, especially in patients with ruptured aneurysms and recent SAH. Concerns remain, however, regarding the durability of treatment, as many aneurysms are only incompletely obliterated after endovascular treatment, and the risk of aneurysm rerupture and further growth remains undetermined. These concerns are amplified by observations that the risk of suboptimal aneurysmal exclusion is elevated with endovascular treatment compared with surgical aneurysm ligation. In a follow-up study of 127 aneurysms that had been either clipped or coiled, investigators found only one residual aneurysm in the 63 that were surgically clipped; by contrast, the authors noted a "postembolization remnant" in 20 of 64 aneurysms that were coiled (16). In the ISAT trial (where not all patients received follow-up angiograms), angiography performed at about one year posttreatment revealed that complete occlusion of the ruptured aneurysm was achieved more often in the neurosurgery group (370 of 450 follow-up angiograms or 82%), compared with the endo-vascular group (584 of 881 angiograms or 66%).

Suboptimal aneurysmal occlusion may be related to a higher risk of rebleeding. Detailed analysis of the ISAT trial data (15), for example, reveals that the incidence of aneurysmal rebleeding in the first 30 days after endovascular coiling (20 of 1073 or 1.86%) is significantly higher than after neurosurgery (8 of 1070 or 0.75%) (RR, 2.46; 95% CI, 1.09–5.57). Between 30 days and one year after embolization, that risk still remains higher with endovascular treatment, though it is not statistically significant. Although the incidence of late rebleeding (> 1 year) was very low in both groups (further discussed below), it was higher in the endovascular group (7 patients out of 1073) than in the surgical group (2 patients out of 1070) (15). Overall, the risk of rebleeding during the first year remained low in both groups (2.4% for the endovascular group and 1% for the surgical group).

In response to the ISAT rebleeding data, the Cerebral Aneurysm Rerupture After Treatment (CARAT) study was designed to analyze and compare rebleeding rates in patients with aSAH treated either by coil embolization or surgical clipping (17). The study was conducted at nine U.S. centers with recognized experience with either therapeutic modality. The records of patients with aSAH admitted and treated between 1996 and 1998 were reviewed. To study long-term rebleeding rates, patients were followed for a period of time up to nine years.

Overall, 1010 patients (711 treated with surgical clipping and 299 with coil embolization) met inclusion criteria. Patients treated with coil embolization were older, harbored more posterior circulation aneurysms, and tended to have smaller aneurysms. Rebleeding from the index aneurysm during the first year was more common with coil embolization. Rebleeding during the first month after treatment occurred in 2.7% of patients after coil embolization and in 1% of patients after clipping, this difference being statistically significant and consistent with the

Table 1 Rebleeding Rates After Surgical or Endovascular Treatment of Ruptured Intracranial Aneurysms

	Surgery			Endovasular				
	n	rebleeds[a]	%	n	rebleeds[a]	%	RR (95% CI)	p value
ISAT (15)								
< 1 mo	1051	8	0.8	1066	19	1.8	2.46 (1.09–5.57)	
1 mo–1 yr	1047	3	0.3	1057	8	0.8	2.64 (0.70–9.93)	
Total in 1yr	1051	11	1.0	1066	27	2.5		
>1 yr	1046	2	0.2	1051	7	0.7		
CARAT (17)								
< 1 mo	711	7	1.0	299	8	2.7		< 0.03
1 mo–1 yr	485	2	0.4	201	1	0.5		< 0.87
Total in 1 yr	711	9	1.3	299	9	3.0		< 0.04
> 1 yr	439	0	0.0	173	1	0.6		< 0.11

[a]rebleeds from ruptured aneurysm.

Abbreviations: ISAT, International Subarachnoid Aneurysm Trial; CARAT, Cerebral Aneurysm Rerupture after Treatment (CARAT).

findings of the ISAT trial (15). After the first year, rates of rebleeding from the index aneurysm were 0.11% after coil embolization and 0% after surgical clipping.

The CARAT and ISAT trials confirm that a small but definite risk of rebleeding exists in the first month after either endovascular or surgical treatment of ruptured intracranial aneurysms, even in the hands of very experienced operators. This risk is higher with coil embolization (see Table 1). Therefore, the 2% added risk of early rebleeding after coil embolization must be taken into account when making treatment recommendations for ruptured intracranial aneurysms. After the first year, these studies indicate that the risk of rerupture of a ruptured aneurysm treated with either modality is exceedingly low. Thus, concerns about long-term durability of endovascular embolization of ruptured aneurysms appear to be no longer justified.

Combining data from the ISAT and CARAT studies, after the first treatment year, one rerupture occurred during 5771 person-years of follow-up after surgical clipping (annual rate 0.02%) and eight reruptures occurred during 4162 person-years after coiling (annual rate 0.19%). This very low risk of long-term rebleeding must be weighed against the risk of aneurysm retreatment, which is not without complications. Debilitating or potentially life-threatening complications related to retreatment occurred in 11% of patients after coiling and in 17% after surgery (17). Therefore, it is important to refrain from over-retreating embolized aneurysms just for the goal of achieving a perfect angiographic result. Rebleeding from a previously coiled aneurysm one year or more after treatment is a rare occurrence that probably does not justify the risk of retreatment in the majority of cases.

In the CARAT study, retreatment of the index aneurysm within one year was more common in patients who were initially treated by coil embolization (7.7% of patients after endovascular treatment and 1.7% of patients after surgery). There were no retreatments beyond the first year after surgery. In contrast, in patients who had undergone coil embolization, the rate of retreatment was 4.5% in the second year and 1.1% yearly thereafter.

CEREBRAL VASOSPASM AFTER ENDOVASCULAR AND SURGICAL TREATMENT

It is estimated that angiographic narrowing of cerebral arteries or vasospasm occurs in 40% to 70% of patients who suffer SAH, often 7 to 14 days after the initial aneurysm rupture. Symptomatic vasospasm occurs in 17% to 40% of patients with SAH, resulting in delayed ischemic neurologic deficits in approximately half of these patients (18). Despite decades of research into its pathophysiology, prevention and treatment, cerebral vasospasm remains one of the major causes of morbidity and mortality in patients with aSAH. Endovascular treatment in theory might decrease the incidence and severity of vasospasm after aneurysm rupture by avoiding external mechanical manipulation of the intracranial vessels. On the other hand, vasospasm is thought to be caused by breakdown of blood products in the subarachnoid space; therefore, clot removal and washout at surgery might lower its incidence (19,20).

A thorough literature review and meta-analysis of the incidence of vasospasm following surgical or endovascular treatment of aSAH has recently been performed (18). The authors found nine studies in which investigators evaluated overall vasospasm (measured angiographically or by transcranial Doppler), symptomatic vasospasm, and delayed ischemic neurologic deficits due to vasospasm, comparing their incidence in patients who were treated with either surgery or embolization. One of these studies was a randomized prospective analysis (21), three were nonrandomized prospective analyses (22–24), four studies were performed retrospectively (25–28), and one study had prospective and retrospective components (29). Overall, no significant differences were noted between the two treatment modalities on any parameters. However, a recently completed multicentered randomized trial of a novel endothelin receptor antagonist conducted at several large academic North American and European centers showed a dramatically reduced incidence of moderate-to-severe angiographic vasospasm in patients treated endovascularly when compared with patients treated surgically, as assessed by a blinded third-party investigator (30). In the placebo group of the CONSCIOUS (Clazosentan to Overcome Neurological iSChemia and Infarction OccUrring after SAH) trial, moderate-to-severe angiographic vasospasm was observed in more than 80% of patients who underwent clipping and in less than 50% of those who underwent endovascular treatment. This study included only patients who had significant subarachnoid blood burden and were therefore at high risk of developing vasospasm.

INDIVIDUAL PATIENT AND ANEURYSM CHARACTERISTICS FAVORING ONE TREATMENT OVER THE OTHER

One potential limitation of the ISAT study is that only patients whose ruptured aneurysm was judged by both a neurosurgeon and a neurointerventionalist to be equally amenable to surgery or endovascular embolization were entered in the trial. As a result, only 2143 of the 9559 patients (22%) assessed for eligibility at the participating centers during the enrollment period were eventually enrolled. Therefore, the ISAT results cannot necessarily be extended to the population of patients with aSAH as a whole, as most patients had aneurysms that were best treated by one modality or the other. Of these patients not enrolled, 3615 were treated surgically and 2737 were coiled. Information as to what treatment was chosen for the remaining 1064 was not available. Clearly, surgical treatment continues to be beneficial for a significant proportion of patients with aSAH.

In treating the individual patient with a ruptured aneurysm, multiple factors must be taken into account to choose the best therapeutic course, including aneurysm location, size, shape, orientation, and neck-to-dome ratio, as well as tortuosity of the proximal vessels and the parent artery and the presence of calcifications at the neck of the aneurysm. Patient characteristics that are taken into account include the patient's chronologic and biologic age, systemic comorbidities, life expectancy, and neurologic condition (Fig. 2). Additionally, the treating physician must carefully assess local expertise, complication rates, and patient outcomes to offer patients and their families evolving treatment options.

In some centers, the two treatment options (surgical clip or endovascular coil) can be successfully used interchangeably and, at times, in a complementary fashion to protect the patient from aneurysm rerupture while attempting to minimize complications related to treatment. In assessing patient outcome at one center (31), it was found that 71% of patients with ruptured intracranial aneurysms treated by a multidisciplinary team (with expertise in both surgical and endovascular treatment) were able to function independently or with only minor restrictions in their lifestyle at six months (mRS = 0–2).

Aneurysm location is commonly among the most important factors that influence choice of treatment for ruptured aneurysms. For example, basilar bifurcation aneurysms pose significant surgical challenges from a technical point of view, yet they are very easy to embolize, given their orientation in the same direction of flow. Therefore, in most cases, it is apparent that endovascular treatment is superior to surgical clipping of these basilar bifurcation aneurysms (Fig. 3).

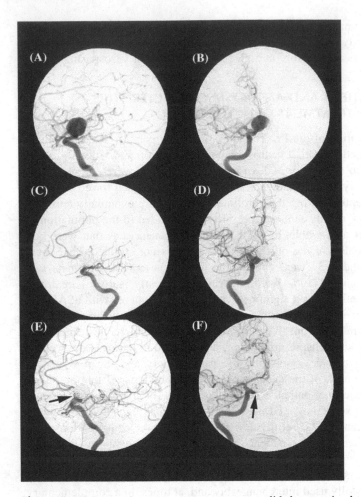

Figure 2 Endovascular treatment represents a valid therapeutic choice in patients with poor neurologic condition. This 60-year-old man presented with a WFNS Grade V SAH from a large aneurysm of the internal carotid artery (**A,B**). He underwent endovascular embolization (**C,D**) and made a good neurologic recovery after a prolonged hospital course. Three-month follow-up angiography (**E,F**) shows recurrent filling of the aneurysm neck (*arrows*). He will undergo repeat cerebral angiography with retreatment if further recanalization is demonstrated. *Abbreviations*: WFNS, World Federation of Neurosurgical Societies; SAH, subarachnoid hemorrhage.

By contrast, MCA aneurysms are currently better treated with direct surgical exclusion. These aneurysms are relatively superficial and can be clipped with minimal brain retraction. All but the largest (''giant'') MCA aneurysms can be completely exposed to allow visualization and control of the entire parent vessel-aneurysm complex. Endovascular embolization, on the other hand, still

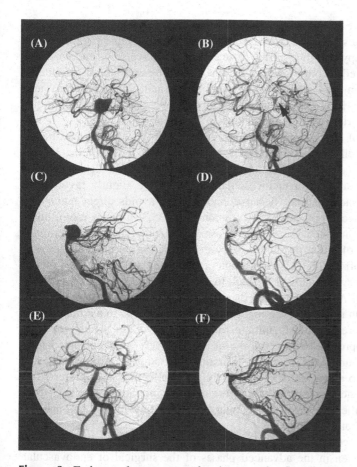

Figure 3 Endovascular treatment has become the first line of treatment for basilar bifurcation aneurysms at most centers. This 52-year-old woman presented with a WFNS Grade III SAH from a large irregular basilar bifurcation aneurysm (**A,C**). Despite the broad neck, this aneurysm was treated successfully with Guglielmi detachable coils (**B,D**). Immediately after treatment, faint filling can still be seen of the top of the aneurysm's dome (**B**, *arrow*). Follow-up cerebral angiography (**E,F**) three months later shows complete aneurysm obliteration with interval thrombosis of the residual dome. *Abbreviations*: WFNS, World Federation of Neurosurgical Societies; SAH, subarachnoid hemorrhage.

has several drawbacks when applied to this subset of aneurysms. MCA aneurysms often have a broad, complex neck that partially incorporates the origin of M2 branches, thus increasing the risk of periprocedural thromboembolic complications (32).

Likewise, in most patients with small, ruptured PCom artery aneurysms, surgery should be considered as the first line of treatment. These aneurysms can be reached with minimal brain retraction and can be permanently secured by clip application with very low surgical morbidity and mortality. Endovascular treatment still carries a higher risk of hemorrhagic and ischemic complications than surgical therapy for this subset of aneurysms. Conversely, endovascular treatment of ruptured PCom artery aneurysms should be considered for elderly patients (older than 70 years), patients with poor neurologic baseline, and patients with large PCom aneurysms, where significant manipulation of the anterior choroidal artery can be anticipated.

Aneurysms of the ACom artery represent a complex condition that is associated with a well-characterized profile of neuropsychologic deficits (33,34). Studies that examined cognitive outcome after ACom aneurysms that have been treated with either surgical or endovascular methods have slightly favored the endovascular approach, perhaps because embolization avoids direct manipulation of the anterior cerebral artery–ACom complex (35,36). Quite often, however, ruptured ACom aneurysms are very small, and the risk is higher with smaller aneurysms of intraprocedural aneurysm perforation during embolization (32,37). The takeoff of the A1 at an acute angle from the bifurcation of the internal carotid artery can make it difficult to obtain a "stable" catheter position within a very small ACom aneurysm; therefore, the elevated risk of perforation during embolization might be even higher in these aneurysms. In a collaborative environment, it is reasonable to initiate treatment for ACom aneurysms with an endovascular approach. However, if the aneurysm is very small and any degree of difficulty is encountered during catheterization or attempted coiling, treatment should be shifted to a surgical approach. Surgical treatment is also preferred in the small ACom aneurysms with which the anatomy of the aneurysm and its relationship with the parent vessels cannot be adequately identified on high-resolution 3-D catheter angiography.

To minimize complications, it is very important to constantly assess the risk/benefit ratio even in the advanced phases of the surgical or endovascular procedure. If risks are higher than originally estimated or unexpected findings are encountered while performing surgery or endovascular embolization, the procedure can be halted and patients can be treated with endovascular embolization after surgical exploration, or vice versa.

FUTURE DIRECTIONS

Introduction of endovascular coiling has significantly changed practice patterns for intracranial aneurysm treatment. In Europe, most intracranial aneurysms are currently treated by endovascular means. A similar trend is emerging in the United States, where more and more aneurysms are being considered for coiling. This trend poses important practical problems and challenges. Most aneurysms left for surgical treatment are those that are the most difficult, with a broad neck. With a decreasing number of aneurysms treated operatively, younger trainees are being exposed less and less to this challenging surgery. This situation already poses significant problems for patients with basilar bifurcation aneurysms not amenable to endovascular treatment, as only a handful of surgeons in North America are performing this procedure on a regular basis, and these surgeons may experience difficulty maintaining an adequate level of skill.

The availability of endovascular treatment as a much less invasive alternative has also changed how we assess patient outcome. Issues such as quality of life, which were neglected in previous surgical publications, are now considered standard for reporting outcome and comparing treatment modalities in randomized trials. As opposed to the recent past, when quite often the approach to patients with aSAH was pessimistic and those who made a "good recovery" were considered the lucky ones, it is now possible to achieve an excellent outcome with return to a normal life in most of those treated. This achievement has been made possible not only through improvement in techniques, but also through a better understanding of the pathophysiology of SAH and its complications, and through improvement in perioperative care and intensive care of patients with these challenging conditions. Also instrumental to improving patient outcome has been the further regionalization of patient care to tertiary care centers, where both surgical and endovascular treatment are available from experienced providers, as studies have shown that outcomes are closely related to hospital and provider volumes (38). It is possible that a new physician figure will emerge who is well versed in surgical and endovascular treatment as well as in the diagnosis, perioperative management, and follow-up of cerebrovascular disease (steps are currently underway in many units in North America to make this possibility a reality).

CONCLUSION

Treatment of intracranial aneurysms has been revolutionized in the past 20 years by the advent and refinement of endovascular techniques. Numerous patient, operator, and aneurysm factors play an important role in deciding whether endovascular or surgical therapy should be employed.

ACKNOWLEDGMENTS

We gratefully acknowledge JoAnna Gass for her assistance in editing this manuscript.

REFERENCES

1. Wang H, Fraser K, Wang D, et al. The evolution of endovascular therapy for neurosurgical disease. Neurosurg Clin N Am 2005; 16(2):223–229, vii.
2. Kanaan Y, Kaneshiro D, Fraser K, et al. Evolution of endovascular therapy for aneurysm treatment. Historical overview. Neurosurg Focus 2005; 18(2):E2.
3. Siddique K, Alvernia J, Fraser K, et al. Treatment of aneurysms with wires and electricity: a historical overview. J Neurosurg 2003; 99(6):1102–1107.

4. Hopkins LN, Lanzino G, Guterman LR. Treating complex nervous system vascular disorders through a "needle stick": origins, evolution, and future of neuro-endovascular therapy. Neurosurgery 2001; 48(3):463–475.

5. Lanzino G, Wakhloo AK, Fessler RD, et al. Efficacy and current limitations of intravascular stents for intracranial internal carotid, vertebral, and basilar artery aneurysms. J Neurosurg 1999; 91(4):538–546.

6. Moret J, Cognard C, Weill A, et al. Reconstruction technique in the treatment of wide-neck intracranial aneurysms. Long-term angiographic and clinical results. Apropos of 56 cases. J Neuroradiol 1997; 24(1):30–44.

7. Lanzino G, Guterman LR, Hopkins LN. Endovascular Treatment of Aneurysms. In: Winn HR, Youmans JR, eds. Youmans Neurological Surgery, 5th ed. Philadelphia: Saunders, 2004:2057–2078.

8. Dandy W. Intracranial aneurysm or the internal carotid artery cured by operation. Ann Surgery 1938; 107:654–659.

9. Todd MM, Hindman BJ, Clarke WR, et al. Mild intraoperative hypothermia during surgery for intracranial aneurysm. N Engl J Med 2005; 352(2):135–145.

10. Vinuela F, Duckwiler G, Mawad M. Guglielmi detachable coil embolization of acute intracranial aneurysm: perioperative anatomical and clinical outcome in 403 patients. J Neurosurg 1997; 86(3):475–482.

11. McDougall CG, Halbach VV, Dowd CF, et al. Endovascular treatment of basilar tip aneurysms using electrolytically detachable coils. J Neurosurg 1996; 84(3):393–399.

12. Vanninen R, Koivisto T, Saari T, et al. Ruptured intracranial aneurysms: acute endovascular treatment with electrolytically detachable coils—a prospective randomized study. Radiology 1999; 211(2):325–336.

13. Koivisto T, Vanninen R, Hurskainen H, et al. Outcomes of early endovascular versus surgical treatment of ruptured cerebral aneurysms. A prospective randomized study. Stroke 2000; 31(10):2369–2377.

14. Molyneux A, Kerr R, Stratton I, et al. International Subarachnoid Aneurysm Trial (ISAT) of neurosurgical clipping versus endovascular coiling in 2143 patients with ruptured intracranial aneurysms: a randomised trial. Lancet 2002; 360(9342): 1267–1274.

15. Molyneux AJ, Kerr RS, Yu LM, et al. International subarachnoid aneurysm trial (ISAT) of neurosurgical clipping versus endovascular coiling in 2143 patients with ruptured intracranial aneurysms: a randomised comparison of effects on survival, dependency, seizures, rebleeding, subgroups, and aneurysm occlusion. Lancet 2005; 366(9488):809–817.

16. Raftopoulos C, Mathurin P, Boscherini D, et al. Prospective analysis of aneurysm treatment in a series of 103 consecutive patients when endovascular embolization is considered the first option. J Neurosurg 2000; 93(2):175–182.

17. The CARAT Investigators. Rates of delayed rebleeding from intracranial aneurysms are low after surgical and endovascular treatment. Stroke 2006; 37(6):1437–1442.

18. de Oliveira JG, Beck J, Ulrich C, et al. Comparison between clipping and coiling on the incidence of cerebral vasospasm after aneurysmal subarachnoid hemorrhage: a systematic review and meta-analysis. Neurosurg Rev 2007; 30(1):22–30 (discussion 30–21).

19. Hansen-Schwartz J. Cerebral vasospasm: a consideration of the various cellular mechanisms involved in the pathophysiology. Neurocrit Care 2004; 1(2):235–246.

20. Amin-Hanjani S, Ogilvy CS, Barker FG II. Does intracisternal thrombolysis prevent vasospasm after aneurysmal subarachnoid hemorrhage? A meta-analysis. Neurosurgery 2004; 54(2):326–334 (discussion 334–325).

21. Koivisto T, Vanninen E, Vanninen R, et al. Cerebral perfusion before and after endovascular or surgical treatment of acutely ruptured cerebral aneurysms: a 1-year prospective follow-up study. Neurosurgery 2002; 51(2):312–325 (discussion 325–316).

22. Dehdashti AR, Mermillod B, Rufenacht DA, et al. Does treatment modality of intracranial ruptured aneurysms influence the incidence of cerebral vasospasm and clinical outcome? Cerebrovasc Dis 2004; 17(1):53–60.

23. Goddard AJ, Raju PP, Gholkar A. Does the method of treatment of acutely ruptured intracranial aneurysms influence the incidence and duration of cerebral vasospasm and clinical outcome? J Neurol Neurosurg Psychiatry 2004; 75(6):868–872.

24. Gruber A, Ungersbock K, Reinprecht A, et al. Evaluation of cerebral vasospasm after early surgical and endovascular treatment of ruptured intracranial aneurysms. Neurosurgery 1998; 42(2):258–267 (discussion 267–258).

25. Charpentier C, Audibert G, Guillemin F, et al. Multivariate analysis of predictors of cerebral vasospasm occurrence after aneurysmal subarachnoid hemorrhage. Stroke 1999; 30(7):1402–1408.

26. Hoh BL, Curry WT, Jr., Carter BS, et al. Computed tomographic demonstrated infarcts after surgical and endovascular treatment of aneurysmal subarachnoid hemorrhage. Acta Neurochir (Wien) 2004; 146(11):1177–1183.

27. Rabinstein AA, Pichelmann MA, Friedman JA, et al. Symptomatic vasospasm and outcomes following aneurysmal subarachnoid hemorrhage: a comparison between surgical repair and endovascular coil occlusion. J Neurosurg 2003; 98(2):319–325.

28. Yalamanchili K, Rosenwasser RH, Thomas JE, et al. Frequency of cerebral vasospasm in patients treated with endovascular occlusion of intracranial aneurysms. AJNR Am J Neuroradiol 1998; 19(3):553–558.

29. Hoh BL, Topcuoglu MA, Singhal AB, et al. Effect of clipping, craniotomy, or intravascular coiling on cerebral vasospasm and patient outcome after aneurysmal subarachnoid hemorrhage. Neurosurgery 2004; 55(4):779–786 (discussion 786–779).

30. MacDonald RL, Kakarieka A, Mayer SA, et al. Prevention of cerebral vasospasm after aneurysmal subarachnoid hemorrhage with Clazosentan, an endothelin receptor antagonist: 801. Neurosurgery 2006; 59(2):453.

31. Lanzino G, Fraser K, Kanan Y, et al. Treatment of ruptured intracranial aneurysms since the International Subarachnoid Aneurysm Trial: practice utilizing clip ligation and coil embolization as individual or complementary therapies. J Neurosurg 2006; 104(3):344–349.

32. Raymond J, Roy D. Safety and efficacy of endovascular treatment of acutely ruptured aneurysms. Neurosurgery 1997; 41(6):1235–1245 (discussion 1245–1236).

33. Damasio AR, Graff-Radford NR, Eslinger PJ, et al. Amnesia following basal forebrain lesions. Arch Neurol 1985; 42(3):263–271.

34. DeLuca J, Diamond BJ. Aneurysm of the anterior communicating artery: a review of neuroanatomical and neuropsychological sequelae. J Clin Exp Neuropsychol 1995; 17(1):100–121.

35. Chan A, Ho S, Poon WS. Neuropsychological sequelae of patients treated with microsurgical clipping or endovascular embolization for anterior communicating artery aneurysm. Eur Neurol 2002; 47(1):37–44.

36. Fontanella M, Perozzo P, Ursone R, et al. Neuropsychological assessment after microsurgical clipping or endovascular treatment for anterior communicating artery aneurysm. Acta Neurochir (Wien) 2003; 145(10):867–872 (discussion 872).
37. Ricolfi F, Le Guerinel C, Blustajn J, et al. Rupture during treatment of recently ruptured aneurysms with Guglielmi electrodetachable coils. AJNR Am J Neuroradiol 1998; 19(9):1653–1658.
38. Cross DT III, Tirschwell DL, Clark MA, et al. Mortality rates after subarachnoid hemorrhage: variations according to hospital case volume in 18 states. J Neurosurg 2003; 99(5):810–817.

15

Diagnosis and Medical Management of Vasospasm and Delayed Cerebral Ischemia

Olga Helena Hernandez, MD, Fellow

Neurocritical Care, Case Medical Center, Case Western Reserve University, Cleveland, Ohio, U.S.A.

Jose I. Suarez, MD, Director[a] and Professor[b]

*[a]Vascular Neurology and Neurocritical Care,
[b]Neurology and Neurosurgery, Baylor College of Medicine,
Houston, Texas, U.S.A.*

Cerebral vasospasm is a reversible reduction of the caliber of the intracranial arteries that is triggered by the presence of blood in the subarachnoid space (so-called subarachnoid hemorrhage, SAH) and leads to decreased cerebral blood flow (CBF). The result is cerebral ischemia with permanent neurologic deficits, death, or both. Any intracranial artery that is surrounded by a large amount of blood for a sufficient length of time is prone to developing vasospasm (1). SAH can be traumatic or nontraumatic. The most common cause of nontraumatic SAH is aneurysmal rupture. Cerebral aneurysms are most commonly located in the arteries that form the circle of Willis or their branches, which may explain why these are the arteries that develop vasospasm most often. Vasospasm has also been associated with tuberculosis, purulent meningitis, ophthalmoplegic migraine, myelography, electroconvulsive therapy, eclampsia, and nonruptured aneurysms (1). However, the pathophysiology of the arterial narrowing in these cases is different and will not be discussed in this chapter (1).

In general, cerebral vasospasm begins three days after SAH, is maximal seven or eight days later, and clears by day 14. If the vasospasm is detected only by cerebral angiography, it is called an *angiographic vasospasm,* but if it is associated with a neurologic deficit, it is called *symptomatic vasospasm.* Cerebral vasospasm is the most common cause of delayed cerebral ischemia or delayed ischemic deficit (DID) after SAH. Thus, DID secondary to cerebral vasospasm continues to be the most common and severe complication of SAH.

In the last 50 years, the pathophysiology of vasospasm has been better recognized and understood, not only because it carries a high rate of complications, but also because it is potentially preventable and treatable.

HISTORY

Cerebral vasospasm was first described by Gull in 1859 (2). He noticed the association between vasospasm and DID in a 30-year-old woman who died after a middle cerebral artery (MCA) aneurysm ruptured. In 1925, Florey induced local spasm in the cerebral arteries of cats (3). Ecker and Riemenschneider described the angiographic findings of vasospasm after SAH in 1951 (4). In 1958, Johnson and his collaborators gave the first surgical option to prevent cerebral spasm by using mechanical blood removal (5). Subsequently, in 1975, Fisher described that one-third of patients who survived SAH developed symptoms related to vasospasm typically between days 3 and 13 (6). Katada et al. described the relation between the quantity of blood observed in a head CT and the subsequent onset of vasospasm in 1977 (7), and in 1982, Aaslid et al. introduced the Transcranial Doppler (TCD) ultrasound to evaluate the spasm in cerebral blood vessels (8).

George Allen, in 1979, found that nimodipine reversed the spasm in dogs and then conducted the first multicentric study in humans (9). Balloon angioplasty was introduced in the 1980s in the Soviet Union as a way to reverse angiographic vasospasm (10). Such an outline of these historic milestones is but a sample of the interest generated since vasospasm was found to be associated with SAH. In spite of multiple studies and efforts to prevent or control vasospasm, research in this area has not been completely successful, and neither vasospasm nor its pathophysiology is well understood.

EPIDEMIOLOGY

Aneurysmal SAH accounts for 2% to 5% of strokes, with an incidence of 10.5 per 100,000 people per year (11). Mortality and morbidity increase with the amount of blood, but in general the average case fatality rate is 51%, and one-third of survivors require care for the rest of their lives (12). The incidence of vasospasm is lower than that of SAH. In general, at least two-thirds of the angiographies performed between days 4 and 12 in patients after SAH have some degree of narrowing, and historically it has been estimated that one-third of these patients develop neurologic symptoms or DID. Of these, approximately one-third die from their deficits, another third are left disabled, and the last third have favorable recoveries (1). Various series report that 22% to 40% of patients with SAH experience symptomatic vasospasm and at the same time have associated increases in morbidity (34%) and mortality (30%). In general, cerebral vasospasm-induced DID doubles the mortality after SAH (1,11,12).

RISK FACTORS

Amount of Blood on Head CT Scanning

Takemae et al. were the first to demonstrate that cerebral vasospasm could be present in over 80% of patients at day 4 after SAH if they had areas of high density of blood in the basal cisterns and the sylvian fissures on head CT scanning (13). Fisher et al. then concluded that a sufficient quantity of blood in the subarachnoid space is the only predictor of vasospasm onset (14). They also categorized this certain predictor into four groups, according to the localization and quantity of blood in the CT performed between the day 4 and day 5 of SAH. According to this report that included 47 patients, those with grade I or II very rarely developed vasospasm, but grade III was found to strongly predict angiographic and symptomatic vasospasm. This radiographic scale became known as the Fisher scale. In spite of being a scale widely utilized by neurosurgeons, the usefulness of the Fisher scale in predicting vasospasm has remained controversial. Subsequent studies demonstrated that intraventricular bleeding was also a strong predictor of vasospasm and that the inter-rater variability of the scale is poor (15). A recent study proposed a modified Fisher scale to predict vasospasm (Table 1) (16). Such a version may be more reliable.

Table 1 Original Fisher Scale and Modified Fisher Scale

Fisher grade	Features
1	No or focal, thin SAH
2	Diffuse, thin SAH
3	Focal or diffuse, thick SAH
4	Focal or diffuse, thick SAH, with significant ICH or IVH.
Modified Fisher grade	
0	No SAH or IVH
1	Focal or diffuse, thin SAH, no IVH
2	Focal or diffuse, thin SAH, with IVH
3	Focal or diffuse, thick SAH[a], no IVH
4	Focal or diffuse thick SAH[a], with IVH

[a]Thick refers to the fact that a hemorrhage fills one or more cisterns or fissures. A total of 10 cisterns are evaluated: frontal interhemispheric fissure, quadrigeminal cistern, both suprasellar cisterns, both ambient cisterns, both basal sylvian cisterns, and both lateral sylvian Fissures. *Abbreviations*: SAH, subarachnoid hemorrhage; ICH, intracerebral hemorrhage; IVH, intraventricular hemorrhage.

Antifibrinolytics

Since 1970, it has been postulated that antifibrinolytic agents may increase DID following SAH. Such a finding was corroborated in a study in which the administration of tranexamic acid, as a measure of rebleeding prevention, increased the incidence of DID (24% vs. 15%) despite decreased rebleeding rates (9% in the experimental group vs. 24% in the control group) (17).

Other Factors

Cerebral vasospasm-induced DID is more common in patients with structural disturbances of their vasculature, such as carotid stenosis, presence of small communicating blood vessels, or compromised terminal arteries, and in patients with hypotension, dehydration, poor cardiac output, anemia, and hypoxia (18). A definitive relationship between age, hypertension, or gender and DID has not been established. However, smokers are more likely to develop vasospasm and DID (19).

Timing of Aneurysm Treatment

An analysis of 443 patients with aneurysmal SAH between 1971 and 1978 found that patients who had surgical repair on the day of hemorrhage or in the following two days had better results, with less vasospasm-associated morbidity and mortality. The contrary occurred with those patients operated on between days 4 and 7 of the SAH (20). Subsequently, the International Cooperative Study Group examined the timing of surgery and reported that no relationship existed between the moment of surgery and the development of vasospasm, other than the fact that delayed surgeries were correlated with complications such as hydrocephalus and rebleeding and early surgeries were correlated with a greater frequency of cerebral edema (21). The same group also showed that with surgery and removal of the clots it was possible to diminish the incidence of vasospasm (22).

Today, despite lower associated risks with surgery—due to better microsurgical techniques, instruments, and improvements in anesthetic procedures—very few patients with SAH return to a similar premorbid lifestyle, and many remain with cognitive problems and defects. Improved postsurgery care in neurointensive care units has not been able to change this outcome. However, endovascular treatment of ruptured aneurysms may be associated with better outcomes compared with surgery in patients with clinical equipoise; that is, the ruptured aneurysm is amenable to treatment by either technique (23,24).

PATHOPHYSIOLOGY

Animal models of SAH have overwhelmingly shown that the oxyhemoglobin of erythrocytes triggers events that lead to vasospasm (25,26). The accumulated blood following SAH is hemolyzed and degraded, leading to the production of free radicals, potent culprits of vascular damage. In turn, this leads to the initiation of an inflammatory cascade, with activation of leukocytes and platelets and subsequent overexpression of other inflammatory agents. The down-regulation of nitric oxide and prostacyclin production and overexpression of potent vasoconstrictors, such as endothelin-1, have also been shown to play a very important role. Likewise, the nervous reflex pathways are also activated. Thus, it is likely that a multitude of pathways and mechanisms are responsible for the development of vasospasm (1,27).

DIAGNOSIS

The associated symptoms of vasospasm are at their highest point on day 7 or 8 after SAH and are rare during the first three days or after day 13. The onset of symptoms can be either sudden or gradual. Specific symptoms include increasing headache, neck stiffness, or increased temperature. The most common clinical presentation is progressive confusion, delirium, or changed level of consciousness, with or without focal symptoms (1,28).

It is important to keep in mind that many pathologic entities may mimic symptomatic vasospasm. It is therefore necessary to follow through with a detailed neurologic exam and with a new head CT, besides conducting blood tests and other imaging modalities, in order to detect the cause of a patient's clinical deterioration (Table 2) (28).

Transcranial Doppler Ultrasound

In clinical use since the 1980s, transcranial Doppler (TCD) ultrasound takes advantage of the principle that mean cerebral blood flow velocity (MCBFV) is

Table 2 Differential Diagnoses of Delayed Neurologic Deficit after Subarachnoid Hemorrhage

System	Causes
Metabolic/Systemic	Electrolyte imbalances (hyponatremia or hypernatremia); arterial blood gases abnormalities (hypoxemia or hypercarbia); renal or hepatic dysfunction; hypothyroidism; sepsis
Cardiovascular	Hypotension (hypovolemia, sepsis, cardiac dysfunction, including pump failure or cardiac dysrhythmias)
Infections	Any systemic or central nervous system infection with or without sepsis or septic shock; fever
Neurologic	Aneurysmal rebleeding; epidural hemorrhage; subdural hemorrhage; intraventricular hemorrhage; hydrocephalus; postoperative hemorrhagic complications; ventriculitis, seizures; post-ictal state; cerebral vasospasm; embolic stroke
Miscellaneous	Medication allergic reaction; noninfectious fever

inversely proportional to changes in vessel diameter. It should be performed between day 3 and up to two weeks after SAH, given that this is the window for vasospasm to occur.

In the initial studies, it was found that the average MCBFV for the MCA was 62 cm/sec, with a range between 33 and 90 cm/sec (8). Later, the same group found that mild angiographic vasospasm of the MCA correlated with MCBFVs greater than 120 cm/sec and that severe vasospasm correlated with MCBFVs greater than 200 cm/sec (29). Another group conducted daily TCD ultrasounds in 50 patients with ruptured aneurysms and with elective clipping of unruptured aneurysms. They found that MCBFVs less than 100 cm/sec in the MCA have an insufficient degree of narrowing in the angiography to cause symptoms; however, MCBFVs greater than 200 cm/sec were associated with great risk of developing symptoms (30). A study of 102 patients with SAH reported that TCD ultrasound had a sensitivity of 80% when diagnosing vasospasm (31), while others found that TCD ultrasound had a sensitivity of 59% and a specificity of 100% for the detection of vasospasm (32). A systematic review reported sensitivity for vasospasm of MCA of 67% [confidence interval (CI) 48% to 87%] and specificity of 99% (CI, 98% to 100%); it was concluded that TCD ultrasound has a high specificity for vasospasm and can be very useful for detecting patients who are at risk of developing vasospasm (33). These results were replicated when it was shown that TCD ultrasound can detect up to 93% of cases with vasospasm, even if the most distal vessels or the vertically oriented branches of the MCA cannot be insonated (34). In many studies, the correlation between the elevation of MCBFVs and the degree of vasospasm on cerebral angiography has not been good (8,32,35). For this reason, it is still controversial as to whether TCD ultrasound is a good tool with which to monitor and follow patients who are at risk for cerebral vasospasm. To clarify some of these unknowns and to try to improve the correlation between angiographic vasospasm and TCD ultrasound, other parameters have been investigated. Lindegaard et al. measured the diameter of the proximal segments of the MCA and found an inverse relationship between this diameter and the MCBFVs obtained by TCD ultrasound. They also measured the ratio between the MCBFV of the proximal MCA to that of the MCBFVs of the extracranial internal carotid artery. An increase of 3 or more in this so-called *Lindegaard ratio* may indicate vasospasm. As such, this is a useful marker of vasospasm, as it differentiates between hyperemia and vasospasm. Generally, when the index is greater than 6, there is almost always a correlation with angiographic vasospasm (36).

Another unresolved question regarding the usefulness of TCD ultrasound in following patients with SAH was dealt with by investigators who reviewed data from 199 patients, of whom 55 had symptomatic vasospasm. They found a TCD ultrasound sensitivity of 73% and specificity of 80% to detect abnormalities in the symptomatic vascular territory (37). The sensitivity was even better for the detection of vasospasm in the MCA compared with other insonated vessels. In addition, they showed how the angiographic improvement was also correlated with the improvement in MCBFVs and, apart from elevated MCBFVs and the Lidegaard ratio, the rate of MCBFV increase was also important. MCBFV increases of greater than 50 cm/sec within 25 hours correlated with DID. Consequently, they concluded that daily TCD ultrasounds can help to identify patients who are at risk of vasospasm and DID and can even help in their follow-up after endo-vascular therapy (37). However, it is worth noting that, although some studies have supported these findings (38,39), others have failed to demonstrate a good correlation between TCD ultrasound and cerebral angiography (40,41).

The role of TCD ultrasound in the detection of vasospasm in the posterior circulation is less clear. In a recent cohort study, it was shown that vasospasm in the posterior circulation was associated with a high rate of complications due to compromise of the brain stem (42). Thus, it is important that steps be taken to improve the diagnosis of vasospasm in this area. A specificity of 100% was reported for the detection of vasospasm in the vertebral and basilar arteries, when velocities of 80 and 95 cm/sec were found, respectively (43). A group that further developed a ratio of intracranial basilar artery to extracranial vertebral artery velocities found that an index greater than 2 is 100% sensitive in the diagnosis of vasospasm and that if the index is less than 2, it is 95% specific (44). Further confirmation of this ratio comes from a recent study of 123 patients (45).

In conclusion, despite its limitations (i.e., operator dependency, poor cranial windows in some patients, inability to insonate deep vessels), it seems that TCD ultrasound is an easy, economic, and useful method for monitoring and diagnosing patients who are at risk of developing vasospasm after SAH (46).

Head CT Scanning

As mentioned above, the greatest risk factor for developing vasospasm is the amount of subarachnoid blood seen in the initial head CT; this has been shown in various studies (7,14,16,47,48). A variety of head CT-scanning techniques and other perfusion modalities has been more recently used for diagnosis and management of patients with SAH. Head CT angiography, which is commonly used to identify the source of SAH, has also been evaluated for the diagnosis of vasospasm. However, it has not been shown to be a reliable method and cannot, for now, substitute for traditional cerebral angiography (49). Findings on xenon-enhanced CT scanning have been correlated with the presence of cerebral ischemia in patients with vasospasm and have been useful for defining improvement of CBF after treatment of vasospasm (50,51). Single-photon emission CT imaging may also be useful but has not been extensively tested on patients with SAH. Generally, it has been found that the zones of hypoperfusion on single-photon emission CT correlate with DID (52).

Lastly, two other promising imaging techniques include head CT perfusion and MRI of the head. Head CT perfusion may allow for the differentiation between reversible and nonreversible ischemia. Some preliminary evidence suggests that head CT perfusion may correlate quite well with cerebral angiography for detecting cerebral vasospasm (53). Thus, some investigators have recommended that head CT perfusion scans be routinely used as another tool to diagnose and monitor for vasospasm (54). Perfusion- and diffusion-weighted MR imaging has also been evaluated to detect early ischemia in patients with vasospasm following SAH (55). Currently, we cannot conclude that any of these mentioned imaging techniques is ideal, as most of the data are preliminary and the techniques themselves are very costly. Nonetheless, they are very promising and deserve further investigation for the management and monitoring of patients with vasospasm due to SAH (56).

Cerebral Angiography

Cerebral angiography, via transfemoral approach, is the criterion standard for the diagnosis of vasospasm, and when performed in patients with DID, angiographic vasospasm may be found in up to 80% of patients. The current recommendations for repeat cerebral angiographies after SAH include the following: in all instances when DID does not improve after hemodynamic optimization, immediately after DID has been detected, when hemodynamic optimization poses a risk to patients, and in all patients with new neurologic deficits of unclear etiology. In general, a 0.5% to 1% risk of morbidity and mortality, including ischemic stroke, is associated with cerebral angiography (1,57). A major advantage of this method is that angiographic treatment (e.g. angioplasty, stenting, administrating vasodilating drugs) can be initiated with little delay after diagnosis (1).

TREATMENT

Currently, few options exist for the prevention or management of cerebral vasospasm-induced DID (Fig. 1). In general, either L-type calcium channel blockers, such as nimodipine, hypervolemia, hypertension, and hemodilution (HHH therapy), or endovascular therapies, such as balloon angioplasty and the direct application of vasodilating agents, can be used (1,58,59).

General Management

Some general measures should be taken with all patients with SAH; they are summarized in Table 3. They serve to optimize CBF, reduce metabolic demand, and prevent secondary brain injury.

L-type Calcium Channel Blockers

Oral nimodipine has been used for many years (9), and sufficient evidence supports its use in patients with SAH. Nimodipine reduces DID, cerebral infarction, and poor outcome. The recommended dosage of nimodipine is 60 mg, four times per day,

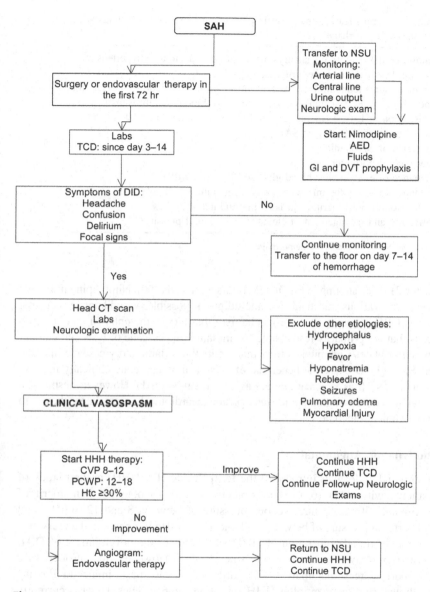

Figure 1 Monitoring and treatment of vasospasm. *Abbreviations*: SAH, subarachnoid hemorrhage; NSU, neurosurgical unit; TCD, transcranial Doppler ultrasound; AED, antiepileptic drugs; GI, gastrointestinal; DVT, deep venous thrombosis; DID, delayed ischemic deficit; HHH, hemodilution, hypertension, hypervolemia; CVP, central venous pressure; PCWP, pulmonary-capillary wedge pressure; Htc, hematocrit.

Table 3 General Measure that May Impact Upon Outcome of Patients with Subarachnoid Hemorrhage

---

Prevention of risk factors for aneurysm formation and rupture: hypertension, smoking, heavy alcohol use, drug use

Reduction of subarachnoid blood burden: intraoperative irrigation, surgical clot removal, ventricular or lumbar drain to remove bloody cerebrospinal fluid

Administration of L-type calcium channel blockers: nimodipine 60 mg PO every 4 hr up to day 21 post-SAH

Maintenance of euvolemia

Maintenance of normotension

Maintenance of euglycemia (blood glucose 80–110 mg/dL)

Maintenance of normothermia (core body temperature < 37.5°C)

Normalization of hematocrit, or at least maintained at > 30%

Identification and management of elevated intracranial pressure

---

Abbreviation: SAH, subarachnoid hemorrhage.

orally for 21 days, starting in the first 96 hours after SAH (60). Nimodipine improves outcome by various mechanisms, including a possible vasodilator effect that improves CBF, a neuroprotective mechanism that blocks the entry of calcium into the cells that are primarily responsible for initiating the cascade of lysis and cellular death, and a platelet-inhibitory effect that limits the inflammatory cascade initiated by the SAH (1). Because the beneficial effects of nimodipine are clinically modest, other agents, such as IV nicardipine, have been studied (61). However, despite the fact that it reduces angiographic vasospasm, nicardipine has not been shown to improve clinical outcome.

Hemodynamic Augmentation

Origitano and colleagues introduced the term "triple H" (HHH) in their study of 43 patients with SAH (62). Their objectives were to obtain a hematocrit of approximately 30%, a central venous pressure of between 8 and 12 mmHg, and systolic arterial pressure of between 130 and 150 mmHg in nonclipped aneurysms. The prophylactic administration of HHH (i.e., prior to the development of DID) had not been shown to improve outcome (63–65). However, uncontrolled case series reports suggest that up to 70% of patients with vasospasm-induced DID may show clinical improvement after HHH initiation (66,67). Thus, HHH is currently used in SAH patients who show evidence of DID related to cerebral vasospasm.

HHH is based on the basic principles of the Hagen–Poisieulle equation:

$$Q = (\Delta P \pi r^4)/(8 \times L \times \eta)$$

where Q is blood flow, ΔP is the change in pressure, r is the vessel radius, L is the length, and η is viscosity.

If the radius is fixed, pressure and viscosity changes are the variables that may be manipulated to improve blood flow. The fundamental understanding is that a high circulation volume increases the perfusion pressure and decreases blood viscosity. The application of this equation is obviously an oversimplification of brain vessel physiology, as cerebral arteries are not rigid tubes and CBF follows a non-Newtonian physics. Nonetheless, understanding the Hagen–Poisieulle equation may facilitate management of patients with cerebral vasospasm following SAH.

Various IV fluids (colloids or crystalloids) have been utilized to successfully expand the blood volume, but the objective is the same: an increase in volume, and in turn, an increase in cardiac output and arterial pressure, while a reduction in serum viscosity is achieved. Hypertension is sometimes achieved by simply expanding the volume. At other times, administration of vasopressors such as dopamine, phenylephrine, or norepinephrine may be required. It is not generally clear how much arterial pressure should be increased, but it has been recommended that systolic blood pressure be maintained at between 140 and 200 mmHg.

HHH is associated with several risks (28,58). Some patients have experienced a worsening of cerebral edema or intracranial pressure, development of pulmonary edema, or adult respiratory distress syndrome, reduced capacity to carry oxygen, and other risks associated with hypertension, such as rebleeding, cardiac dysrhythmia, or myocardial infarction. Therefore, it is important to monitor these patients and chart their progress in a neurointensive care unit (1,67).

Investigational Treatment Modalities

Several preliminary, investigational treatments have been reported. However, no definitive controlled, randomized, phase III clinical trials have been conducted. Because such emerging therapies have shown some promise, they will be briefly discussed below.

Magnesium

A few studies have reported on the continuous infusion of magnesium sulfate for the prevention of vasospasm after SAH. In 283 patients, a favorable trend for reduction of poor outcome was found in those who were treated with magnesium sulfate (68). This finding has been supported by other reports that have found lower morbidity and shorter in-hospital stays associated with magnesium sulfate infusions (69–71).

Statins

Small studies have suggested that the administration of statins, particularly simvastatin and pravastatin, may reduce the incidence and duration of cerebral vasospasm, reduce mortality, and improve CBF autoregulation after SAH (72–74). These results are encouraging and provide evidence that statins may prove to be an integral part of the management of SAH (75).

Lumbar Drains

The lumbar drainage of CSF has also been used as a means to reduce the incidence of vasospasm following SAH. In an uncontrolled study of 167 patients, this method was associated with reduced risk of clinical vasospasm, and its consequences compared to historic controls (76).

Many other medications have been studied with the goal of preventing vasospasm and DID, but none have shown positive results (77,78). In any case, research is ongoing with the hope that future medications may help to improve and prevent complications associated with SAH and vasospasm.

CONCLUSION AND FUTURE DIRECTIONS

Vasospasm and DID continue to be among the main reasons for poor neurologic outcome and death after SAH. Even though novel drug and therapies have been developed, treatment of vasospasm-induced DID is often unsuccessful, and many patients are left dependent. Most survivors remain with many neuropsychiatric problems, including memory loss and poor executive functions.

Continued research in the area of prevention and management of vasospasm after SAH is not only warranted, but essential. Today, many promising therapies to tackle the pathophysiology of vasospasm are being explored with the hope that they will find a clinical application in the near future.

REFERENCES

1. Macdonald RL, Weir B. Cerebral vasospasm. San Diego: Academic Press, 2001.
2. Gull W. Cases of aneurism of the cerebral vessels. Guys Hosp Rep 1859; 5:281–304.
3. Florey H. Microscopical observations on the circulations of the blood in the cerebral cortex. Brain 1925; 48:43–64.
4. Ecker A, Riemenschneider PA. Arteriographic demonstration of spasm of the intracranial arteries with special reference to saccular arterial aneurysms. J Neurosurg 1951; 8:660–667.
5. Johnson R, Potter JF, Reid RG. Arterial spasm and subarachnoid hemorrhage: mechanical considerations. J Neurol Neurosurg Psych 1958; 21:68.
6. Fisher CM. Clinical syndromes in cerebral thrombosis, hypertensive hemorrhage, and ruptured or saccular aneurysm. Clin Neurosurg 1975; 22:117–147.
7. Katada K, Kanno T, Sano H, et al. Computed tomography of ruptured intracranial aneurysm in acute stage. No Shinkei Geka 1977; 5:955–963.
8. Aaslid R, Markwalder TM, Nornes H. Noninvasive Transcranial Doppler ultrasound, recording of flow velocity in basal cerebral arteries. J Neurosurg 1982; 57:769–774.
9. Allen GS, Ahn HS, Preziosi TJ. Cerebral arterial spasm—a controlled trial of nimodipine in patients with subarachnoid hemorrhage. N Engl J Med 1983; 308:619–624.
10. Zubkov YN, Nikiforov BM, Shustin VA. Ballon catheter technique for dilatation of constricted cerebral arteries after aneurysmal SAH. Acta Neurochir 1984; 70:65–69.
11. Linn FH, Rinkel GJ, Algra A, et al. Incidence of subarachnoid hemorrhage: role of region, year, and rate of computed tomography: a meta-analysis. Stroke 1996; 27:625–629.

12. Hop JW, Rinkel GJ, Algra A, et al. Case-fatality rates and functional outcome alter subarachnoid hemorrhage: a systematic review. Stroke 1997; 28:660–664.

13. Takemae T, Mizukami M, Kim H, et al. Computed tomography of ruptured intracranial aneurysms in acute stage—Relationship between vasospasm and high density on CT scan. Brain Nerve 1978; 30:861–866.

14. Fisher CM, Kistler JP, Davis JM. Relation of cerebral vasospasm to subarachnoid hemorrhage visualized by computerized tomographic scanning. Neurosurgery 1980; 6:1–9.

15. Claassen J, Bernardini GL, Kreiter K, et al. Effect of cisternal and ventricular blood on risk of delayed cerebral ischemia after subarachnoid hemorrhage: the Fisher scale revisited. Stroke 2001; 32:2012–2020.

16. Frontera JA, Claassen J, Schmidt JM, et al. Prediction of symptomatic vasospasm after subarachnoid hemorrhage: the modified Fisher scale. Neurosurgery 2006; 59:21–27.

17. Vermeulen M, Lindsay KW, Cheah MF, et al. Antifibrinolytic treatment in subarachnoid hemorrhage. N Engl J Med 1984; 311:432–437.

18. Ohman J, Servo A, Heiskanen O. Risk factors for cerebral infarction in good-grade patients after aneurysmal subarachnoid hemorrhage and surgery: a prospective study. J Neurosurg 1991; 74:14–20.

19. Weir B, Kongable GL, Kasell NF, et al. Cigarette smoking as a cause of aneurysmal subarachnoid hemorrhage and risk of vasospasm: a report of the Cooperative Aneurysmal Study. J Neurosurg 1998; 89:405–411.

20. Sano K, Saito I. Timing and indication of surgery for ruptured intracranial aneurysms with regard to cerebral vasospasm. Acta Neurochir 1978; 41:49–60.

21. Torner J, Kassell NF, Haley EC. The timing of surgery and vasospasm. Neurosurg Clin North Am 1990; 1:335–347.

22. Torner J, Kassell NF, Haley EC. The timing of surgery and focal ischemic deficits from vasospasm. In: Sano K, Takakura K, Kassell NF, et al., eds. Cerebral Vasospasm. Tokyo: University of Tokyo Press, 1990:287–291.

23. Molyneux A, Kerr R, Stratton I, et al. International Subarachnoid Aneurysm Trial (ISAT) of neurosurgical clipping versus endovascular coiling in 2143 patients with ruptured intracranial aneurysms: a randomized trial. Lancet 2002; 360:1267–1274.

24. Molyneux AJ, Kerr RS, Yu L-M, et al. International Subarachnoid Aneurysm Trial (ISAT) of neurosurgical clipping versus endovascular coiling in 2143 patients with ruptured intracranial aneurysms: a randomized comparison of effects on survival, dependency, seizures, rebleeding, subgroups, and aneurysm occlusion. Lancet 2005; 366:809–817.

25. Mayberg MR, Okada T, Bark DH. The role of hemoglobin in arterial narrowing after subarachnoid hemorrhage. J Neurosurg 1990; 72:634–640.

26. Macdonald RL, Weir BK, Runzer TD, et al. Etiology of cerebral vasospasm in primates. J Neurosurg 1991; 75:415–424.

27. Hansen-Schwartz J. Cerebral Vasospasm. A consideration of the various cellular mechanisms involved in the pathophysiology. Neurocrit Care 2004; 2:235–246.

28. Macdonald RL. Management of cerebral vasospasm. Neurosurg Rev 2006; 29:179–193.

29. Aaslid R, Huber P, Nornes H. Evaluation of cerebrovascular spasm with transcranial Doppler ultrasound. J Neurosurg 1984; 60:37–41.

30. Hutchison K, Weir B. Transcranial Doppler studies in aneurysm patients. Can J Neurol Sci 1989; 16:411–416.

31. Seiler RW, Grolimund P. Transcranial Doppler evaluation of cerebral vasospasm. In: Wilkins RH, ed. Cerebral Vasospasm. New York: Raven Press, 1988.

32. Sloan MA, Haley EC, Kassell NF, et al. Sensitivity and specificity of transcranial Doppler ultrasonography in the diagnosis of vasospasm following subarachnoid hemorrhage. Neurology 1989; 39(11):14–18.

33. Lysakowski C, Walder B, Costanza MC, et al. Transcranial Doppler versus angiography in patients with vasospasm due to a ruptured cerebral aneurysm: a systematic review. Stroke 2001; 32:2292–2298.

34. Newell DW, Grady MS, Eskridge JM, et al. Distribution of angiographic vasospasm after subarachnoid hemorrhage: implications for diagnosis by transcranial Doppler ultrasonography. Neurosurgery 1990; 27:574–577.

35. Ekelund A, Saveland H, Rommer B, et al. Is transcranial Doppler sonography useful in detecting late cerebral ischaemia after aneurysmal subarachnoid hemorrhage? Br J Neurosurg 1996;10:19–25.

36. Lindegaard KF, Nornes H, Bakke SJ, et al. Cerebral vasospasm diagnosis by means of angiography and blood velocity measurements. Acta Neurochir (Wien) 1989; 100:12–24.

37. Suarez JI, Qureshi AI, Yahia AB, et al. Symptomatic vasospasm diagnosis after subarachnoid hemorrhage: evaluation of Transcranial Doppler ultrasound and cerebral angiography as related to compromised vascular distribution. Crit Care Med 2002; 30:1348–1355.

38. Vora YY, Suarez-Almazor M, Steinke DE, et al. Role of transcranial Doppler monitoring in the diagnosis of cerebral vasospasm after subarachnoid hemorrhage. Neurosurgery 1999; 44:1237–1247.

39. Sekhar LN, Wechsler LR, Yonas H, et al. Value of transcranial Doppler examination in the diagnosis of cerebral vasospasm after subarachnoid hemorrhage. Neurosurgery 1988; 22:813–821.

40. Grosset DG, Straiton J, McDonald I, et al. Use of transcranial Doppler sonography to predict development of a delayed ischemic deficit after subarachnoid hemorrhage. J Neurosurg 1993; 78:183–187.

41. Grosset DG, McDonald I, Cockburn M, et al. Prediction of delayed neurological deficit after subarachnoid haemorrhage: a CT blood load and Doppler velocity approach. Neuroradiology 1994; 36:418–421.

42. Sviri GE, Lewis DH, Correa R, et al. Basilar artery vasospasm and delayed posterior circulation ischemia after aneurysmal subarachnoid hemorrhage. Stroke 2004; 35:1867–1872.

43. Sloan MA, Burch CM, Wozniak MA, et al. Transcranial Doppler detection of verte-brobasilar vasospasm following subarachnoid hemorrhage. Stroke 1994; 25:2187–2197.

44. Soustiel JF, Shik V, Shreiber R, et al. Basilar vasospasm diagnosis: investigation of a modified "Lindegaard Index" based on imaging studies and blood velocity measurements of the basilar artery. Stroke 2002; 33:72–77.

45. Sviri GE, Ghodke B, Britz GW, et al. Transcranial Doppler grading criteria for basilar artery vasospasm. Neurosurgery 2006; 59:360–366.

46. White H, Venkatesh B. Applications of transcranial Doppler in the ICU: a review. Intensive Care Med 2006; 32:981–994.

47. Adams HP, Kassell NF, Torner JC. Usefulness of computed tomography in predicting the outcome after subarachnoid hemorrhage: a preliminary report of the Cooperative Aneurysm Study. Neurology 1985; 35:1263–1267.

48. Tazawa T, Mizukami M, Usami T, et al. Relationship between contrast enhancement on computed tomography and cerebral vasospasm in patients with subarachnoid hemorrhage. Neurosurgery 1983; 12:643–648.

49. Takagi R, Hayashi H, Kobayashi H, et al. Evaluation of three-dimensional CT angiography (3D CTA) for the diagnosis of cerebral vasospasm. Nippon Igaku Hoshasen Gakkai Zasshi 1997; 57:64–66.
50. Firlik AD, Kaufmann AM, Jungreis CA, et al. Effect of transluminal angioplasty on cerebral blood flow in the management of symptomatic vasospasm following aneurysmal subarachnoid hemorrhage. J Neurosurg 1997; 86:830–839.
51. Yonas H, Sekhar L, Johnson DW, et al. Determination of irreversible ischemia by xenon-enhanced computed tomographic monitoring of cerebral blood flow in patients with symptomatic vasospasm. Neurosurgery 1989; 24:368–372.
52. Davis SM, Andrews JT, Lichtenstein M, et al. Correlations between cerebral arterial velocities, blood flow, and delayed ischemia after subarachnoid hemorrhage. Stroke 1992; 23:492–497.
53. Hoeffner EG, Case I, Jain R, et al. Cerebral perfusion CT: technique and clinical applications. Radiology 2004; 231:632–644.
54. Moftakhar R, Rowley HA, Turk A, et al. Utility of computed tomography perfusion in detection of cerebral vasospasm in patients with subarachnoid hemorrhage. Neurosurg Focus 2006; 21(3):E6.
55. Rordorf G, Koroshetz WJ, Copen WA, et al. Diffusion- and perfusion-weighted imaging in vasospasm after subarachnoid hemorrhage. Stroke 1999; 30:599–605.
56. Lad SP, Guzman R, Kelly ME, et al. Cerebral perfusion imaging in vasospasm. Neurosurg Focus 2006; 21(3):E7.
57. Mehta B. Cerebral arteriography. In: Welch KM, Caplan LR, Reis DJ, et al., eds. Cerebrovascular Disease. San Diego: Academic Press, 1997:611–614.
58. Suarez JI, Tarr RW, Selman WR. Aneurysmal subarachnoid hemorrhage. N Engl J Med 2006; 354:387–396.
59. Weyer GW, Nolan CP, Macdonald RL. Evidence-based cerebral vasospasm management. Neurosurg Focus 2006; 21(3):E8.
60. Rinkel GJ, Feigin VL, Algra A, et al. Calcium antagonists for aneurysmal subarachnoid haemorrhage. Cochrane Database Syst 2005; Rev:CD000277.
61. Haley EC, Jr., Kassell NF, Torner JC. A randomized controlled trial of high-dose intravenous nicardipine in aneurysmal subarachnoid hemorrhage. A report of the Cooperative Aneurysm Study. J Neurosurg 1993; 78:537–547.
62. Origitano TC, Karesh SM, Reichman OH, et al. Sustained increased cerebral blood flow with prophylactic hypertensive hypervolemic hemodilution ("triple-H" therapy) after subarachnoid hemorrhage. Neurosurgery 1990; 27:729–739.
63. Egge A, Waterloo K, Sjoholm H, et al. Prophylactic hyperdynamic postoperative fluid therapy after aneurysmal subarachnoid hemorrhage: a clinical, prospective, randomized, controlled study. Neurosurgery 2001; 49:593–605.
64. Lennihan L, Mayer SA, Fink ME, et al. Effect of hypervolemic therapy on cerebral blood flow after subarachnoid hemorrhage: a randomized controlled trial. Stroke 2000; 31:383–391.
65. Rinkel GJE, Feigin VL, Algra A, et al. Hypervolemia in aneurysmal subarachnoid hemorrhage. Stroke 2005; 36:1104–1105.
66. Romner B, Reinstrup P. Triple H therapy after aneurysmal subarachnoid hemorrhage. A review. Acta Neurochir Suppl 2001; 77:237–241.
67. Liu-DeRyke X, Rhoney DH. Cerebral Vasospasm after aneurysmal subarachnoid hemorrhage: an overview of pharmacologic management. Pharmacotherapy 2006; 26(2):182–203.

68. van den Bergh WM, Algra A, van Kooten F, et al. Magnesium sulfate in aneurysmal subarachnoid hemorrhage: a randomized controlled trial. Stroke 2005; 36:1011–1015.
69. Prevedello DM, Cordeiro JG, de Morais AL, et al. Magnesium sulfate: role as possible attenuating factor in vasospasm morbidity. Surg Neurol 2006; 65(suppl 1): S1–S20.
70. Schmid-Elsaesser R, Kunz M, Zausinger S, et al. Intravenous magnesium versus nimodipine in the treatment of patients with aneurysmal subarachnoid hemorrhage: a randomized study. Neurosurgery 2006; 58(6):1054–1065.
71. Van den Bergh WM, Mess SM, Rinkel GJ. Intravenous magnesium versus nimodipine in the treatment of patients with aneurysmal subarachnoid hemorrhage: a randomized study. Neurosurgery. 2006; 59(5):E1152.
72. Lynch JR, Wang H, McGirt MJ, et al. Simvastatin reduces vasospasm after aneurysmal subarachnoid hemorrhage: results of a pilot randomized clinical trial. Stroke 2005; 36:2024–2026.
73. Tseng MY, Czosnyka M, Richards H, et al. Effects of acute treatment with pravastatin on cerebral vasospasm, autoregulation, and delayed ischemic deficits after aneurysmal subarachnoid hemorrhage: a phase II randomized placebo-controlled trial. Stroke 2005; 36:1627–1632.
74. Tseng MY, Phil M, Czosnyka M, et al. Effects of acute treatment with statins on cerebral autoregulation in patients after aneurysmal subarachnoid hemorrhage. Neurosurg Focus 2006; 21(3):E10.
75. Mocco J, Zacharia BE, Komotar RJ, et al. A review of current and future medical therapies for cerebral vasospasm following aneurysmal subarachnoid hemorrhage. Neurosurg Focus 2006; 21(3):E9.
76. Klimo P, Jr., Kestle JR, MacDonald JD, et al. Marked reduction of cerebral vasospasm with lumbar drainage of cerebrospinal fluid after subarachnoid hemorrhage. J Neurosurg 2004; 100(2):215–224.
77. van den Bergh WM, MASH Study Group, Algra A, et al. Randomized controlled trial of acetylsalicylic acid in aneurysmal subarachnoid hemorrhage: the MASH Study. Stroke 2006; 37:2326–2330.
78. Dorsch NW, Kassell NF, Sinkula MS. Meta-analysis of trials of tirilazad mesylate in aneurysmal SAH. Acta Neurochir Suppl 2001; 77:233–235.

Pharmacologic Cerebroprotection in Aneurysmal Subarachnoid Hemorrhage

Yekaterina Axelrod, MD, Assistant Professor[a,b]
Salah Keyrouz, MD[*]**, Fellow**[d]
Michael Diringer, MD, FCCM, Professor[a,b,c] **and Director**[d]
Department of [a]*Neurology,* [b]*Neurosurgery, and* [c]*Anesthesia;*
[d]*Neurology and Neurosurgery Intensive Care Unit,*
Washington University School of Medicine, St. Louis, Missouri, U.S.A.

INTRODUCTION

Acute aneurysmal subarachnoid hemorrhage (aSAH) is a complex multifaceted disorder that evolves over days to weeks. The initial hemorrhage can be devastating; it is fatal in approximately 25% of patients. Those who survive the initial bleed are at risk for a host of secondary insults, including rebleeding, hydrocephalus, and delayed ischemic deficits (DIDs). The management of SAH patients focuses on the anticipation, prevention, and management of these secondary complications.

DIDs usually become evident 5 to 10 days after the initial hemorrhage, which makes the potential for neuroprotective agents to be of benefit particularly appealing, as they may be administered prior to the onset of ischemic symptoms. Although DIDs are frequently attributed to "vasospasm," several factors appear to interact to produce them; they are likely a result of some combination of three key factors: severe narrowing of the large intracranial arteries (leading to reduced perfusion pressure), intravascular volume depletion, and a disturbed autoregulatory

Present affiliation: Assistant Professor, Department of Neurology, University of Arkansas for Medical Sciences, Little Rock, Arkansas, U.S.A.

function in the distal cerebral circulation. In the presence of clinical symptoms, cerebral blood flow (CBF) can fall to the point at which the compensatory rise in oxygen extraction can no longer maintain adequate oxygen delivery to meet the metabolic needs of the brain.

Neuroprotective agents could potentially improve outcome by ameliorating reduced CBF, by a direct protective effect on the ischemic tissue, or both. Demonstrating a clinical benefit of neuroprotective agents in aSAH is particularly challenging. The complex nature of the disease and the multiple factors that influence outcome make it difficult to discover the effect of an intervention that might influence only one of the factors. This high level of clinical variability requires very large numbers of patients with a relatively uncommon disease to be enrolled into trials to establish the benefit of an intervention.

CALCIUM CHANNEL ANTAGONISTS

A rise in intracellular calcium concentration in the vascular smooth muscle cells due to influx via the L-type calcium channels plays a crucial role in the pathogenesis of cerebral vasospasm and subsequent ischemia (1). By blocking the channels, calcium channel antagonists reduce the intracellular calcium influx and prevent vasoconstriction. In addition, some "neuroselective" calcium channel blockers act at the level of the neurons by preventing calcium influx following ischemia (2). These agents have been widely used since the mid-1980s as neuroprotective agents following aSAH to reduce the impact of cerebral vasospasm and DID.

Nimodipine is the most rigorously studied agent among all calcium channel blockers (3–10) and is the only approved medication for the treatment of cerebral vasospasm in North America and Europe. The exact mechanism of its neuroprotection is still unknown. This drug is selective for the cerebral vessels; it increases CBF and dilates the pial vessels in experimental models (1). However, it does not affect the frequency or appearance of angiographic vasospasm in humans (3,7,9). Nimodipine has been shown to inhibit platelet thromboxane release, reducing platelet aggregation, thereby producing a theoretical benefit in ischemia (11). Limitation of neuronal intracellular calcium entry during ischemia may be one of the possible mechanisms; or a yet unknown direct cerebral protective mechanism may play a role.

Nimodipine is a safe, well-tolerated calcium channel antagonist that is administered via the gastrointestinal tract for 14–21 days after aSAH. Numerous prospective trials (3–10) demonstrated that it reduces both the incidence of DID and poor outcome (death and severe disability) at three months following aSAH of all grades. The largest study was the British aneurysm nimodipine trial (9). This randomized, double-blinded, multicentered trial enrolled 554 patients with aSAH within 96 hours of symptom onset and compared nimodipine to placebo. A 34% reduction in the incidence of cerebral infarctions was observed with nimodipine administered for 21 days; poor outcome at three months was reduced by 40%. Two meta-analyses (12,13) of nimodipine efficacy showed that it improved the odds of good or fair outcome after aSAH, reduced the odds of morbidity and mortality related to clinical vasospasm, and reduced the frequency of infarcts. No significant difference in overall mortality was seen. Of note, nimodipine did not seem to have a significant effect on angiographic vasospasm (14) or on CBF (3).

Nicardipine belongs to the same family of calcium channel blockers as nimodipine. The ability of intravenous (IV) nicardipine to reduce the impact of vasospasm was tested in a large prospective trial. Even though the drug reduced the incidence of clinical vasospasm, it failed to change the overall outcome (15). This lack of demonstrated benefit may have been confounded by more frequent use of hemodynamic treatments for vasospasm in the placebo arm. IV administration was associated with hypotension in some patients (16).

Intra-arterial infusions are also used to directly dilate cerebral arteries affected by vasospasm (14,17) and have been shown to reduce transcranial-Doppler (TCD) mean peak systolic velocities in treated vessels (17). When administered intrathecally in a nonblinded and noncontrolled fashion, nicardipine reduced the incidence of both symptomatic and angiographic spasm and improved good clinical outcome at one month following aSAH (18). However, side effects were common; headache occurred in 18%, and meningitis occurred in 4% of patients.

The investigation of nicardipine prolonged-release implants is gaining momentum following encouraging preclinical data (19). In a preliminary report about 20 patients who underwent nicardipine implant placement into the thick subarachnoid clots at the time of surgical aneurysm clipping, none of the vessels near the pellets developed vasospasm, and only one patient developed a cerebral infarction (20). No complications were reported. In a more recent retrospective series published by the same authors, the incidence of DID after pellet implantation was 6%; at three months, 89% of patients were independent (21). In a small, single-centered randomized study of nicardipine pellet placement, 16 patients received implants and no additional calcium channel antagonists. The incidence of angiographic vasospasm in the study group was significantly reduced to 7% from 73%, mortality dropped to 6% from 38%, and clinical long-term outcomes were more favorable (22).

Diltiazem tested in phase I and II studies showed no effect on amelioration of vasospasm (23). The use of oral diltiazem was reported in the treatment of 123 aSAH patients. Incidence of DID was 19.5%, and a favorable outcome, defined as Glasgow Outcome Scale score of 4 or 5, was achieved in almost 75% of patients. These results obtained in a noncontrolled series do not permit any conclusions regarding the role of diltiazem in management of aSAH (24).

MAGNESIUM

Hypomagnesemia is found on admission in patients following stroke (25) and in over one-third of individuals with aSAH (25). In one study, hypomagnesemia occurring between days 2 and 12 after aSAH independently predicted development of DID (26); yet no similar association was found in another retrospective study (27).

Magnesium is actively transported across the blood-brain barrier; its concentration is higher in the cerebrospinal fluid than in serum (28). It is a physiologic antagonist of calcium, relaxes vascular smooth muscles, inhibits calcium-mediated activation of intracellular enzymes, and antagonizes calcium entry into the cells via the voltage-gated channels (29). In addition, magnesium inhibits release of excitatory amino-acids and blocks NMDA receptors during hypoxic-ischemic insults. It also increases CBF in animals with stroke (30). Magnesium is very appealing as a neuroprotective agent because of the ease of administration, the ability to maintain steady state and measure concentration in body fluids (31,32), and its low cost and favorable safety profile. Interest is bolstered by the success of magnesium administration in preventing and treating eclampsia, the vascular pathophysiology of which superficially resembles that of aSAH-induced vasospasm (33–35).

A wealth of experimental data exists regarding magnesium-related neuroprotection in stroke and aSAH. Magnesium administration led to a reduction of infarct volume in a rodent model of focal cerebral ischemia (36,37). In animal models, magnesium pretreatment diminished MRI cerebral lesion volume in the acute period after aSAH (38). In addition, both topical and IV administration of magnesium helps to dilate vasospastic vessels (39). In stroke or aSAH patients, magnesium has been shown to be practical and safe (31,32,40–42).

To date, three randomized controlled pilot studies that have enrolled a total of 209 patients treated with magnesium showed a small trend toward a better outcome (32,41,42). In a randomized double-blinded pilot study that compared magnesium sulfate to saline infusion, investigators showed a trend toward less symptomatic vasospasm in the magnesium arm (41). Another study noted a trend toward reduced DID and poor outcome in a controlled trial of continuous magnesium sulfate infusion (42). A small, single-centered trial compared the effect of magnesium in preventing DID to that of IV nimodipine (43); however, the study was underpowered to detect a clinical difference between the two treatment modalities. A large, prospective, multicentered, placebo-controlled trial of magnesium in patients with aSAH that is investigating clinical outcome is in progress (44). In a study comparing magnesium and prophylactic hypervolemia/hemodilution to hypervolemia/hemodilution alone, the incidence of vasospasm was no different (45). It is interesting to note that a TCD study showed no improvement in elevated mean blood flow velocities in the middle cerebral arteries of patients who had clinical vasospasm after receiving a bolus infusion of magnesium sulfate (46).

NITRIC OXIDE DONORS AND ENDOTHELIN-1 ANTAGONISTS

Physiology of Nitric Oxide and Endothelin-1

Nitric oxide (NO) and endothelin-1 (ET-1) have intricate, crucial roles in controlling the cerebral vasomotor tone. NO is a free radical gas formed by the enzyme NO synthase from L-arginine. Its identity as endothelium-derived relaxing factor was discovered in 1987 (47). Tonic release of NO is an important regulator of resting CBF; inhibition of NO synthase constricts cerebral arteries and decreases CBF (48–50). ET-1 was identified in 1988 (51); it is a peptide with three iso-forms: ET-1, ET-2, and ET-3. ET-1 is the major isoform generated in the endothelium of the blood vessels and is the most important player in vascular tone regulation. ET-1 is thought to have effects through two receptor subtypes, ET_A and ET_B. Both are found on the vascular *smooth muscle* cells, where they mediate vasoconstriction. ET_B receptors found on cerebral, aortic, pulmonary, and renal vascular *endothelial* cells also participate in vasodilatation via NO and prostacyclin liberation (52–55).

Given the interdigitating roles of these two agents in the regulation of basal cerebral vasomotor tone, an impairment of the balanced action of NO and ET-1 is thought to contribute to the development of vasospasm following aSAH (56–58). Preclinical and early clinical use of NO donors and ET-1 antagonists in aSAH suggests a potential therapeutic role in the future, pending the outcomes of larger controlled trials.

Nitric Oxide Donors

In animal models of aSAH, intra-arterial and intrathecal administration of NO donors reversed angiographic vasospasm (59–61), increased CBF, and decreased cerebral vascular resistance (59), without causing systemic side effects. However, similar infusion of L-arginine, a natural NO donor, did not influence the incidence or degree of cerebral vasospasm in a primate aSAH model (62).

In patients with aSAH and cerebral vasospasm, intraventricular adminis-tration of sodium nitroprusside (SNP) as an NO donor has been attempted (63–66). This experience yielded inconsistent effects of variable duration on CBF, with a high frequency of adverse events. Intrathecal SNP was used as a therapy of last resort in patients with severe refractory vasospasm. Six of 13 patients exhibited improved cerebral hemodynamics (64). In another study, partial-to-complete reversal of angiographic vasospasm was demonstrated in 10 aSAH patients after SNP administration (65). Two patients who were symptomatic because of vas-ospasm recovered strength in their extremities. Vomiting was the commonest adverse effect seen in seven patients, while three patients had mild fluctuation in blood pressure. In another study, clinical and angiographic vasospasm was reversed with excellent outcome following intrathecal SNP administration with nausea being the most frequent side effect (63). The high frequency of nausea and vomiting prompted one author to recommended elective endotracheal intubation prior to this procedure (67).

Finally, transdermal nitroglycerin has been used in a small cohort of aSAH patients. Even though no difference in terms of DID and TCD velocities was observed between the nitroglycerin group (9 patients) and the control group (8 patients), CBF measured by CT perfusion was increased in the nitroglycerin group despite a drop in systemic blood pressure (68). Nitroglycerin paste was applied to five patients with vasospasm while they were in the angiographic suite, with mild-to-moderate improvement in angiographic vasospasm and minimal changes in blood and intracranial pressures (69).

Endothelin-1 Antagonists

In vitro and in vivo use of various ET_A antagonists in animal models of aSAH administered intrathecally or intravenously significantly decreased the degree of vasospasm (70–77). A selective ET_A-receptor antagonist, clazosentan, has been recently tested in a phase IIa trial in which it was administered as an IV infusion for 14 days. A reduction in the incidence and severity of angiographic vasospasm was reported (78). Most recently, three doses of clazosentan (1, 5, and 15 mg/hr) were tested in a phase IIb randomized controlled clinical trial of 413 patients with aSAH (79). Moderate-to-severe angiographic spasm at day 9 was significantly reduced in a dose-dependent fashion from 66% in the placebo group to 36% in the high-dose clazosentan group. Of note, administration of the drug was associated with hypotension, pulmonary edema, and adult respiratory distress syndrome. Even though no effect on outcome occurred, as measured by modified Rankin scale at three months, a trend toward reduction of morbidity and mortality was observed. A phase III outcome trial of clazosentan is planned.

Another compound, TAK-044, was tested in a phase II trial. Unlike others tested so far, it is an $ET_{A/B}$ antagonist. DID occurred in 29.5% of patients who received active treatment and in 36.6% of patients who received placebo (Relative risk, 0.8; 95% confidence interval, 0.61–1.06). The drug has been very well tolerated (80).

GLUCOCORTICOSTEROIDS

As aSAH and subsequent vasospasm are thought to be associated with the inflammatory cascade, potent anti-inflammatory agents such as glucocorticosteroids could conceivably benefit patients at risk for vasospasm. Neuroprotective effects of corticosteroids have been seen in animal models of aSAH (81–86), in which investigators reported attenuation of vasospasm (82,85,86) and positive effect on CBF (83). Very limited data are available in human trials. One randomized placebo-controlled trial of IV hydrocortisone conducted in Japan (87) was reviewed by the Cochrane group (88), who concluded that too few patients ($n = 140$) were enrolled to make a recommendation. In another small clinical trial that recruited 21 aSAH patients with large amounts of subarachnoid blood, IV methylprednisolone was given at high doses for one week. When compared to historic controls, only five patients in the study group (versus 9 in the control group) developed vasospasm (89). Lastly, an attempt to prevent vasospasm in 55 aSAH patients who underwent surgical clipping was made by irrigation of the operative site with methylprednisolone. These patients, when compared to controls (irrigation with lactated Ringer solution), were less likely to develop vasospasm or die (90). The frequency of good outcome was also higher.

TIRILAZAD

Tirilazad mesylate is a non–glucocorticoid steroid that exhibits neuroprotective effects that appear to be mediated via inhibition of lipid peroxidation. While experimental data in primate models of aSAH were encouraging with remarkable attenuation of vasospasm (91–93), clinical results did not demonstrate benefit. This agent was tested in five large, randomized placebo-controlled trials that enrolled over 4000 acute aSAH patients, all of whom also received nimodipine. The first trial, which looked at safety, showed a trend toward better outcome at three months with a 2-mg/kg/day dose, whereas administration of the highest dose (6 mg/kg/day) was associated with increased clinical vasospasm and mortality (94). The next two trials (95,96) failed to show any significant benefits on angiographic or clinical vasospasm; however, in one trial (95), mortality rates and clinical outcome at 3 months were better, especially in male poor-grade aSAH patients. These results and an observation of different gender-related pharmacokinetics of the drug encouraged conduction of two more trials of a higher tirilazad dose (15 mg/kg/day) in female patients (97,98). One of these demonstrated a significantly lower rate of symptomatic spasm without any change in mortality (97), whereas in the other, while the rate of symptomatic vasospasm was not different in the study group, mortality was lower in patients with Hunt and Hess grades IV–V (98). A meta-analysis of the four latter trials concluded that overall mortality was decreased in patients treated with tirilazad, but this effect was most evident in patients with poor neurologic grades (99).

STATINS

Initially developed as cholesterol-lowering agents, statins (3-hydroxy-3-methylglutaryl coenzyme A reductase inhibitors) appear to have much wider applications because of their broad range of various properties. After promising results in animal models of aSAH (100,101), where simvastatin reduced vasospasm and improved neurologic outcome, a great clinical interest arose for use of statins in aSAH patients. One proposed mechanism of neuroprotection is related to the upregulation of the NO synthase pathway (102,103) with subsequent improvement in the CBF (104). Morphologically, not only was luminal patency increased, but perivascular granulocyte migration was also decreased after treatment with simvastatin (101).

In a retrospective cohort study, statin use prior to admission for aSAH increased the risk for TCD and angiographic vasospasm but not clinical vasospasm. In a multivariate analysis, where statin exposure was replaced with statin discontinuation, the latter did not increase the risk for vasospasm (105). In another multivariate analysis of 115 patients admitted with aSAH, including 15 who had been taking statins for at least one month, an 11-fold reduction in the odds ratio of subsequent vasospasm was independently associated with current statin therapy (106). A recent review of effects of statin discontinuation in clinical and experimental studies (107) suggested that a proinflammatory, prothrombotic state with impaired endothelium function after an acute ischemic event (cardiac or cerebral) might also occur after abrupt cessation of statins; therefore, discontinuation of current statin therapy for more than 24 hours may be harmful.

Two small, randomized placebo-controlled studies to evaluate the effect of statins in patients suffering aSAH have been performed (108,109). In one, 40 patients were randomized to receive 40 mg of pravastatin in addition to nimodipine (108). A 42% relative reduction in the incidence of TCD-defined, severe vasospasm was seen in the pravastatin group. Mortality was also significantly lower (2% versus 8% in the placebo group). In the second trial, 19 SAH patients received 80 mg of simvastatin for 14 days; the incidence of vasospasm in the study arm was 26% compared to 60% in the placebo arm ($n = 20$) (109).

HYPOTHERMIA

Temperature elevations above 38°C have been described in over two-thirds of patients with aSAH (110). Fever after aSAH was independently associated with vasospasm and poor outcome after controlling for severity of hemorrhage or presence of infection (111).

Induced hypothermia has been shown to be neuroprotective in various animal models of local and global ischemia (112–116). The potential mechanisms responsible for its impact include stabilization of the blood-brain barrier, reduction in postischemic hyperperfusion and subsequent edema formation, and a reduction in free radicals and excitatory neurotransmitters. Hypothermia has been studied in aSAH as well. In a rat model of aSAH, moderate hypothermia was able to reverse MRI-defined ischemic deficits, thus creating a basis for further clinical studies (117).

Several small studies of therapeutic hypothermia in poor-grade aSAH patients and refractory cerebral vasospasm have yielded somewhat promising results (118–120). In one metabolic study, the reduction in cerebral metabolic rate for oxygen exceeded the fall in CBF, suggesting a state of luxury perfusion (121).

Hypothermia has been best studied as a neuroprotectant when applied during surgical clipping of aneurysms. Initial trials of moderate hypothermia (33.5°C) had encouraging results (122,123). Yet, an NIH-sponsored, large, prospective, multicentered controlled trial of moderate intraoperative hypothermia (33°C) in patients with good grades, hypothermia showed no benefit to clinical or functional outcome at three months despite the large size of the trial, high-quality follow-up, and high protocol compliance (124). Complex neuropsychiatric evaluations performed in these patients demonstrated no difference in impairment between the study and control groups (125).

CONCLUSIONS

Extensive efforts have been applied to defining a role for neuroprotective agents in cerebral ischemia and aSAH. Unfortunately, to date, no agents have been established as beneficial in ischemic stroke, and only one is FDA-approved for the treatment of aSAH patients. However, new techniques for delivering agents and our growing understanding of the molecular mechanisms involved in ischemia after aSAH have yielded new promising agents. It is important to recognize, though, that many agents have appeared promising in phase II trials but failed the final test by not demonstrating improved clinical outcome in large, controlled trials. Thus, early adoption of promising agents is not warranted.

Oral nimodipine has been established as being beneficial to all grades of SAH patients. It is routinely administered for 21 days. The data on IV nicardipine are mixed, and it can reduce blood pressure at inopportune times. Although an appealing concept, few data exist regarding intra-arterial administration of nimodipine, and more information is essential before its role can be defined. Nicardipine pellet implantation during surgery looks promising in early small studies, but large randomized controlled trials are needed before this approach is adopted.

The studies on magnesium in aSAH have all resulted in positive trends without statistical significance. Although very appealing in terms of use and safety, the data do not support its routine use. The data regarding trilazad are mixed, and outcome trials did not establish a clear benefit.

Two new avenues—endothelin antagonists and statins—are under active development. Phase II clinical trials are very encouraging, and phase III trials are in progress.

REFERENCES

1. Alborch E, Salom JB, Torregrosa G. Calcium channels in cerebral arteries. Pharmacol Ther 1995; 68, 1–34.
2. Won SJ, Kim DY, Gwag BJ. Cellular and molecular pathways of ischemic neuronal death. J Biochem Mol Biol 2002; 35(1), 67–86.
3. Allen GS, Ahn HS, Preziosi TJ, et al. Cerebral arterial spasm: a controlled trial of nimodipine in patients with subarachnoid hemorrhage. N Engl J Med 1983; 308(11): 619–624.
4. Philippon J, Grob R, Dagreou F, et al. Prevention of vasospasm in subarachnoid haemorrhage. A controlled study with nimodipine. Acta Neurochir (Wien) 1986; 82(3–4):110–114.
5. Neil-Dwyer G, Mee E, Dorrance D, et al. Early intervention with nimodipine in subarachnoid haemorrhage. Eur Heart J 1987 Nov; 8 suppl K: 41–47.
6. Jan M, Buchheit F, Tremoulet M. Therapeutic trial of intravenous nimodipine in patients with established cerebral vasospasm after rupture of intracranial aneurysms. Neurosurgery 1988; 23(2):154–157.
7. Petruk KC, West M, Mohr G, et al. Nimodipine treatment in poor-grade aneurysm patients. Results of a multicenter double-blind placebo-controlled trial. J Neurosurg 1988; 68(4):505–517.
8. Ohman J, Heiskanen O. Effect of nimodipine on the outcome of patients after aneurysmal subarachnoid hemorrhage and surgery. J Neurosurg 1988; 69(5):683–686.
9. Pickard JD, Murray GD, Illingworth R, et al. Effect of oral nimodipine on cerebral infarction and outcome after subarachnoid haemorrhage: British aneurysm nimodipine trial. BMJ 1989; 298:636–642.

10. Gilsbach JM, Reulen HJ, Ljunggren B, et al. Early aneurysm surgery and preventive therapy with intravenously administered nimodipine: a multicenter, double-blind, dose-comparison study. Neurosurgery 1990; 26(3):458–464.

11. Juvela S, Kaste M, Hillbom M. Effect of nimodipine on platelet function in patients with subarachnoid hemorrhage. Stroke 1990; 21:1283–1288.

12. Rinkel GJ, Feigin VL, Algra A, et al. Calcium antagonists for aneurysmal subarachnoid haemorrhage. Cochrane Database Syst Rev 2005: CD000277.

13. Barker FG II, Ogilvy CS. Efficacy of prophylactic nimodipine for delayed ischemic deficit after subarachnoid hemorrhage: a metaanalysis. J Neurosurg 1996; 84(3): 405–414.

14. Feigin VL, Rinkel GJ, Algra A, et al. Calcium antagonists in patients with aneurysmal subarachnoid hemorrhage: a systematic review. Neurology 1998; 50:876–883.

15. Haley EC Jr, Kassell NF, Torner JC. A randomized controlled trial of high-dose intravenous nicardipine in aneurysmal subarachnoid hemorrhage. A report of the Cooperative Aneurysm Study. J Neurosurg 1993; 78(4):537–547.

16. Haley EC Jr, Kassell NF, Torner JC, et al. A randomized trial of two doses of nicardipine in aneurysmal subarachnoid hemorrhage. A report of the Cooperative Aneurysm Study. J Neurosurg 1994; 80(5):788–796.

17. Badjatia N, Topcuoglu MA, Pryor JC, et al. Preliminary experience with intra-arterial nicardipine as a treatment for cerebral vasospasm. Am J Neuroradiol 2004; 25:819–826.

18. Shibuya M, Suzuki Y, Enomoto H, et al. Effects of prophylactic intrathecal administrations of nicardipine on vasospasm in patients with severe aneurysmal subarachnoid haemorrhage. Acta Neurochir (Wien) 1994; 131:19–25.

19. Kawashima A, Kasuya H, Sasahara A, et al. Prevention of cerebral vasospasm by nicardipine prolonged-release implants in dogs. Neurol Res 2000; 22:634–641.

20. Kasuya H, Onda H, Takeshita M, et al. Efficacy and safety of nicardipine prolonged-release implants for preventing vasospasm in humans. Stroke 2002; 33:1011–1015.

21. Kasuya H, Onda H, Sasahara A, et al. Application of nicardipine prolonged-release implants: analysis of 97 consecutive patients with acute subarachnoid hemorrhage. Neurosurgery 2005; 56:895–902.

22. Barth M, Capelle HH, Weidauer S, et al. Effect of nicardipine prolonged-release implants on cerebral vasospasm and clinical outcome after severe aneurysmal subarachnoid hemorrhage: a prospective, randomized, double-blind phase IIa study. Stroke 2007; 38(2):330–336.

23. Saunders FW, Marshall WJ. Diltiazem: does it affect vasospasm? Surg Neurol 1986; 26:155–158.

24. Papavasiliou AK, Harbaugh KS, Birkmeyer NJ, et al. Clinical outcomes of aneurysmal subarachnoid hemorrhage patients treated with oral diltiazem and limited intensive care management. Surg Neurol 2001; 55(3):138–146.

25. Altura BT, Memon ZI, Zhang A, et al. Low levels of serum ionized magnesium are found in patients early after stroke which result in rapid elevation in cytosolic free calcium and spasm in cerebral vascular muscle cells. Neurosci Lett 1997; 230:37–40.

26. van den Bergh WM, Algra A, van der Sprenkel JW, et al. Hypomagnesemia after aneurysmal subarachnoid hemorrhage. Neurosurgery 2003; 52:276–281.

27. Collignon FP, Friedman JA, Piepgras DG, et al. Serum magnesium levels as related to symptomatic vasospasm and outcome following aneurysmal subarachnoid hemorrhage. Neurocrit Care 2004; 1:441–448.

28. Fishman RA. Composition of the Cerebrospinal Fluid. In Fishman RA, ed. Cerebrospinal Fluid in Diseases of the Central Nervous System, 2nd ed. Philadelphia: WB Saunders, 1992:26–227.
29. Muir KW. Magnesium for neuroprotection in ischaemic stroke: rationale for use and evidence of effectiveness. CNS Drugs 2001; 15(12):921–930.
30. Chi OZ, Pollak P, Weiss HR. Effects of magnesium sulfate and nifedipine on regional cerebral blood flow during middle cerebral artery ligation in the rat. Arch Int Pharmacodyn Ther 1990; 304:196–205.
31. van den Bergh WM, Albrecht KW, Berkelbach van der Sprenkel JW, et al. Magnesium therapy after aneurysmal subarachnoid haemorrhage a dose-finding study for long-term treatment. Acta Neurochir (Wien) 2003; 145:195–199.
32. Veyna RS, Seyfried D, Burke DG, et al. Magnesium sulfate therapy after aneurysmal subarachnoid hemorrhage. J Neurosurg 2002; 96:510–514.
33. Belfort MA, Anthony J, Saade GR, et al. A comparison of magnesium sulfate and nimodipine for the prevention of eclampsia. N Engl J Med 2003; 348:304–311.
34. Naidu S, Payne AJ, Moodley J, et al. Randomised study assessing the effect of phenytoin and magnesium sulphate on maternal cerebral circulation in eclampsia using transcranial Doppler ultrasound. Br J Obstet Gynaecol 1996; 103:111–116.
35. Sadeh M. Action of magnesium sulfate in the treatment of preeclampsia-eclampsia. Stroke 1989; 20:1273–1275.
36. Izumi Y, Roussel S, Pinard E, et al. Reduction of infarct volume by magnesium after middle cerebral artery occlusion in rats. J Cereb Blood Flow Metab 1991; 11:1025–1030.
37. Marinov MB, Harbaugh KS, Hoopes PJ, et al. Neuroprotective effects of preischemia intraarterial magnesium sulfate in reversible focal cerebral ischemia. J Neurosurg 1996; 85:117–124.
38. van den Bergh WM, Zuur JK, Kamerling NA, et al. Role of magnesium in the reduction of ischemic depolarization and lesion volume after experimental subarachnoid hemorrhage. J Neurosurg 2002; 97:416–422.
39. Ram Z, Sadeh M, Shacked I, et al. Magnesium sulfate reverses experimental delayed cerebral vasospasm after subarachnoid hemorrhage in rats. Stroke 1991; 22:922–927.
40. Boet R, Mee E. Magnesium sulfate in the management of patients with Fisher Grade 3 subarachnoid hemorrhage: a pilot study. Neurosurgery 2000; 47:602–606.
41. Wong GK, Chan MT, Boet R, et al. Intravenous magnesium sulfate after aneurysmal subarachnoid hemorrhage: a prospective randomized pilot study. J Neurosurg Anesthesiol 2006; 18:142–148.
42. van den Bergh WM, Algra A, van Kooten F, et al. Magnesium sulfate in aneurysmal subarachnoid hemorrhage: a randomized controlled trial. Stroke 2005; 36:1011–1015.
43. Schmid-Elsaesser R, Kunz M, Zausinger S, et al. Intravenous magnesium versus nimodipine in the treatment of patients with aneurysmal subarachnoid hemorrhage: a randomized study. Neurosurgery 2006; 58:1054–1065.
44. Anonymous. Major ongoing stroke trials. Stroke 2007; 38(2):e1–e9.
45. Prevedello DM, Cordeiro JG, de Morais AL, et al. Magnesium sulfate: role as possible attenuating factor in vasospasm morbidity. Surg Neurol 2006; 65 (suppl 1), S1:14–1:20.
46. Brewer RP, Parra A, Lynch J, et al. Cerebral blood flow velocity response to magnesium sulfate in patients after subarachnoid hemorrhage. J Neurosurg Anesthesiol 2001; 13:202–206.

47. Palmer RM, Ferrige AG, Moncada S. Nitric oxide release accounts for the biological activity of endothelium-derived relaxing factor. Nature 1987; 327:524–526.

48. Faraci FM. Role of endothelium-derived relaxing factor in cerebral circulation: large arteries vs. microcirculation. Am J Physiol 1991; 261:H1038–H1042.

49. Prado R, Watson BD, Kuluz J, et al. Endothelium-derived nitric oxide synthase inhibition. Effects on cerebral blood flow, pial artery diameter, and vascular morphology in rats. Stroke 1992; 23:1118–1123.

50. You J, Johnson TD, Marrelli SP, et al. P2u receptor-mediated release of endothelium-derived relaxing factor/nitric oxide and endothelium-derived hyperpolarizing factor from cerebrovascular endothelium in rats. Stroke 1999; 30:1125–1133.

51. Yanagisawa M, Kurihara H, Kimura S, et al. A novel potent vasoconstrictor peptide produced by vascular endothelial cells. Nature 1988; 332:411–415.

52. Davenport AP, Maguire JJ. Is endothelin-induced vasoconstriction mediated only by ETA receptors in humans? Trends Pharmacol Sci 1994; 15:9–11.

53. Hosoda K, Nakao K, Hiroshi A, et al. Cloning and expression of human endothelin-1 receptor cDNA. FEBS Lett 1991; 287:23–26.

54. Molenaar P, O'Reilly G, Sharkey A, et al. Characterization and localization of endothelin receptor subtypes in the human atrioventricular conducting system and myocardium. Circ Res 1993; 72:526–538.

55. Ogawa Y, Nakao K, Arai H, et al. Molecular cloning of a non-isopeptide-selective human endothelin receptor. Biochem Biophys Res Commun 1991; 178:248–255.

56. Hirose H, Ide K, Sasaki T, et al. The role of endothelin and nitric oxide in modulation of normal and spastic cerebral vascular tone in the dog. Eur J Pharmacol 1995; 277:77–87.

57. Nishizawa S, Chen D, Yokoyama T, et al. Endothelin-1 initiates the development of vasospasm after subarachnoid haemorrhage through protein kinase C activation but does not contribute to prolonged vasospasm. Acta Neurochir (Wien) 2000; 142:1409–1415.

58. Pluta R. Dysfunction of nitric oxide synthases as a cause and therapeutic target in delayed cerebral vasospasm after SAH. Neurol Res 2006; 28(7):730–737(8).

59. Afshar JK, Pluta RM, Boock RJ, et al. Effect of intracarotid nitric oxide on primate cerebral vasospasm after subarachnoid hemorrhage. J Neurosurg 1995; 83:118–122.

60. Pluta RM, Oldfield EH, Boock RJ. Reversal and prevention of cerebral vasospasm by intracarotid infusions of nitric oxide donors in a primate model of subarachnoid hemorrhage. J Neurosurg 1997; 87:746–751.

61. Wolf EW, Banerjee A, Soble-Smith J, et al. Reversal of cerebral vasospasm using an intrathecally administered nitric oxide donor. J Neurosurg 1998; 89:279–288.

62. Pluta RM, Afshar JK, Thompson BG, et al. Increased cerebral blood flow but no reversal or prevention of vasospasm in response to L-arginine infusion after subarachnoid hemorrhage. J Neurosurg 2000; 92:121–126.

63. Thomas JE, Rosenwasser RH. Reversal of severe cerebral vasospasm in three patients after aneurysmal subarachnoid hemorrhage: initial observations regarding the use of intraventricular sodium nitroprusside in humans. Neurosurgery 1999; 44:48–57.

64. Raabe A, Zimmermann M, Setzer M, et al. Effect of intraventricular sodium nitroprusside on cerebral hemodynamics and oxygenation in poor-grade aneurysm patients with severe, medically refractory vasospasm. Neurosurgery 2002; 50: 1006–1013.

65. Kumar R, Pathak A, Mathuriya SN, et al. Intraventricular sodium nitroprusside therapy: a future promise for refractory subarachnoid hemorrhage-induced vasospasm. Neurol India 2003; 51:197–202.
66. Pachl J, Haninec P, Tencer T, et al. The effect of subarachnoid sodium nitroprusside on the prevention of vasospasm in subarachnoid haemorrhage. Acta Neurochir Suppl 2005; 95:141–145.
67. Mathew J. Airway safety for patients receiving intraventricular sodium nitroprusside therapy. Neurol India 2003; 51:560–561.
68. Reinert M, Wiest R, Barth L, et al. Transdermal nitroglycerin in patients with subarachnoid hemorrhage. Neurol Res 2004; 26:435–439.
69. Lesley WS, Lazo A, Chaloupka JC, et al. Successful treatment of cerebral vasospasm by use of transdermal nitroglycerin ointment (Nitropaste). Am J Neuroradiol 2003; 24 (6):1234–1236.
70. Roux S, Breu V, Giller T, et al. Ro 61–1790, a new hydrosoluble endothelin antagonist: general pharmacology and effects on experimental cerebral vasospasm. J Pharmacol Exp Ther 1997; 283:1110–1118.
71. Vatter H, Zimmermann M, Tesanovic V, et al. Cerebrovascular characterization of clazosentan, the first nonpeptide endothelin receptor antagonist clinically effective for the treatment of cerebral vasospasm. Part I: inhibitory effect on endothelin(A) receptor-mediated contraction. J Neurosurg 2005; 102:1101–1107.
72. Vatter H, Zimmermann M, Tesanovic V, et al. Cerebrovascular characterization of clazosentan, the first nonpeptide endothelin receptor antagonist shown to be clinically effective for the treatment of cerebral vasospasm. Part II: effect on endothelin(B) receptor-mediated relaxation. J Neurosurg 2005; 102:1108–1114.
73. Cirak B, Kiymaz N, Ari HH, et al. The effects of endothelin antagonist BQ-610 on cerebral vascular wall following experimental subarachnoid hemorrhage and cerebral vasospasm. Clin Auton Res 2004; 14:197–201.
74. Wanebo JE, Louis HG, Arthur AS, et al. Attenuation of cerebral vasospasm by systemic administration of an endothelin-A receptor antagonist, TBC 11251, in a rabbit model of subarachnoid hemorrhage. Neurosurg Focus 1997; 3(4) (article).
75. Wanebo JE, Arthur AS, Louis HG, et al. Systemic administration of the endothelin-A receptor antagonist TBC 11251 attenuates cerebral vasospasm after experimental subarachnoid hemorrhage: dose study and review of endothelin-based therapies in the literature on cerebral vasospasm. Neurosurgery 1998; 43:1409–1417.
76. Josko J, Hendryk S, Jedrzejowska-Szypulka H, et al. Effect of endothelin-1 receptor antagonist BQ-123 on basilar artery diameter after subarachnoid hemorrhage (SAH) in rats. J Physiol Pharmacol 2000; 51:241–249.
77. Macdonald RL, Johns L, Lin G, et al. Prevention of vasospasm after subarachnoid hemorrhage in dogs by continuous intravenous infusion of PD156707. Neurol Med Chir (Tokyo) 1998; 38 (suppl):138–145.
78. Vajkoczy P, Meyer B, Weidauer S, et al. Clazosentan (AXV-034343), a selective endothelin A receptor antagonist, in the prevention of cerebral vasospasm following severe aneurysmal subarachnoid hemorrhage: results of a randomized, double-blind, placebo-controlled, multicenter phase IIa study. J Neurosurg 2005; 103:9–17.
79. Macdonald RL, Kassell N, Mayer S, et al. Randomized trial of clazosentan for prevention of vasospasm after aneurysmal subarachnoid hemorrhage. Presented at International Stroke Conference. San Francisco, CA, 2007.

80. Shaw MD, Vermeulen M, Murray GD, et al. Efficacy and safety of the endothelin, receptor antagonist TAK-044 in treating subarachnoid hemorrhage: a report by the Steering Committee on behalf of the UK/Netherlands/Eire TAK-044 Subarachnoid Haemorrhage Study Group. J Neurosurg 2000; 93:992–997.

81. Hall ED, Travis MA. Attenuation of progressive brain hypoperfusion following experimental subarachnoid hemorrhage by large intravenous doses of methyl-prednisolone. Exp Neurol 1988; 99:594–606.

82. Chyatte D. Prevention of chronic cerebral vasospasm in dogs with ibuprofen and high-dose methylprednisolone. Stroke 1989; 20:1021–1026.

83. Yamakawa K, Sasaki T, Tsubaki S, et al. Effect of high-dose methylprednisolone on vasospasm after subarachnoid hemorrhage. Neurol Med Chir (Tokyo) 1991; 31(1): 24–31.

84. Lombardi D, Gaetani P, Marzatico F, et al. Effect of high-dose methylprednisolone on anti-oxidant enzymes after experimental SAH. J Neurol Sci 1992; 111:13–19.

85. Shibata S, Suzuki S, Ohkuma H, et al. Effects of intracisternal methylprednisolone on lipid peroxidation in experimental subarachnoid haemorrhage. Acta Neurochir (Wien) 1999; 141:529–532.

86. Chen D, Nishizawa S, Yokota N, et al. High-dose methylprednisolone prevents vasospasm after subarachnoid hemorrhage through inhibition of protein kinase C activation. Neurol Res 2002; 24:215–222.

87. Hashi K, Takakura K, Sano K, et al. Intravenous hydrocortisone in large doses in the treatment of delayed ischemic neurological deficits following subarachnoid hemorrhage—results of a multi-center controlled double-blind clinical study. No To Shinkei 1988; 40(4):373–382.

88. Feigin VL, Anderson N, Rinkel GJ, et al. Corticosteroids for aneurysmal sub-arachnoid haemorrhage and primary intracerebral haemorrhage. Cochrane Database Syst Rev. 2005; 20(3), CD004583.

89. Chyatte D, Fode NC, Nichols DA, et al. Preliminary report: effects of high dose methylprednisolone on delayed cerebral ischemia in patients at high risk for vaso-spasm after aneurysmal subarachnoid hemorrhage. Neurosurgery 1987; 21:157–160.

90. Suzuki S, Ogane K, Souma M, et al. Efficacy of steroid hormone in solution for intracranial irrigation during aneurismal surgery for prevention of the vasospasm syndrome. Acta Neurochir 1994; 131:184–188.

91. Steinke DE, Weir BK, Findlay JM, et al. A trial of the 21-aminosteroid U74006F in a primate model of chronic cerebral vasospasm. Neurosurgery 1989; 24(2):179–186.

92. Kanamaru K, Weir BK, Findlay JM, et al. A dosage study of the effect of the 21-aminosteroid U74006F on chronic cerebral vasospasm in a primate model. Neurosurgery 1990; 27(1):29–38.

93. Suzuki H, Kanamaru K, Kuroki M, et al. Effects of tirilazad mesylate on vasospasm and phospholipid hydroperoxides in a primate model of subarachnoid hemorrhage. Stroke 1999; 30(2):450–455.

94. Haley EC Jr, Kassell NF, Alves WM, et al. Phase II trial of tirilazad in aneurysmal subarachnoid hemorrhage. A report of the Cooperative Aneurysm Study. J Neurosurg 1995; 82(5):786–790.

95. Kassell NF, Haley EC Jr, Apperson-Hansen C, et al. Randomized, double-blind, vehicle-controlled trial of tirilazad mesylate in patients with aneurysmal sub-arachnoid hemorrhage: a cooperative study in Europe, Australia, and New Zealand. J Neurosurg 1996; 84(2):221–228.

96. Haley EC Jr, Kassell NF, Apperson-Hansen C, et al. A randomized, double-blind, vehicle-controlled trial of tirilazad mesylate in patients with aneurysmal subarachnoid hemorrhage: a cooperative study in North America. J Neurosurg 1997; 86(3):467–474.

97. Lanzino G, Kassell NF, Dorsch NW, et al. Double-blind, randomized, vehicle-controlled study of high-dose tirilazad mesylate in women with aneurysmal subarachnoid hemorrhage. Part I. A cooperative study in Europe, Australia, New Zealand, and South Africa. J Neurosurg 1999; 90(6):1011–1017.

98. Lanzino G, Kassell NF. Double-blind, randomized, vehicle-controlled study of high-dose tirilazad mesylate in women with aneurysmal subarachnoid hemorrhage. Part II. A cooperative study in North America. J Neurosurg 1999; 90(6):1018–1024.

99. Dorsch NW, Kassell NF, Sinkula MS. Metaanalysis of trials of tirilazad mesylate in aneurysmal SAH. Acta Neurochir Suppl 2001; 77:233–235.

100. McGirt MJ, Lynch JR, Parra A, et al. Simvastatin increases endothelial nitric oxide synthase and ameliorates cerebral vasospasm resulting from subarachnoid hemorrhage. Stroke 2002; 33(12):2950–2956.

101. McGirt MJ, Pradilla G, Legnani FG, et al. Systemic administration of simvastatin after the onset of experimental subarachnoid hemorrhage attenuates cerebral vasospasm. Neurosurgery 2006; 58(5):945–951.

102. Laufs U, La Fata V, Liao JK. Inhibition of 3-hydroxy-3-methylglutaryl (HMG)-CoA reductase blocks hypoxia-mediated downregulation of endothelial nitric oxide synthase. J Biol Chem 1997; 272:31725–31729.

103. Amin-Hanjani S, Stagliano NE, Yamada M, et al. Mevastatin, an HMG-CoA reductase inhibitor, reduces stroke damage and upregulates endothelial nitric oxide synthase in mice. Stroke 2001; 32:980–986.

104. Yamada M, Huang Z, Dalkara T, et al. Endothelial nitric oxide synthase-dependent cerebral blood flow augmentation by L-arginine after chronic statin treatment. J Cereb Blood Flow Metab 2000; 20:709–717.

105. Singhal AB, Topcuoglu MA, Dorer DJ, et al. SSRI and statin use increases the risk for vasospasm after subarachnoid hemorrhage. Neurology 2005; 64(6):1008–1013.

106. Endres M, Laufs U. Discontinuation of statin treatment in stroke patients. Stroke 2006; 37(10):2640–2643.

107. McGirt MJ, Blessing R, Alexander MJ, et al. Risk of cerebral vasospasm after subarachnoid hemorrhage reduced by statin therapy: a multivariate analysis of an institutional experience. J Neurosurg 2006; 105(5):671–674.

108. Tseng MY, Czosnyka M, Richards H, et al. Effects of acute treatment with pravastatin on cerebral vasospasm, autoregulation, and delayed ischemic deficits after aneurysmal subarachnoid hemorrhage: a phase II randomized placebo-controlled trial. Stroke 2005; 36(8):1627–1632.

109. Lynch JR, Wang H, McGirt MJ, et al. Simvastatin reduces vasospasm after aneurysmal subarachnoid hemorrhage: results of a pilot randomized clinical trial. Stroke 2005; 36(9):2024–2026.

110. Albrecht RF II, Wass CT, Lanier WL. Occurrence of potentially detrimental temperature alterations in hospitalized patients at risk for brain injury. Mayo Clin Proc 1998; 73(7):629–635.

111. Oliveira-Filho J, Ezzeddine MA, Segal AZ, et al. Fever in subarachnoid hemorrhage: relationship to vasospasm and outcome. Neurology 2001; 56:1299–1304.

112. Karibe H, Zarow GJ, Graham SH, et al. Mild intra-ischemic hypothermia reduces postischemic hyperperfusion, delayed postischemic hypoperfusion, blood-brain barrier disruption, brain edema, and neuronal damage volume after temporary focal cerebral ischemia in rats. J Cereb Blood Flow Metab 1994; 14:620–627.

113. Baker CJ, Fiore AJ, Frazzini VI, et al. Intraischemic hypothermia decreases the release of glutamate in the cores of permanent focal cerebral infarcts. Neurosurgery 1995; 36(5):994–1001.

114. Toyoda T, Suzuki S, Kassell NF, et al. Intraischemic hypothermia attenuates neutrophil infiltration in the rat neocortex after focal ischemia-reperfusion injury. Neurosurgery 1996; 39(6):1200–1205.

115. Chopp M, Knight R, Tidwell CD, et al. The metabolic effects of mild hypothermia on global cerebral ischemia and recirculation in the cat: comparison to normothermia and hyperthermia. J Cereb Blood Flow Metab 1989; 9(2):141–148.

116. Luan X, Li J, McAllister JP II, et al. Regional brain cooling induced by vascular saline infusion into ischemic territory reduces brain inflammation in stroke. Acta Neuropathol (Berl) 2004; 107(3):227–234.

117. Piepgras A, Elste V, Frietsch T, et al. Effect of moderate hypothermia on experimental severe subarachnoid hemorrhage, as evaluated by apparent diffusion coefficient changes. Neurosurgery 2001; 48:1128–1135.

118. Nagao S, Irie K, Kawai N, et al. Protective effect of mild hypothermia on symptomatic vasospasm: a preliminary report. Acta Neurochir Suppl 2000; 76:547–550.

119. Nakamura T, Tatara N, Morisaki K, et al. Cerebral oxygen metabolism monitoring under hypothermia for severe subarachnoid hemorrhage: report of eight cases. Acta Neurol Scand 2002; 106(5):314–318.

120. Nagao S, Irie K, Kawai N, et al. The use of mild hypothermia for patients with severe vasospasm: a preliminary report. J Clin Neurosci 2003; 10(2):208–212.

121. Kawamura S, Suzuki A, Hadeishi H, et al. Cerebral blood flow and oxygen metabolism during mild hypothermia in patients with subarachnoid haemorrhage. Acta Neurochir (Wien) 2000; 142(10):1117–1121.

122. Hindman BJ, Todd MM, Gelb AW, et al. Mild hypothermia as a protective therapy during intracranial aneurysm surgery: a randomized prospective pilot trial. Neurosurgery 1999; 44(1):23–32.

123. Karibe H, Sato K, Shimizu H, et al. Intraoperative mild hypothermia ameliorates postoperative cerebral blood flow impairment in patients with aneurysmal subarachnoid hemorrhage. Neurosurgery 2000; 47(3):594–599.

124. Todd MM, Hindman BJ, Clarke WR, et al. Intraoperative Hypothermia for Aneurysm Surgery Trial (IHAST) Investigators. Mild intraoperative hypothermia during surgery for intracranial aneurysm. N Engl J Med 2005; 352(2):135–145.

125. Anderson SW, Todd MM, Hindman BJ, et al. Effects of intraoperative hypothermia on neuropsychological outcomes after intracranial aneurysm surgery. Ann Neurol 2006; 60(5):518–527.

17

Use of Anticonvulsants and Corticosteroids in SAH

Panayiotis N. Varelas, MD, PhD, Director[a] and Senior Staff[b]

*[a]Neuro-ICU, [b]Departments of Neurology and Neurosurgery,
Henry Ford Hospital, Detroit, Michigan, U.S.A.*

Lotfi Hacein-Bey, MD, Professor

*Departments of Radiology and Neurological Surgery,
Loyola University, Chicago, Illinois, U.S.A.*

INTRODUCTION

Nontraumatic subarachnoid hemorrhage (SAH) accounts for 2% to 5% of all strokes, affects women more than men, and peaks in the sixth decade of life (1). The most frequent cause of SAH is a ruptured intracranial aneurysm, although in 20% of cases a different cause may be identified. Despite progress in diagnosis and management, prognosis of this lethal disease remains dismal, with an average case fatality of 51% and only one-third of survivors living independently (2).

Patients with SAH may develop many complications during their long course in the hospital, including rebleeding, hydrocephalus, seizures, vasospasm with or without permanent ischemic strokes, hyponatremia, stunned myocardium and cardiac arrhythmias, and pulmonary edema (1). This chapter contains a review of the role of two families of medications—antiepileptics and corticosteroids—in the treatment of SAH.

ANTIEPILEPTIC MEDICATIONS AND SAH

Some studies suggest that antiepileptic drugs (AEDs) should be used in patients with SAH for several reasons. The most common reason is prophylaxis, i.e., preventing seizure-induced rerupture of a cerebral aneurysm, which may occur during the diagnostic or therapeutic acute phase. AED treatment may also prevent seizure-induced worsening of intracranial pressure or cerebral blood flow in patients with vasospasm or cerebral edema. The argument against the prophylactic use of AEDs, however, is that some data suggest a negative influence of AEDs (e.g., phenytoin) on motor and cognitive recovery after stroke (3) or head trauma (4).

Several studies have examined the timing of seizures and the need and effectiveness of AED use in patients with SAH. A chart review at a major health center found that most seizures occurred prior to admission (25.3%) and that seizures that occurred after admission (4.1%) were not prevented by AEDs in 75% of patients. None of the in-hospital seizing patients had recurrent seizures after discharge, but 14% of patients (all with prehospital seizures and half on AEDs) had seizures after discharge. Thus, seizures after SAH are arguably unpreventable, and because the incidence of in-hospital seizures (4%) is lower than the incidence of adverse effects from AEDs (7%), long-term treatment may not be beneficial (5).

In a prospective study from Portugal, new-onset seizures after SAH occurred in 16 of 253 (6.3%) patients and were more common in those with hemiparesis, Hunt and Hess grade 4 or 5, Fisher grade III or IV, and when an aneurysm was found by angiography. Rebleeding was more frequent in patients with seizures but did not correlate temporally with the seizures. All patients with new-onset seizures were prescribed phenytoin 300 mg/day, and one-fourth (4/16) had recurrent seizures. Such a recurrence rate prompted the authors to recommend prescribing AEDs during hospitalization to patients with new-onset seizures but argued against long-term prophylactic treatment (6).

In another retrospective study from Australia, new-onset seizures post-SAH correlated with a large amount of blood on computer tomography (CT) of the head and were independent predictors for both late seizures and disability at six weeks. On the basis of these results, the authors recommended early anti-epileptic treatment for any patient who had a large amount of blood on CT and long-term treatment for those with onset seizures (7). However, not all authors agree with this recommendation. In older studies, early seizures were not predictive of later recurrence, which brings into question the necessity of long-term AED use (8).

The method of seizure detection also plays an important role, with routine electroencephalogram (EEG) considered inferior to continuous EEG. A study of 233 patients with SAH from Columbia-Presbyterian Hospital, New York, identified 101 patients who were stuporous or comatose. All patients received fosphenytoin prophylactically. Twenty-six of those patients were monitored with continuous EEG, and eight were diagnosed as having nonconvulsive status epilepticus (NCSE), an average of 18 days (range, 5–38 days) after SAH. A Hunt and Hess grade of IV or V, older age, ventricular drainage, and cerebral edema on CT were identified as risk factors for NCSE. NCSE was successfully terminated in five patients (63%) after additional fosphenytoin administration or loading of phenobarbital or valproic acid or infusion of midazolam, but only one experienced clinical improvement, which was transient; all eight patients eventually died after a period of prolonged coma. Therefore, NCSE could be detected with continuous EEG in 8% of patients with SAH and otherwise unexplained coma or neurologic deterioration and was highly refractory to therapy, with a dismal prognosis (9).

In a subsequent study, the same group of investigators reported that 9% of patients had in-hospital seizures or NCSE after SAH, but these seizures, unlike those related to focal pathology (subdural hematoma or cerebral infarction), were not predictive of subsequent epilepsy development. After discharge, 4% of patients had one seizure and another 7% had two or more seizures. In the same study, the authors mention the unpublished results from a survey by the American Association of Neurological Surgeons, wherein 24% of participants admitted to routinely treating SAH patients with AEDs for three months, regardless of whether in-hospital seizures occurred or not; they further suggest that prophylactic treatment after discharge is not warranted in the absence of cerebral infarction or subdural hematoma (10).

In addition to the direct effect of SAH on seizure incidence, the mode of treatment of an aneurysm (surgical or endovascular) may be a contributing factor to occurrence of early postprocedural seizures or epilepsy. The relative efficacy of AEDs with each form of aneurysm treatment is unknown. Earlier studies reported a 10% to 25% incidence of epilepsy after aneurysm surgery (11). In a retrospective Finnish study of 177 patients who were surgically treated for ruptured aneurysms, all patients were started on phenytoin treatment during surgery and maintained for two to three months or longer (if they developed seizures); late seizures developed in 25 (14%) patients and were recurrent in 21 (12%). The authors concluded that patients with low preoperative grades have a very low risk for epilepsy and that treatment with phenytoin can be discontinued by three months postsurgery if no high-risk factors are present, such as a high preoperative Hunt and Hess grade, middle cerebral artery aneurysm location, complications of SAH (hematoma, vasospasm with infarction, shunt-dependent hydrocephalus), or persistent neurologic deficits (hemiparesis, dysphasia, visual field defects) (11). Another, older prospective study of 100 consecutive patients followed for four years after aneurysm surgery determined no need for prophylactic phenytoin (12). In this series only 3% of patients developed postoperative epilepsy, and seizure incidence did not differ between the groups with or without antiepileptic prophylaxis.

More recent studies of surgical treatment, however, report a lower rate of early seizures of 1.9% to 5% (13–15). In a retrospective analysis of 217 surgically treated patients, 17 (7.8%) patients had new-onset seizures. Only one

(3.8%) of 26 patients with perioperative seizures had late epilepsy at follow-up. Moreover, 21 (9.7%) patients had at least one seizure episode after the first postoperative week, while late epilepsy developed in 15 (6.9%). All patients were treated with prophylactic phenytoin (and if phenytoin was not tolerated, they were treated with carbamazepine or valproic acid) until the first outpatient visit two to three weeks postsurgery, at which time the dose was tapered if no late seizures had occurred (15). These results could be contrasted with those of another group that did not administer prophylactic AEDs in their prospective study of 121 operated patients unless epilepsy (two or more seizures) developed. Eight of their patients had seizures during the perioperative period, but only one subsequently developed epilepsy. These authors reported an overall 7% risk for epilepsy and another 2.5% for a single seizure at 12 months and concluded that prophylactic AEDs are not justified after aneurysmal surgery (16).

On the basis of these results, a large retrospective study was conducted at Columbia-Presbyterian Hospital in New York to evaluate perioperative, short-term, antiepileptic prophylaxis after craniotomies for aneurysms (14). All the patients were loaded and maintained on AEDs, which were then stopped within seven days of surgery (on average after 3.1 days from surgery or after 5.3 days of average total treatment duration). Postoperative seizures occurred in 5.4% of patients (4.5% for those with ruptured aneurysms and 6.9% for those with unruptured aneurysms). Early postoperative seizures (within 14 days from surgery) occurred in 1.9% of patients (1.5% with ruptured and 2.6% with unruptured aneurysms) and late postoperative seizures occurred in 3.5% (3% with ruptured and 4.4% with unruptured aneurysms). Two-thirds of early postoperative seizures occurred in patients with significant intracranial complications, such as hematomas or infarcts. Only one-third of patients had therapeutic antiepileptic levels when the early seizures occurred, but all were reloaded and maintained on treatment for one year without any further seizures. Late seizures developed in 8 of 11 patients within three months of surgery and were easily controlled with AEDs. In the multivariate analysis, no association was seen between total or postoperative duration of treatment and risk of early or late seizures. They concluded that patients with early postoperative seizures should always be evaluated for ongoing intracranial pathology. The authors also recommended loading the patients the day before surgery but not using antiepileptics after surgery for more than seven days if patients are at a low perioperative risk for seizures.

With the advent of endovascular aneurysm therapy, one would expect a lower risk for seizures because of a lack of additional injury from a craniotomy. This hypothesis was examined in a prospective study from Oxford, England, in which 243 patients treated with Guglielmi detachable coils were followed for up to 7.7 years (17). Only three patients were epileptics, already on AEDs when they developed SAH, and 33 other patients (12%) received prophylactic treatment after they bled. Ictal seizures (within 24 hours from ictus) occurred in 26 of 243 (11%) patients and were independently predicted by loss of consciousness, middle cerebral artery aneurysm location, and antiepileptic treatment. Seven of 233 (3%) patients developed late seizures, including three with preexisting epilepsy and only four (1.7%) with de novo seizures. None of the patients with late seizures presented during the periprocedural period (i.e., within 30 days), and none with ictal seizures experienced late seizures. Only half of them (0.85%) had recurrent seizures that required long-term AEDs. Late seizures were independently predicted by a history of epilepsy before SAH, cerebrospinal fluid shunting or drainage procedure, and antiepileptic medications. This latter finding could probably be explained by the fact that patients who experienced ictal seizures were started on AEDs before referral. The authors concluded that periprocedural seizure prophylaxis is not necessary and that the low incidence of de novo late seizures justifies not recommending long-term prophylactic AEDs after coiling.

The one-year clinical outcomes from the International Subarachnoid Aneurysm Trial (ISAT) were recently published. In this mainly European study, 2143 patients with ruptured intracranial aneurysms were randomly assigned to neurosurgical clipping ($n = 1070$) or endovascular coiling ($n = 1073$). One of the secondary outcomes evaluated in the study was the risk of developing seizures. Seizures occurred in the endovascular group in three patients before the first treatment, in 16 after the procedure and before discharge, in 27 between discharge and one year, and in 14 after the first year. In the neurosurgical group, seizures occurred in 11, 33, 44, and 24 patients, respectively. Therefore, a highly significant reduction in seizures was seen in the endovascular group compared with the neurosurgical group after the first procedure (relative risk, 0.52; 95% confidence interval, 0.37–0.74). The implications of these results on the treatment with AEDs after SAH as related to choice of aneurysm therapy remain unclear.

Lastly, the use of AEDs for seizure prophylaxis after SAH must be contrasted with emerging evidence that these drugs, particularly older-generation AEDs, are not benign and may lead to adverse effects or outcomes. The usefulness of prophylactic AEDs (phenytoin, phenobarbital, carbamazepine) was examined in 3552 patients entered in four prospective randomized double-blind, placebo-controlled trials conducted between 1991 and 1997. Adjusting for baseline differences, the authors reported elevated temperatures at day 8 and worse outcome at three months with AED use (18). Another group studied 527 SAH patients and calculated a "phenytoin burden" for each by multiplying the average serum level of phenytoin by the time between the first and last measurements, up to a maximum of 14 days from ictus. These authors reported that phenytoin burden was associated with poor functional outcome at 14 days (but not at 3 months) and remained significant (odds ratio, 1.6 per quartile; 95% confidence interval, 1.2–2.1; $p < 0.001$) after adjustment for other variables. Higher quartiles of phenytoin burden were also associated with worse scores for cognitive status via telephone interview at both hospital discharge and three months (19). These reports must be contrasted with emerging evidence that newer AEDs (e.g., levetiracetam) may have neuroprotective effects in SAH animal models (20).

STEROIDS AND SAH

The rationale for the use of steroids in acute SAH is the significant inflammatory process present in the meninges, the ventricles, and the vascular wall (which may lead to vasospasm). Following SAH, concentrations of eicosanoids (prostaglandins and thromboxanes) are markedly increased in human cisternal and lumbar cerebrospinal fluid compared with normal lumbar cerebrospinal fluid. With intraventricular hemorrhage after SAH, these levels are also severalfold higher than normal, but the most dramatic increase is found following rebleeding. These eicosanoid concentrations are sufficient to have cerebrovascular and neuromodulatory effects (21) and through the ensuing meningeal inflammation may eventually lead to hydrocephalus. Genes encoding inflammatory processes have also been found to be upregulated, and mRNA for interleukins and intercellular adhesion molecules are elevated in arteries exposed to subarachnoid blood (22).

Data from both animal and clinical studies are available regarding steroid use after SAH (23). The first experiments with hydrocortisone or prednisolone-phosphate in dogs to evaluate their effect on adhesions and hydrocephalus were conducted in the 1960s and showed that the soluble form led to seizures and that the insoluble form was well tolerated (24). Similarly, investigation of post-hemorrhagic hydrocephalus in cats after intraventricular blood injection showed that intramuscular methylprednisolone for four days reduced hydrocephalus, but intraventricular administration was not effective (25). Other experiments looked at the incidence of vasospasm after steroid treatment. Adventitial hyperpermeability, which occurs after SAH and leads to easy penetration of vasoactive substances into the vascular wall, was prevented by intrathecal administration of methylprednisolone in an SAH rat model (26). Both cortisol and methylprednisolone led to marked vasodilation after topical application in a canine model of vasospasm, although intra-arterial (40 mg) or IV (10 mg/kg) injection of the latter failed to show beneficial effect. In a monkey vasospasm model of the circle of Willis, application of methylprednisolone also aborted spasm (27). In another canine model of induced vasospasm after injection of autologous blood in the cisterna magna, treatment with high-dose IV methylprednisolone (30 mg/kg) and ibuprofen (12.5 mg/kg) reduced meningismus, accelerated the rate of neurologic recovery, and prevented degeneration of vessel wall smooth muscle (28). In a similar SAH model in cats, IV administration of methylprednisolone (30 mg/kg) resulted in restoration of reduced cerebral blood flow in the caudate nucleus subsequent to the hemorrhage and improved the vascular resistance. This effect was not correlated with any decrease in the elevated intracranial pressure or any increase in the reduced cerebral perfusion pressure. Interestingly, in that experiment, a 15 mg/kg dose of the drug showed only a modest effect on cerebral blood flow, while a 60 mg/kg dose, although initially effective, lost its effect during the later stages of the experiment. This larger dose, however, was the only dose that reduced the posthemorrhage increased intracranial pressure (29). Subsequent experiments in rats showed that high-dose IV methylprednisolone (30 mg/kg q8 hr) decreased the ex vivo release of eicosanoids (prostaglandin D2 and E2, prostacyclin, and leukotriene C4) (30), enhanced the Na,K-ATPase activity, decreased the products of lipid peroxidation, (31) and restored the superoxide dismutase and glutathione peroxidase activities (32) following induced SAH. Most recently, in an SAH rabbit model, it was shown that the SAH–induced alterations in the density of three of four smooth muscle cell proteins in the basilar artery tunica media were prevented by intramuscular dexamethasone treatment (5.6 mg/kg for 3 daily doses); two of these proteins (alpha-actin and the actin-binding protein h-caldesmon) are directly related to contraction of the muscle (22).

Human studies have also been conducted to evaluate the usefulness of steroids in SAH. On the basis of the assumption that chronic vasospasm is an inflammatory vasculopathy, 21 post–SAH patients at high risk for vasospasm were treated within 72 hours with high-dose IV methylprednisolone (30 mg/kg immediately prior to surgery, then 30 mg/kg q6 hr for 12 doses, then 15 mg/kg q6 hr for 4 doses, then 7.5 mg/kg q6 hr for 4 doses, then 3 mg/kg q6 hr for 4 doses, then 1.5 mg/kg q12 hr for 2 doses). These patients were compared to a cohort of 21 well-matched control patients. Treated patients had reduced incidence and severity of delayed cerebral ischemia (24% vs. 43%), no serious side effects, half the mortality (14% vs. 29%), and better "excellent outcome" (71% vs. 33%), compared with those who were not treated (33). In an uncontrolled series from Japan, 18 of 21 patients who received large amounts of steroids for symptomatic vasospasm showed improvement in their symptoms. The effect was more pronounced in those patients with mild-to-moderate spasm and less with those in severe spasm. One patient developed gastrointestinal bleeding (34). Another study from Japan reported on a series of 55 patients with SAH who were subjected to partial clot removal during early craniotomy (before day 3) and intracranial irrigation with a Hartman solution containing 1 mg/mL methylprednisolone after the aneurysm clipping. These patients fared better than 68 controls who were treated with regular Hartman solution irrigation [11% vasospasm vs. 29% for the controls, better Glasgow Outcome Scale (GOS) upon discharge in the steroid-treated patients] (26). However, because of significant concerns regarding side effects with these large doses of steroids, another study was conducted, randomizing 171 patients with SAH, 107 of whom were assigned to an IV dose of 48 mg of dexamethasone followed by 8 mg q2 hr for three days, and 64 of whom were control patients. Although no difference was observed in the incidence of gastrointestinal hemorrhage or diabetes, the treated patients had a significant 10.2% increase in infections, mostly urinary tract infections (35). In another case series from Japan, 48 patients with SAH received IV high-dose diltiazem combined with dextran and hydrocortisone. The steroid dose was 400 mg q6 hr for three days, then 400 mg q8 hr for three days, then 400 mg q12 hr for three days, then 200 mg q12 hr for three days, and, finally, 200 mg/day for three days. Symptomatic vasospasm occurred in only five patients (10.4%), with four patients recovering and only one left with a severe neurologic deficit (36). The most recent study, a retrospective study from Germany, evaluated 242 patients with SAH. Patients were divided into four groups based on the World Federation of Neurological Surgeons (WFNS) grades (I–III vs. IV and V) on admission and the amount of dexamethasone administered (≥ 12 mg/day for 5 days and then slow weaning over 5 days, or a smaller dose). Rehemorrhage was observed significantly less frequently in the WFNS I–III group with the high steroid dose (3% vs. 13%). Clinically relevant vasospasm was not different between the groups, but hydrocephalus was. In the group with WFNS I–III and high steroid dose, 19% developed hydrocephalus, which was less than the 37% incidence in the comparable group with low-dose steroid ($p = 0.011$). A difference was also found in the higher WFNS patients (IV and V), in whom 16% of the high steroid dose group developed hydrocephalus versus 57% in the low-dose group ($p = 0.006$). The rate of infection did not differ between the groups, and the percentage of patients with favorable GOS at six months was significantly higher in the groups with high dexamethasone dose, regardless of WFNS grade (23).

Results of clinical trials that evaluated the synthetic nonglucocorticoid 21-aminosteroid (lazaroid) tirilazad mesylate are controversial. The drug was developed as a cytoprotective inhibitor of oxygen radical-induced lipid peroxidation and, in animal models of SAH, was shown to cause improvement in vasospasm (37). Tirilazad was tested in a large randomized double-blinded, vehicle-controlled study in Europe, Australia, and New Zealand (38) and was found to reduce mortality and improve the rates of good recovery (based on the GOS at 3 months) when used at 6 mg/kg/day IV (38). These results were not corroborated in a parallel study conducted in North America, which showed significant rates of mortality reduction only for men with WFNS grades IV and V (39). The explanation was that plasma concentrations of tirilazad and its first-order metabolite are substantially reduced in women. Therefore, similar large-scale multicentered studies were conducted again with a higher dose of tirilazad (15 mg/kg/day IV) in women only. In the study from Europe, Australia, New Zealand, and South Africa, although a significant reduction in the incidence of symptomatic vasospasm was observed in the treatment group, mortality and GOS at three months were not different (40). The parallel North American study showed significantly reduced mortality in patients with WFNS grades IV and V only but no difference in favorable GOS at three months, symptomatic vasospasm, or vasospasm severity (41). In conclusion, tirilazad may show some benefit in men (and at higher doses in women) admitted with the worst neurologic grades after SAH.

Lastly, steroids have been used to treat the frequently occurring, excessive natriuresis after SAH. Two randomized unblinded studies have evaluated the use of the mineralocorticoid fludrocortisone. In the first, fludrocortisone significantly reduced the frequency of a negative sodium balance during the first six days and nonsignificantly diminished the decrease in plasma volume in the treated group (42). In a later Japanese study, fludrocortisone (0.3 mg/day) reduced the mean sodium and water intake, the urinary sodium excretion, and urine volume, and effectively prevented a negative shift in sodium and water balance, compared with the untreated group. A decrease in serum potassium level within the range of 2.8–3.5 mEq/L was transiently noted in 73.3% of treated patients but was easily corrected (43). Another steroid, hydrocortisone, at a dose of 300 mg q6 hr for 10 days and gradual tapering for another four days, has been used in another randomized unblinded Japanese study to evaluate its usefulness in sodium retention. This daily 1200-mg dose is equivalent to 0.3-mg fludrocortisone per day, but has the advantage of easier control of the drug effects because of the much shorter elimination half-life of the former. Treated patients showed lower sodium excretion, higher serum sodium level, no hyponatremia, lower urine volume, lower fluid infusion volume for hypervolemic treatment, and higher central venous pressure, without serious side effects, compared with the untreated group (44).

CONCLUSION

The use of anticonvulsants in aneurysmal SAH has been based more on empirical practice than on an evidence-based approach, which, considering the significant side effects of traditional AEDs (phenytoin, phenobarbital, carbamazepine), may be a cause for concern. As data emerge from clinical studies, with the advent of new less-invasive treatments for cerebral aneurysms along with newer categories of AEDs (some possibly with neuroprotective effects), the role of anticonvulsants in SAH will become clearer.

As for steroids, despite ample intuitive justification in fighting the formidable inflammation that accompanies SAH, laboratory evidence, and data from scant clinical studies, a general cautious approach continues, justified by the many side effects of these drugs. Initial hopes generated by 21-aminosteroids such as tirilazad have been tempered by modest and unclear clinical results. It is hoped that modulators of the eicosanoic acid response in SAH may prove beneficial (45).

REFERENCES

1. Suarez JI, Tarr RW, Selman WR. Aneurysmal subarachnoid hemorrhage. N Engl J Med 2006; 354:387–396.
2. Hop JW, Rinkel GJ, Algra A, et al. Case-fatality rates and functional outcome after subarachnoid hemorrhage: a systematic review. Stroke 1997; 28:660–664.
3. Goldstein LB. Potential effects of common drugs on stroke recovery. Arch Neurol 1998; 55:454–456.
4. Dikmen SS, Temkin NR, Miller B, et al. Neurobehavioral effects of phenytoin prophylaxis of posttraumatic seizures. JAMA 1991; 265:1271–1277.
5. Rhoney DH, Tipps LB, Murry KR, et al. Anticonvulsant prophylaxis and timing of seizures after aneurysmal subarachnoid hemorrhage. Neurology 2000; 55:258–265.
6. Pinto AN, Canhao P, Ferro JM. Seizures at the onset of subarachnoid haemorrhage. J Neurol 1996; 243:161–164.
7. Butzkueven H, Evans AH, Pitman A, et al. Onset seizures independently predict poor outcome after subarachnoid hemorrhage. Neurology 2000; 55:1315–1320.

8. Sundaram MB, Chow F. Seizures associated with spontaneous subarachnoid hemorrhage. Can J Neurol Sci 1986; 13:229–231.
9. Dennis LJ, Claassen J, Hirsch LJ, et al. Nonconvulsive status epilepticus after subarachnoid hemorrhage. Neurosurgery 2002; 51:1136–1143 (discussion 1144).
10. Claassen J, Peery S, Kreiter KT, et al. Predictors and clinical impact of epilepsy after subarachnoid hemorrhage. Neurology 2003; 60:208–214.
11. Keranen T, Tapaninaho A, Hernesniemi J, et al. Late epilepsy after aneurysm operations. Neurosurgery 1985; 17:897–900.
12. Sbeih I, Tamas LB, O'Laoire SA. Epilepsy after operation for aneurysms. Neurosurgery 1986; 19:784–788.
13. Ohman J. Hypertension as a risk factor for epilepsy after aneurysmal subarachnoid hemorrhage and surgery. Neurosurgery 1990; 27:578–581.
14. Baker CJ, Prestigiacomo CJ, Solomon RA. Short-term perioperative anticonvulsant prophylaxis for the surgical treatment of low-risk patients with intracranial aneurysms. Neurosurgery 1995; 37:863–870 (discussion 870–871).
15. Lin CL, Dumont AS, Lieu AS, et al. Characterization of perioperative seizures and epilepsy following aneurysmal subarachnoid hemorrhage. J Neurosurg 2003; 99: 978–985.
16. Bidzinski J, Marchel A, Sherif A. Risk of epilepsy after aneurysm operations. Acta Neurochir (Wien) 1992; 119:49–52.
17. Byrne JV, Boardman P, Ioannidis I, et al. Seizures after aneurysmal subarachnoid hemorrhage treated with coil embolization. Neurosurgery 2003; 52:545–552 (discussion 550–552).
18. Rosengart AJ, Novakovic R, Dezheng H, et al. Impact of prophylactic anticonvulsive use on outcome in subarachnoid hemorrhage. Stroke 2004; 35:250.
19. Naidech AM, Kreiter KT, Janjua N, et al. Phenytoin exposure is associated with functional and cognitive disability after subarachnoid hemorrhage. Stroke 2005; 36:583–587.
20. Wang H, Gao J, Lassiter TF, et al. Levetiracetam is neuroprotective in murine models of closed head injury and subarachnoid hemorrhage. Neurocritical care 2006; 5: 71–78.
21. Pickard JD, Walker V, Brandt L, et al. Effect of intraventricular haemorrhage and rebleeding following subarachnoid haemorrhage on CSF eicosanoids. Acta Neurochir (Wien) 1994; 129:152–157.
22. Gomis P, Tran-Dinh YR, Sercombe C, et al. Dexamethasone preventing contractile and cytoskeletal protein changes in the rabbit basilar artery after subarachnoid hemorrhage. J Neurosurg 2005; 102:715–720.
23. Schurkamper M, Medele R, Zausinger S, et al. Dexamethasone in the treatment of subarachnoid hemorrhage revisited: a comparative analysis of the effect of the total dose on complications and outcome. J Clin Neurosci 2004; 11:20–24.
24. Oppelt WW, Rall DP. Production of convulsions in the dog with intrathecal corticosteroids. Neurology 1961; 11:925–927.
25. Wilkinson HA, Wilson RB, Patel PP, et al. Corticosteroid therapy of experimental hydrocephalus after intraventricular-subarachnoid haemorrhage. J Neurol Neurosurg Psychiatry 1974; 37:224–229.
26. Suzuki S, Ogane K, Souma M, et al. Efficacy of steroid hormone in solution for intracranial irrigation during aneurysmal surgery for prevention of the vasospasm syndrome. Acta neurochirurgica 1994; 131:184–188.

27. Fox JL, Yasargil MG. The relief of intracranial vasospasm: an experimental study with methylprednisolone and cortisol. Surg Neurol 1975; 3:214–218.
28. Chyatte D, Rusch N, Sundt TM, Jr. Prevention of chronic experimental cerebral vasospasm with ibuprofen and high-dose methylprednisolone. J Neurosurg 1983; 59:925–932.
29. Hall ED, Travis MA. Attenuation of progressive brain hypoperfusion following experimental subarachnoid hemorrhage by large intravenous doses of methylprednisolone. Exp Neurol 1988; 99:594–606.
30. Gaetani P, Marzatico F, Renault B, et al. High-dose methylprednisolone and "ex vivo" release of eicosanoids after experimental subarachnoid haemorrhage. Neurol Res 1990; 12:111–116.
31. Marzatico F, Gaetani P, Buratti E, et al. Effects of high-dose methylprednisolone on Na(+)-K+ ATPase and lipid peroxidation after experimental subarachnoid hemorrhage. Acta Neurol Scand 1990; 82:263–270.
32. Lombardi D, Gaetani P, Marzatico F, et al. Effect of high-dose methylprednisolone on anti-oxidant enzymes after experimental SAH. J Neurol Sci 1992; 111:13–19.
33. Chyatte D, Fode NC, Nichols DA, et al. Preliminary report: effects of high dose methylprednisolone on delayed cerebral ischemia in patients at high risk for vasospasm after aneurysmal subarachnoid hemorrhage. Neurosurgery 1987; 21:157–160.
34. Yasukawa K, Kamijou Y, Momose G, et al. [The experiences of a large amount of steroid therapy for symptomatic vasospasm after subarachnoid hemorrhage: clinical analysis of 21 cases]. No Shinkei Geka 1994; 22:17–22.
35. Karnik R, Valentin A, Prainer C, et al. [Steroid therapy in subarachnoid hemorrhage]. Wien Klin Wochenschr 1990; 102:1–4.
36. Kawano T, Kazekawa K, Nakashima S, et al. Combined drug therapy with diltiazem, dextran, and hydrocortisone (DDH therapy) for late cerebral vasospasm after aneurysmal subarachnoid hemorrhage: Assessment of efficacy and safety in an open clinical study. Int J Clin Pharmacol Ther 1995; 33:513–517.
37. Zuccarello M, Marsch JT, Schmitt G, et al. Effect of the 21-aminosteroid U-74006F on cerebral vasospasm following subarachnoid hemorrhage. J Neurosurgery 1989; 71:98–104.
38. Kassell NF, Haley EC Jr., Apperson-Hansen C, et al. Randomized, double-blind, vehicle-controlled trial of tirilazad mesylate in patients with aneurysmal subarachnoid hemorrhage: a cooperative study in Europe, Australia, and New Zealand. J Neurosurgery 1996; 84:221–228.
39. Haley EC Jr., Kassell NF, Apperson-Hansen C, et al. A randomized, double-blind, vehicle-controlled trial of tirilazad mesylate in patients with aneurysmal subarachnoid hemorrhage: a cooperative study in North America. J Neurosurg 1997; 86:467–474.
40. Lanzino G, Kassell NF, Dorsch NW, et al. Double-blind, randomized, vehicle-controlled study of high-dose tirilazad mesylate in women with aneurysmal subarachnoid hemorrhage. Part I. A cooperative study in Europe, Australia, New Zealand, and South Africa. J Neurosurg 1999; 90:1011–1017.
41. Lanzino G, Kassell NF. Double-blind, randomized, vehicle-controlled study of high-dose tirilazad mesylate in women with aneurysmal subarachnoid hemorrhage. Part II. A cooperative study in North America. J Neurosurg 1999; 90:1018–1024.
42. Hasan D, Lindsay KW, Wijdicks EF, et al. Effect of fludrocortisone acetate in patients with subarachnoid hemorrhage. Stroke 1989; 20:1156–1161.

43. Mori T, Katayama Y, Kawamata T, et al. Improved efficiency of hypervolemic therapy with inhibition of natriuresis by fludrocortisone in patients with aneurysmal subarachnoid hemorrhage. J Neurosurgery 1999; 91:947–952.

44. Moro N, Katayama Y, Kojima J, et al. Prophylactic management of excessive natriuresis with hydrocortisone for efficient hypervolemic therapy after subarachnoid hemorrhage. Stroke 2003; 34:2807–2811.

45. Hacein-Bey L, Harder DR, Meier HT, et al. Reversal of delayed vasospasm by TS-011 in the dual hemorrhage dog model of subarachnoid hemorrhage. AJNR Am J Neuroradiol 2006; 27:1350–1354.

18

Management of Electrolyte and Metabolic Derangements in Subarachnoid Hemorrhage

Tarik Hanane, MD, Fellow
Eelco F. M. Wijdicks, MD, Professor
Mayo Clinic College of Medicine, Rochester, Minnesota, U.S.A.

Electrolytes and metabolic disorders occur frequently in the acute period following subarachnoid hemorrhage (SAH) and may worsen the manifestations of the initial brain injury. Disorders of sodium and water metabolism occur in approximately one-third of patients and are associated with increased morbidity and mortality. Hyponatremia is the most common electrolyte abnormality after SAH and is correlated with an increase in symptomatic vasospasm and poor outcome. Hyperglycemia has been reported in 30% of patients after SAH and is associated with poor outcome. Other electrolyte derangements are common but less specific to SAH. There has been better understanding of electrolyte and metabolic disturbances and new clinical parameters that impact on our day to day care are discussed. Some changes are small and seemingly inconsequential. Others may be true paradigm shifts in our approach to aneurysmal subarachnoid hemorrhage. The pathophysiology, causes, diagnostic evaluation, and treatment of the most frequent electrolyte and metabolic derangements in patients with SAH will be reviewed in this chapter.

DISORDERS OF SODIUM AND WATER HOMEOSTASIS

Hyponatremia

Hyponatremia is the most common electrolyte abnormality after aneurysmal SAH (aSAH). Serum sodium concentrations below 134 mmol/L have been reported in 30% to 40% of patients with SAH admitted to the neurocritical care unit (1–3). Severe hyponatremia (serum sodium level below 125 mmol/L) is rarely seen in SAH; therefore, other major complications of SAH such as rebleeding, hydrocephalus, or vasospasm should be sought before attributing a worsening neurologic status to hyponatremia (4). Hyponatremia frequently occurs within the first week after the initial hemorrhage and its emergence is typically in the same time period of cerebral vasospasm and suggest a close relationship between the two (5). The risk of developing hyponatremia is significantly increased in patients with enlargement of the third ventricle (6) and the presence of suprasellar or intraventricular blood (7). A higher incidence of hyponatremia has been reported in patients with SAH after rupture of an anterior communicating artery (ACA) aneurysm, and this was tentatively explained by ACA vasospasm causing hypothalamic dysfunction (8). However, a recent study showed that the location of the aneurysm has no effect on the incidence of development of hyponatremia (9). It has also been found that those patients with no identifiable aneurysm or who did not have an intervention had lower incidence of hyponatremia than patients who underwent surgical repair. Interestingly, patients who had endovascular coiling of aneurysms had similar occurrence of hyponatremia as those treated with craniotomy and clipping (9).

Hyponatremia is associated with increased morbidity and mortality in hospitalized patients (10). In-hospital mortality can be as high as 60-fold increase in patients with the disorder but these correlations-found in medically critically ill patients cannot be extrapolated to patients with ruptured cerebral aneurysms (11). Left untreated, hyponatremia may result in cerebral edema, seizures, coma, and death. Delayed cerebral ischemia is the leading cause of morbidity and mortality after aSAH, and hyponatremia in patients with SAH is strongly associated with delayed ischemic neurologic deficits that result from cerebral vasospasm (5). The incidence of cerebral infarction in hyponatremic patients was significantly higher in comparison with patients with normal serum sodium values (61% vs. 21%), and it remained high even if no fluid restriction was applied (1). The mortality rate was higher in patients with hyponatremia and cerebral ischemia (5). Hyponatremia is also associated with an increase in duration of hospital stay and seizures in post-SAH patients (9), but in contrast to hypernatremia, is not a predictor of mortality following SAH (9,12,13).

The etiology of hyponatremia after SAH has been a matter of controversy. The two most common noniatrogenic causes are syndrome of inappropriate secretion of antidiuretic hormone (SIADH) and cerebral salt wasting (CSW). Unlike many previous reports that considered CSW to be the major etiology, a recent retrospective study of 316 patients with SAH found that SIADH was the most frequent cause (62.9%), followed by hypovolemia (21%) and CSW (6.5%) (9).

Pathophysiology

Hyponatremia following SAH may be due to SIADH or CSW. They are phys-iologically different, and the approach to treatment of these two disorders varies markedly. The mainstay treatment of SIADH is fluid restriction, while CSW is treated with water and salt replacement. Hence, the understanding of the pathogenesis of hyponatremia associated with SAH is critical for accurate diagnosis and treatment (14).

CSW. Hyponatremia was initially attributed to SIADH (15). However, later evidence suggested that hyponatremia was associated with intravascular volume contraction and negative sodium balance. The first work to challenge the notion of SIADH in intracranial disease (16,17) was supported by a prospective study of sodium balance and changes in plasma volume that used an isotope dilution technique in the first week after SAH in 21 patients (18). The study demonstrated that in most patients with hyponatremia, the plasma volume was decreased and a negative sodium balance preceded the hyponatremia. Serum ADH levels were elevated on admission and declined in the first week regardless of the presence of hyponatremia. For example in a study of 44 patients with SAH, hyponatremia in 21 of 26 patients treated with fluid restriction (presumptive SIADH) resulted in cerebral infarction. In these patients hyponatremia was more likely the result of CSW, with fluid restriction worsening hyponatremia causing misery perfusion in already clamped arteries from vasospasm (5). A prospective study of 19 patients who were treated by hypervolemic therapy to prevent volume contraction still had detectable levels of ADH during a hypoosmolar state suggesting additional dis-turbance in ADH regulation (19). However, it is important to remember that factors other than hypovolemia, such as pain, nausea, and drugs, could stimulate nonosmolar release of ADH making it very difficult to accurately study ADH levels in critically ill neurologic patients.

The mechanism by which SAH causes renal salt wasting in not well understood. The probable site of impaired sodium absorption in CSW is the proximal nephron. Clinical data suggest that interruptions in sympathetic input to the kidneys (14) and/or presence of circulating plasma natriuretic peptides are the most probable processes involved (2,20–28). Decreased sympathetic tone to the kidneys leads to increased natriuresis and volume depletion by depressing proximal renal sodium absorption and altering renin and aldosterone release. The latter mechanism may account for the absence of hypokalemia in CSW despite the volume contraction (14).

The possible role of natriuretic peptides in CSW has been extensively studied. Early studies have noticed a marked elevation of plasma atrial natriuretic peptide (ANP) concentrations in patients with SAH, and it was speculated that ANP might be responsible for natriuresis and diuresis. How-ever, no significant correlation between hyponatremia and plasma ANP levels was found (22). Others speculated that hyponatremia develops only in patients with persistent elevation of serum ANP levels (21,29). Several reports have questioned the fact that ANP alone would account for the hyponatremia observed after SAH and suggested the existence of another potent natriuretic factor (30). More recently, increasing evidence has been reported that brain natriuretic peptide (BNP) plays a role in the pathogenesis in CSW. For some authors, BNP might be the major factor responsible for the excessive natriuresis in SAH (20). BNP plasma levels, in contrast to ANP levels, were found to be consistently increased in aneurysmal SAH and closely associated with hyponatremia and natriuresis (20,25,28).

Natriuretic peptide group includes three structurally related peptides: ANP, BNP and C-type natriuretic peptide (CNP) (31). ANP is primarily produced in the cardiac atria in response to wall stretch. BNP, so called because it was identified in brain tissue, is activated when the cardiac ventricles stretch receptors are stimulated. All the three natriuretic peptides, particularly CNP, are produced in the brain and act by inhibiting the salt appetite and thirst, reinforcing their natriuretic and diuretic effects at the periphery. Both ANP and BNP secretion may result in renal salt wasting by increasing glomerular filtration rate, directly impairing renal tubular sodium reabsorption, antagonizing the action of vasopressin in the collecting ducts, and inhibiting the renin-angiotensin-aldosterone system and sympathetic autonomic outflow to the kidneys (14,31,32). CNP, in contrast to ANP and BNP, has little effect on salt and water excretion (31,33).

How these natriuretic peptides are released in CSW and which organ is responsible (brain vs. heart) remain controversial. It was suggested that the brain, in response to increase in intracranial pressure, releases BNP as a protective measure (20) that may be induced by a lesion to the hypothalamus caused by SAH (20,26,28). However, another study relates the increase of BNP levels to augmented cardiac production triggered by stress-induced noradrenaline (25). It was recently found that both ANP and BNP are excessively secreted in all patients after SAH, irrespective of the severity of the disease and activation of stress hormones. It is also theorized that natriuretic peptides are probably released by the heart in response to transient left ventricular disturbance (23).

Cerebral vasospasm (CVS) is frequently (~50–70%) observed after SAH (5). CVS is thought to be exacerbated by excessive natriuresis and volume depletion, leading to reduction in cerebral blood flow (26). Plasma BNP, but not ANP levels, have been found to increase progressively and significantly in patients with severe CVS, compared with patients with asymptomatic CVS or without vasospasm (26). The chronologic relationship between elevated BNP levels and the occurrence of delayed ischemic neurologic deficits was answered recently (24). BNP levels did not significantly increase until after the onset of ischemic symptoms, raising the question as to whether BNP elevation is the cause or the result of CVS (24). Another plausible hypothesis is that a common mediator, perhaps endothelin, may induce both vascular changes responsible for the vasospasm and the release of natriuretic peptides (26).

Clinical Manifestations

Most patients with serum sodium concentration above 120 mmol/L are asymptomatic, except when the decline has developed rapidly (34). Symptoms are usually vague and nonspecific: headache, anorexia, nausea, muscle cramps, and lethargy (35). Major neurologic symptoms are largely due to the development of cerebral edema and correlate with the acuteness and magnitude of hyponatremia. They include tonic-clonic seizures and can progress to permanent brain damage, apnea, and death from brain swelling (34). Osmotic demyelination syndrome is a rare and devastating complication of treatment of hyponatremia that occurs when serum sodium is corrected too rapidly (36,37). Although the exact pathogenesis of this syndrome is unknown, it appears to be more common with chronic hyponatremia, when the brain has adapted to hypotonicity by decreasing intracellular osmolytes to limit the degree of cerebral edema. Demyelination typically involves the pons and can involve other extrapontine areas (36). Symptoms usually develop within a week of the correction of hyponatremia. The classic presentation includes behavioral changes, pseudobulbar palsy, and spastic quadriparesis with "locked-in syndrome." The diagnosis is usually confirmed by CT or, more accurately, by MRI (38).

Evaluation of Hyponatremia

Hyponatremia is defined as serum sodium concentration below 135 mmol/L and is usually associated with hypoosmolality; however, normal and high plasma osmolality can occur. Hence, the first step in a patient with hyponatremia is to measure plasma osmolality or tonicity (Fig. 1).

Hyponatremia with a normal plasma osmolality, or pseudohyponatremia, is a laboratory artifact seen in patients with severe hyperlipidemia, hyperproteinemia (multiple myeloma, Waldenström macroglobunemia) (39) or use of IV immunoglobulins (40). This condition occurs when the flame photometry uses the whole plasma rather than aqueous phase to measure the sodium concentration. With the widespread use of ion-specific electrodes, pseudohyponatremia is now rarely encountered (35).

Hypertonic hyponatremia or translocational hyponatremia occurs when an osmotically active solute is present in the extracellular compartment, which causes water shift from the intracellular to the extracellular space, thereby diluting serum sodium. The use of hypertonic mannitol and hyperglycemia are the two major causes. The serum sodium should decrease by approximately 1.6 mEq/L for every 100-mg/dL increase in plasma glucose concentration. However, for very high serum glucose concentrations (>400 mg/dL), the use of a correction factor of 2.4 is recommended (41).

Hypotonic hyponatremia or true hyponatremia is a disorder of water homeostasis that develops when an excess of water relative to sodium in the extracellular fluid is present. Except for rare conditions when water intake

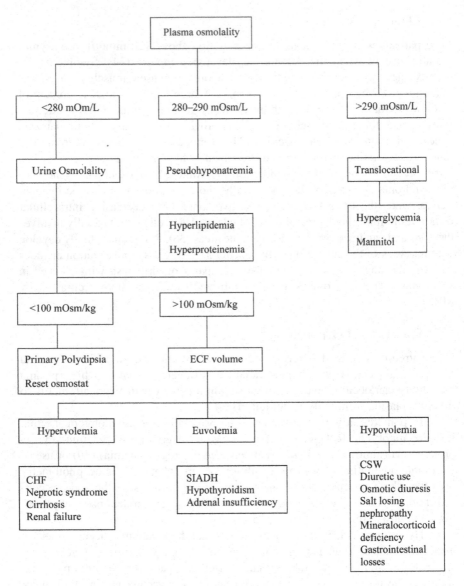

Figure 1 Diagnostic algorithm for hyponatremia. *Abbreviations*: ECF, extracellular fluid; CHF, congestive heart failure; SIADH, syndrome of inappropriate secretion of antidiuretic hormone; CSW, cerebral salt wasting.

exceeds the normal renal water excretory capacity, such as in primary polydipsia and reset osmostat, the principal abnormality is impaired renal water excretion.

Measuring the urine osmolality helps to determine if water excretion is impaired or normal. A level below 100 mOsm/kg suggests that ADH is appropriately suppressed and indicates either primary polydipsia or reset osmostat. In the vast majority of patients with hyponatremia, water excretion by the kidney is impaired and urine osmolality is inappropriately high (Uosm above 200 mOsm/kg).

The next step in treating patients with hyponatremia is to classify them on the basis of volume status; they can be hypovolemic, euvolemic, or hypervolemic.

Hypovolemic hyponatremia occurs when the total body sodium deficit exceeds water deficit. Hypovolemia, irrespective of serum sodium concentration, stimulates ADH release, which is an appropriate response to intravascular volume depletion. Hypovolemia may result from renal or extrarenal losses of solutes and water. Urine sodium concentration helps to differentiate between the renal and extrarenal causes. High urine sodium concentration suggests urinary sodium loss such as via salt wasting syndromes (CSW, mineralocorticoid or corticosteroids insufficiency), recent use of diuretics, osmotic diuresis (e.g., mannitol) or metabolic alkalosis. Urine sodium concentration below 20 mEq/L indicates gastrointestinal or skin losses or fluid sequestration (third spacing).

Hypervolemic hyponatremia occurs when the increase in total body water exceeds the increase in total body sodium; it is seen in congestive heart failure, nephrotic syndrome, or cirrhosis. These conditions are associated with a decrease in effective arterial blood volume, which leads to activation of aortic and carotid baroreceptors, stimulation of ADH and aldosterone release, and increased activity of the sympathetic nervous system.

Euvolemic hyponatremia develops when total body water is increased but the sodium content has not changed. SIADH is the most common diagnosis. Renal and endocrine diseases (hypothyroidism or hypoadrenalism) and other nonosmotic stimuli of ADH such as pain, nausea, and drugs should be ruled out before making the diagnosis.

SIADH Versus CSW

In that both SIADH and CSW are common in SAH, share many clinical and laboratory features, and can sometimes overlap, distinction between these two disorders can be a challenge but is crucial, as it has important implications for the treatment of hyponatremia.

The primary pathogenesis of SIADH is nonphysiologic release of ADH from the posterior pituitary, which results in enhanced renal water absorption, leading to expansion of the extracellular fluid, dilutional hyponatremia, and inappropriately concentrated urine. Signs of hypervolemia are generally not seen because only one-third of water remains in the extracellular fluid. In addition, the renal sodium handling remains normal, leading to increased urinary sodium secretion. Diagnosis of SIADH requires the following features: (*i*) hyponatremia and hypoosmolality, (*ii*) inappropriately concentrated urine (above 100 mOsm/kg), (*iii*) persistent high urine sodium concentration (>40 mmol/L), (*iv*) normovolemia, and (*v*) normal renal, adrenal, and thyroid function (42).

CSW, unlike SIADH, is a volume-depleted state that result from urinary sodium wasting (14). The excessive natriuresis is mediated at least in part by increased circulating natriuretic peptides but not by volume expansion, as in SIADH. The laboratory features are similar to those of SIADH, including hyponatremia, inappropriately concentrated urine, and high urine sodium concentration. The only factor by which to differentiate between the two is the determination of the volume status. Extracellular fluid volume is decreased in CSW, whereas it is usually increased in SIADH (14). Physical findings (orthostatic hypotension, skin turgor, dry mucous membranes, flat neck veins) and evidence of hemoconcentration (elevated hematocrit, albumin) are important clues for volume depletion; however, they lack specificity and sensitivity (43). More invasive procedures such as central venous pressure measurement and pulmonary artery catheterization are sometimes necessary for more accurate assessment of the volume status.

Treatment

Accurate diagnosis of the hyponatremic patient with SAH is crucial because it dramatically alters the therapeutic approach.

CSW. Patients with CSW are usually volume depleted as a consequence of excessive natriuresis. Fluid restriction, which is usually the first-line therapy for SIADH, could be detrimental to these patients, as it will worsen the symptoms of hypovolemia and increase the risk of cerebral vasospasm and infarction. Treatment should always be aimed at restoring normovolemia, aggressively avoiding a negative fluid balance, and curtailing natriuresis (44). Ideally, the volume status should be evaluated by immediate invasive measurement of central venous pressure; in severe cases, pulmonary artery catheterization with monitoring of pulmonary capillary wedge may be necessary (45). Restoration of normovolemia can be achieved with either crystalloid or colloids (albumin 5%) (46). The appropriate fluid type will depend on the sodium concentration and the patient's symptoms. Isotonic (0.9%) saline is the solution of choice in normonatremic or mildly hyponatremic patients (45). Severe hyponatremia requires the use of hypertonic (1.5%, 3%) solutions (47). Fludrocortisone (0.4 mg/day in two divided doses) is sometimes added to induce a positive sodium balance in patients with resistant hyponatremia (48,49). However, the effect is short lived because of the "mineralocorticoid escape" phenomenon (50).

SIADH. The primary treatment for asymptomatic and chronic SIADH is fluid restriction (14). The goal is to achieve a negative fluid balance to raise serum sodium concentration to normal. In most cases, SIADH is self-limited, and free water restriction may be the definitive therapy. In resistant cases, pharmacologic agents such as demeclocycline and lithium, which directly interfere with the effect of ADH on the collecting tubules, can be used (51,52). However, their efficacy is less predictable, and they have multiple side effects. Arginine-vasopressin (AVP) receptor antagonists represent a novel therapy that is under investigation (53). They specifically target V2 receptors or V1a and V2 receptors. V2 receptors are present in the renal medulla and regulate free water reabsorption (53). By blocking V2 receptors, these antagonists produce a selective water diuresis without interfering with sodium and potassium excretion, which could have a beneficial effect in patients with SIADH (54,55). In addition, AVP-receptor antagonists were shown to have a protective effect against cerebral vasospasm in a rat model of SAH (56).

Severe symptomatic patients with SIADH often require salt administration. The osmolality of the fluid given must exceed the urine osmolality; otherwise correction of hyponatremia will not occur (14). Therefore, isotonic saline infusions should not be administered because they will lead to a further reduction in the plasma sodium concentration (14). Hypertonic (1.5%, 3%) saline should instead be used.

Regardless of the etiology of hyponatremia, serum sodium levels should be corrected slowly to prevent osmotic demyelination (35). The recommended rate of correction of hyponatremia should not exceed 8 to 10 mmol/L in the first 24 hours. In severely symptomatic patients, therapy is targeted toward resolution of symptoms, with an initially slightly faster rate (1–2 mmol/L/hr) over the first few hours, but without exceeding the recommended rates. Formulas used to calculate the sodium requirement have been discussed extensively elsewhere (35).

Hypernatremia

Hypernatremia represents a common clinical problem and has been noted in approximately 20% of patients during the acute period after SAH (12,13). Severe hypernatremia (serum sodium > 155 mmol/L) occurs in only 2% of patients (10). In a prospective study of 298 patients with SAH, hypernatremia was independently associated with increased mortality and poor outcomes at three months. No correlation was found between elevated serum sodium levels and symptomatic vasospasm (13). Adverse cardiac outcomes were also increased. In study of 214 SAH patients, hypernatremia was independently linked to left ventricular ejection fraction of less than 50%, elevated troponin, and pulmonary edema. These patients should be closely monitored for cardiac dysfunction (57).

Hypernatremia always represents a state of hyperosmolality (58). The appropriate physiologic response is (*i*) thirst stimulation to increase water intake and (*ii*) increase in ADH release to prevent free water loss. This regulatory system is very efficient; it maintains plasma osmolality within the range of 1% to 2%, even if sodium and water intake vary widely. Therefore, for hypernatremia to persist, one or both of the compensatory mechanisms must be impaired.

Hypernatremia in the NICU usually results from inadequate water intake or increased free water loss. However, a large exogenous sodium administration in hypertonic solutions can cause hypernatremia through a primary sodium gain (58). In a recent study, the etiology of hypernatremia in patients with SAH was mainly secondary to iatrogenic causes (12); only 4% of hypernatremia cases were due to diabetes insipidus (DI), the rest was the result of cerebral edema treatment with mannitol or hypertonic saline. The development of DI in SAH may be due to destruction of hypothalamic nuclei by brain edema, intracerebral hematoma, or vasospasm resulting in impaired vasopressin secretion (10).

Hypernatremia causes a shift of water out of cerebral cells and subsequent intracellular dehydration. The clinical manifestations of hypernatremia are mostly neurologic, and as with hyponatremia, they depend on acuteness and magnitude of rise of serum sodium levels. The symptoms of acute hypernatremia appear only when serum osmolality reaches 400 mOsm/kg of water and include altered mental status, generalized tonic-clonic seizures and coma. Brain shrinkage induced by hypernatremia can cause rupture of bridging veins and possibly subdural hematomas in susceptible patients. Chronic hypernatremia is usually less symptomatic because of cellular adaptation that limits cerebral shrinkage (58).

Evaluation of Hypernatremia

Clinical assessment of the patient's volume status, urine output, and urine osmolality is essential in determining the etiology of hypernatremia (Fig. 2). Hypovolemic hypernatremia is usually present when water loss exceeds sodium loss. Common causes are excessive sweating, gastrointestinal losses, diuretic use, or osmotic diuresis. Hypervolemia is seen instead in patients with primary sodium gain, such as administration of hypertonic saline.

The appropriate renal response to hypernatremia is to excrete a small volume of maximally concentrated urine (urine osmolality > 800 mOsm/L). The presence of polyuria with hypotonic urine (<300 mOsm/L) suggests an abnormality in vasopressin release by the hypothalamus (complete central DI) or impaired collecting tubule response to vasopressin (complete nephrogenic DI). Administration of desmopressin acetate (DDAVP) may help to differentiate between central DI (positive response) and nephrogenic DI (no response). Usually, the defect is partial, and urine osmolality is between 300 and 800 mOsm/L.

Osmotic diuresis is also associated with polyuria, but in this case, the cause is known and daily urine solute excretion greater than 900 mOsm is diagnostic.

Treatment

Hypernatremic dehydration is best corrected by judicious use of IV fluids. Colloids can be used in certain clinical situations of overt shock. The rate of correction of hypernatremia depends on the rate of its development and whether neurologic symptoms are present. If symptoms are present and hypernatremia is acute, rapid correction over the first hours is appropriate but without exceeding 1 mEq/L/hr (58). Free water deficit should be replaced slowly, with a goal to decrease plasma sodium concentration by 0.5 mEq/L/hr or 10 mEq/L/day. If hypernatremia is corrected too promptly, water can move into the cells, causing cerebral edema and neurologic damage. Careful assessment of fluid balance, body

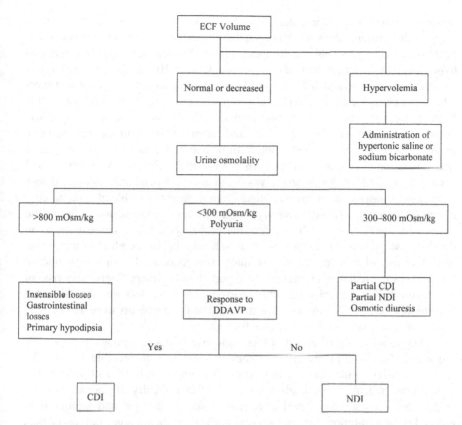

Figure 2 Diagnostic algorithm for hypernatremia. *Abbreviations*: ECF, extracellular fluid; DDAVP, desmopressin acetate; CDI, central diabetes insipidus; NDI, nephrogenic diabetes insipidus.

weight, urine specific gravity, and sodium concentration is required during the course of treatment. The appropriate treatment of acute central DI consists of administration of DDAVP at the usual dose of 0.5 to 2 mcg IV every three hours (4).

HYPERGLYCEMIA

Hyperglycemia is common after SAH and mild increases has been reported in 30% of patients with SAH at anytime during hospitalization (12). Many factors predispose critically ill patients to become hyperglycemic, as it represents a stress response to injury in these patients. Stress-induced hyperglycemia is attributed to excessive elevation of counter-regulatory hormones (Glucagon, cortisol, growth hormone, and catecholamines together increase hepatic gluconeogenesis and promote hepatic glycogenolysis.), effect of cytokines, insulin resistance, and preexisting diabetes. Elevated blood levels on admission have been shown to be a good marker of severity of illness (59). Tentative evidence also suggests that hyperglycemia has a detrimental effect in SAH (60,61). A prospective cohort study of 281 patients with SAH analyzed the association between persistent elevated serum glucose levels and complications (61). The results demonstrated that hyperglycemia (average peak daily glucose level >105 mg/dL) after SAH is associated with increased ICU length of stay, poor functional outcome and mortality at three months after SAH, and serious hospital complications (congestive heart failure, respiratory failure, pneumonia, and brain stem compression or herniation). A link between hyperglycemia and cerebral vasospasm was reported in a previous study, in which blood glucose levels above 215 mg/dL were associated with an increased risk of vasospasm (62). In another retrospective study of 352 patients with aSAH, hyperglycemia was found to be independently associated with symptomatic vasospasm. However, significant differences in blood glucose concentrations were only found between patients with asymptomatic and symptomatic vasospasm, suggesting that hyperglycemia probably does not cause patients to develop vasospasm but may worsen brain ischemia making cerebral infarct worse (63). The risk of vasospasm, in this study, was associated with lower glucose levels (>140 mg/dL) than previously reported (62). Interestingly, the risk of vasospasm was not significant with levels higher than 180 mg/dL (64). One hypothesis offered by the authors was that most of these patients were treated with insulin, which may have a neuroprotective effect.

The relationship of elevated blood glucose levels and poor outcomes has important clinical implications, as hyperglycemia is a correctable factor. The role of intensive insulin therapy in medical and surgical critically ill patients has been established. A recent landmark trial of 1548 critically ill patients demonstrated that patients who receive intensive insulin therapy had significantly reduced in-hospital mortality, bloodstream infections, acute renal failure, critical illness polyneuropathy, and days of mechanical ventilation (65). Intensive insulin therapy has also been found to reduce seizures, intracranial pressure, and duration of mechanical ventilation in various patients with isolated brain injury, including SAH (66). The exact underlying mechanisms of the clinical benefits of intensive insulin therapy remain unclear. However, it has been suggested that normoglycemia, rather than a direct effect of insulin, accounts for the benefits observed with intensive insulin therapy (67,68). Most intensive care units including neuroscience intensive care units operate a nurse driven insulin protocol with very little hypoglycemic or other adverse events. The effect of this measure remains unknown in neurologically ill patients.

OTHER ELECTROLYTE DISTURBANCES

Potassium

Potassium is the major intracellular cation. The total body potassium content in a normal adult is approximately 3000 to 4000 mEq. Only 2% is present in the extracellular compartment (3.5–4 mEq/L) compared with the intracellular compartment ($\sim$150 mEq/L). This gradient is maintained mainly by the Na^+/K^+

adenosine triphosphatase pump, which actively transports K^+ inside the cell in exchange for Na^+ in a 2:3 ratio (69). The regulation of transcellular shift of potassium across cell membranes maintains homeostasis by limiting rapid changes of plasma potassium concentrations. Acid-base disturbances and hormones influence the movement of potassium in and out of the cells. Metabolic acidosis, insulin, and catecholamines promote cellular uptake of potassium and hypokalemia, while, alkalosis, insulin deficiency, and β-adrenergic blockade promote potassium movement out the cells and hyperkalemia (69). Potassium intake of a normal person on a typical western diet is 1 mmol/kg body weight. Maintaining overall balance requires matching potassium intake with excretion. The kidneys are the major routes by which the body eliminates excess potassium. Control of renal potassium secretion occurs in the principal cells in the distal convoluted tubule and the cortical collecting duct. The major physiologic determinants of K^+ secretion are aldosterone and the plasma potassium concentration.

Potassium disturbances are common in the critical care setting and may be associated with life-threatening complications, primarily cardiac dysrhythmias.

Hypokalemia is defined as a plasma potassium concentration of less than 3.5 mEq/L. The clinical manifestations vary greatly among individual patients and the severity of potassium depletion. Marked symptoms seldom develop unless plasma potassium is less than 3 mEq/L. Severe hypokalemia is associated with progressive muscle weakness leading to complete paralysis, hypoventilation, rhabdomyolysis, and life-threatening cardiac dysrhythmias. The electrocardiographic (ECG) changes are ST depression, broad flat T wave, increased U waves, QRS and QT interval prolongation and finally ventricular dysrhythmias that lead to cardiac arrest (70). The most common causes of potassium depletion in the neurologic intensive care setting result from increased excretion. Diuretics (furosemide, thiazides), osmotic agents (mannitol), and mineralocorticoids (fludrocortisone, to expand intravascular volume) are commonly used in patients after SAH, and all promote potassium depletion. Other causes include shifts of potassium into cells (alkalemia, insulin therapy, stress-induced catecholamine surge) and lower gastrointestinal losses.

Oral potassium supplementation is the safest way to correct hypokalemia. Little correlation exists between plasma potassium concentration and total body potassium deficit. In general, a decrement of 1 mEq/L represents a 200 to 300-mEq/L deficit (71). Hypomagnesemia is a frequent reason for treatment failure and should also be corrected (72). Severe hypokalemia with symptoms should be treated with IV replacement therapy with potassium chloride. The rate of correction should not exceed 20 mEq/hr, although higher rates can be used with life-threatening cardiac dysrhythmias and paralysis (73).

Hyperkalemia is defined as serum potassium concentration of greater than 5 mEq/L. The most important clinical manifestations are also neuromuscular and cardiac. Tall, peaked T waves and shortening of the QT interval are the initial changes seen on ECG, followed by widening of the QRS complex and eventual loss of P wave and sine wave pattern. Transcellular shift of potassium out of the cells is associated only with transient hyperkalemia. Metabolic acidosis represents the most common cause of shift-related hyperkalemia (69). Persistent elevation of plasma potassium concentration is usually because of inadequate renal potassium clearance due to renal failure or hypoaldosteronism or resistance to aldosterone activity. Hyperkalemia should be treated emergently if muscle weakness or typical ECG changes are present. The treatment is directed at antagonizing the cardiac effects of hyperkalemia with calcium chloride and shifting potassium into the cells with IV insulin and glucose or sodium bicarbonate (in case of significant acidosis). Removal of potassium from the body can be achieved with cation exchange resins and with the use of loop diuretics. Hemodialysis is often required for patients with renal failure and those with life-threatening hyperkalemia who are unresponsive to medical treatments (70).

Calcium

Hypocalcemia is a frequent finding in critically ill patients, occurring in up to 88% of severely ill patients admitted to the ICU and correlates with the severity of illness and mortality (74). Approximately 40% of calcium is bound to serum proteins, principally albumin. Hypoalbuminemia is the primary cause of low total calcium concentration in severely ill patients. In this scenario, corrected serum calcium for albumin and ionized free calcium are normal. Alkalemia also increases calcium binding to negatively charged proteins and decreases the fraction of ionized calcium. Other causes include sepsis, hypomagnesemia, hyperphosphatemia, renal failure, chelating agents such as citrate anticoagulant in transfused blood, and anticonvulsant drugs (phenytoin, phenobarbital), which increase liver metabolism of vitamin D (75). However, despite careful assessment, no cause is found in 50% of cases (76). The clinical presentation depends on the severity of hypocalcemia and the rapidity of onset. Neuromuscular excitability varies from paresthesias to severe tetany and seizures. Bradycardia, heart failure with hypotension, and dysrhythmias can be seen with severe hypocalcemia. The classic ECG finding consists of prolongation of the QT interval. Hypocalcemia in critically ill patients is usually transient and mild and rarely requires treatment (75). Patients with asymptomatic, mild, hypocalcemia are treated with oral calcium supplements, and infusion of elemental calcium is reserved for severe or symptomatic patients. Hypomagnesemia should also be sought and corrected.

Magnesium

Hypomagnesemia is common in critically ill patients. The reported prevalence can be as high as 65% in patients admitted to the ICU (77–79), and it has been associated with increased mortality and worse outcome, including in patients with acute brain injury (78). Hypomagnesemia is also a frequent finding in patients after SAH. In a prospective study of 107 patients admitted within 48 hours after aSAH, low serum magnesium levels (0.7 mmol/L) were found in 38% of patients on admission and in 54% of patients admitted within 12 hours after SAH. The occurrence of delayed cerebral ischemia was higher in patients with hypomagnesemia than in those with normal serum magnesium level (80). The role of magnesium therapy as a neuroprotective agent in SAH has been shown recently. Patients with SAH who were given a standard dose of magnesium sulfate (64 mmol/L/day) had reduced risks of delayed cerebral ischemia and poor outcome (81,82). The pathogenesis of hypomagnesemia after SAH has not been studied.

Hypomagnesemia is frequently asymptomatic and only identified by measurement of the serum magnesium level. It is often associated with depletion of other electrolytes such as hypokalemia, hypocalcemia, and metabolic alkalosis, and most of the clinical manifestations are related to changes in concentration of other ions. Hypomagnesemia can be induced by two major mechanisms: increased gastrointestinal losses and increased renal losses associated most frequently with diuretics (both loop diuretics and thiazides), volume expansion, chronic alcohol use, and antibiotics (83).

Treatment with IV magnesium sulfate is preferred in symptomatic critically ill patients or in patients with severe magnesium deficiency. The underlying disease should also be corrected if possible.

Phosphorus

Derangements in the metabolism of phosphate are common in the neurologic ICU. Common causes of hypophosphatemia include intracellular shift (respiratory alkalosis, refeeding syndrome, insulin), decreased intestinal absorption, and renal losses. Various factors combine to put patients with SAH at risk for increased renal excretion of phosphorus; osmotic diuresis (mannitol) or excessive diuretic therapy, excessive polyuria due to SIADH, and CSW are all contributing factors. Hypophosphatemia is clinically asymptomatic unless the serum phosphorus level is below 1 mg/dL. Clinical manifestations consist of diffuse skeletal muscle weakness, including respiratory muscles with respiratory failure and ventilatory dependence, congestive cardiomyopathy, hemolysis, and rhabdomyolysis. IV phosphate replacement is required in all cases of severe hypophosphatemia (<1 mg/dL) or the presence of symptoms. Oral supplementation may be adequate in moderate hypophosphatemia.

CONCLUSION

As expected in any critically ill patient electrolyte derangements are commonly encountered following severe forms of SAH. Frequent and close monitoring of electrolytes in the critical care setting are paramount for timely recognition and therapeutic interventions. Changes in serum sodium in SAH do indicate a more serious endocrinopathy and failure to recognize its association with hypovolemia could put the patient at risk of symptomatic vasospasm and eventually cerebral infarction. Therapies that can control the intravascular volume are needed and may target the atrial natriuretic family as a whole. The impact of strict glucose control in SAH on outcome is not yet known. There has been a paradigm shift in this particular area from a laissez faire attitude—simply explaining hypergly-cemia as a stress response—to an aggressive clinical intervention with control of even slightly elevated blood glucose values. Whether other electrolyte disorders seen in SAH need more scrutiny is not known.

REFERENCES

1. Hasan D, Wijdicks EF, Vermeulen M. Hyponatremia is associated with cerebral ischemia in patients with aneurysmal subarachnoid hemorrhage. Ann Neurol 1990; 27(1):106–108.
2. Kurokawa Y, Uede T, Ishiguro M, et al. Pathogenesis of hyponatremia following subarachnoid hemorrhage due to ruptured cerebral aneurysm. Surg Neurol 1996; 46(5):500–5077 (discussion 7–8).
3. Fox JL, Falik JL, Shalhoub RJ. Neurosurgical hyponatremia: the role of inappropriate antidiuresis. J Neurosurg 1971; 34(4):506–514.
4. Wijdicks EF. The clinical practice of critical care neurology. New York: Oxford University Press, 2003.
5. Wijdicks EF, Vermeulen M, Hijdra A, et al. Hyponatremia and cerebral infarction in patients with ruptured intracranial aneurysms: is fluid restriction harmful? Ann Neurol 1985; 17(2):137–140.
6. Wijdicks EF, Vandongen KJ, Vangijn J, et al. Enlargement of the third ventricle and hyponatraemia in aneurysmal subarachnoid haemorrhage. J Neurol Neurosurg Psychiatry 1988; 51(4):516–520.
7. Diringer MN, Lim JS, Kirsch JR, et al. Suprasellar and intraventricular blood predict elevated plasma atrial natriuretic factor in subarachnoid hemorrhage. Stroke 1991; 22(5):577–581.
8. Sayama T, Inamura T, Matsushima T, et al. High incidence of hyponatremia in patients with ruptured anterior communicating artery aneurysms. Neurol Res 2000; 22(2):151–155.
9. Sherlock M, O'Sullivan E, Agha A, et al. The incidence and pathophysiology of hyponatraemia after subarachnoid haemorrhage. Clin Endocrinol (Oxf) 2006; 64(3): 250–254.
10. Takaku A, Shindo K, Tanaka S, et al. Fluid and electrolyte disturbances in patients with intracranial aneurysms. Surg Neurol 1979; 11(5):349–356.
11. Anderson RJ, Chung HM, Kluge R, et al. Hyponatremia: A prospective analysis of its epidemiology and the pathogenetic role of vasopressin. Ann Intern Med 1985; 102(2):164–168.
12. Wartenberg KE, Schmidt JM, Claassen J, et al. Impact of medical complications on outcome after subarachnoid hemorrhage. Crit Care Med 2006; 34(3):617–623.
13. Qureshi AI, Suri MF, Sung GY, et al. Prognostic significance of hypernatremia and hyponatremia among patients with aneurysmal subarachnoid hemorrhage. Neurosurgery 2002; 50(4):749–755 (discussion 55–6).

14. Palmer BF. Hyponatremia in patients with central nervous system disease: SIADH versus CSW. Trends Endocrinol Metab 2003; 14(4):182–187.
15. Doczi T, Bende J, Huszka E, et al. Syndrome of inappropriate secretion of antidiuretic hormone after subarachnoid hemorrhage. Neurosurgery 1981; 9(4):394–397.
16. Nelson PB, Goodman M, Maroon JC, et al. Factors in predicting outcome from operation in patients with prolactin-secreting pituitary adenomas. Neurosurgery 1983; 13(6):634–641.
17. Nelson PB, Seif S, Gutai J, et al. Hyponatremia and natriuresis following subarachnoid hemorrhage in a monkey model. J Neurosurg 1984; 60(2):233–237.
18. Wijdicks EF, Vermeulen M, ten Haaf JA, et al. Volume depletion and natriuresis in patients with a ruptured intracranial aneurysm. Ann Neurol 1985; 18(2):211–216.
19. Diringer MN, Wu KC, Verbalis JG, et al. Hypervolemic therapy prevents volume contraction but not hyponatremia following subarachnoid hemorrhage. Ann Neurol 1992; 31(5):543–550.
20. Berendes E, Walter M, Cullen P, et al. Secretion of brain natriuretic peptide in patients with aneurysmal subarachnoid haemorrhage. Lancet 1997; 349(9047):245–249.
21. Isotani E, Suzuki R, Tomita K, et al. Alterations in plasma concentrations of natriuretic peptides and antidiuretic hormone after subarachnoid hemorrhage. Stroke 1994; 25(11):2198–2203.
22. Diringer M, Ladenson PW, Stern BJ, et al. Plasma atrial natriuretic factor and subarachnoid hemorrhage. Stroke 1988; 19(9):1119–1124.
23. Espiner EA, Leikis R, Ferch RD, et al. The neuro-cardio-endocrine response to acute subarachnoid haemorrhage. Clin Endocrinol (Oxf) 2002; 56(5):629–635.
24. McGirt MJ, Blessing R, Nimjee SM, et al. Correlation of serum brain natriuretic peptide with hyponatremia and delayed ischemic neurological deficits after subarachnoid hemorrhage. Neurosurgery 2004; 54(6):1369–1373 (discussion 73–4).
25. Tomida M, Muraki M, Uemura K, et al. Plasma concentrations of brain natriuretic peptide in patients with subarachnoid hemorrhage. Stroke 1998; 29(8):1584–1587.
26. Sviri GE, Feinsod M, Soustiel JF. Brain natriuretic peptide and cerebral vasospasm in subarachnoid hemorrhage. Clinical and TCD correlations. Stroke 2000; 31(1): 118–122.
27. Wijdicks EF, Ropper AH, Hunnicutt EJ, et al. Atrial natriuretic factor and salt wasting after aneurysmal subarachnoid hemorrhage. Stroke 1991; 22(12):1519–1524.
28. Wijdicks EF, Schievink WI, Burnett JC Jr. Natriuretic peptide system and endothelin in aneurysmal subarachnoid hemorrhage. J Neurosurg 1997; 87(2):275–280.
29. Kurokawa Y, Uede T, Honda O, et al. [Pathogenesis of hyponatremia observed in the treatment of acute subarachnoid hemorrhage]. No To Shinkei 1992; 44(10):905–911.
30. Okuchi K, Fujioka M, Fujikawa A, et al. Rapid natriuresis and preventive hypervolaemia for symptomatic vasospasm after subarachnoid haemorrhage. Acta Neurochir (Wien) 1996; 138(8):951–956 (discussion 6–7).
31. Levin ER, Gardner DG, Samson WK. Natriuretic peptides. N Engl J Med 1998; 339(5):321–328.
32. Wijeyaratne CN, Moult PJ. The effect of alpha human atrial natriuretic peptide on plasma volume and vascular permeability in normotensive subjects. J Clin Endocrinol Metab 1993; 76(2):343–346.
33. Igaki T, Itoh H, Suga S, et al. C-type natriuretic peptide in chronic renal failure and its action in humans. Kidney Int Suppl 1996; 55:S144–S147.

34. Arieff AI, Guisado R. Effects on the central nervous system of hypernatremic and hyponatremic states. Kidney Int 1976; 10(1):104–116.
35. Adrogue HJ, Madias NE. Hyponatremia. N Engl J Med 2000; 342(21):1581–1589.
36. Laureno R, Karp BI. Myelinolysis after correction of hyponatremia. Ann Intern Med 1997; 126(1):57–62.
37. Laureno R. Central pontine myelinolysis following rapid correction of hyponatremia. Ann Neurol 1983; 13(3):232–242.
38. Martin PJ, Young CA. Central pontine myelinolysis: clinical and MRI correlates. Postgrad Med J 1995; 71(837):430–432.
39. Vaswani SK, Sprague R. Pseudohyponatremia in multiple myeloma. South Med J 1993; 86(2):251–252.
40. Lawn N, Wijdicks EF, Burritt MF. Intravenous immune globulin and pseudohyponatremia. N Engl J Med 1998; 339(9):632.
41. Hillier TA, Abbott RD, Barrett EJ. Hyponatremia: evaluating the correction factor for hyperglycemia. Am J Med 1999; 106(4):399–403.
42. Schwartz WB, Bennett W, Curelop S, et al. A syndrome of renal sodium loss and hyponatremia probably resulting from inappropriate secretion of antidiuretic hormone. 1957. J Am Soc Nephrol 2001; 12(12):2860–2870.
43. Chung HM, Kluge R, Schrier RW, et al. Clinical assessment of extracellular fluid volume in hyponatremia. Am J Med 1987; 83(5):905–908.
44. Palmer BF. Hyponatraemia in a neurosurgical patient: Syndrome of inappropriate antidiuretic hormone secretion versus cerebral salt wasting. Nephrol Dial Transplant 2000; 15(2):262–268.
45. Rabinstein AA, Wijdicks EF. Hyponatremia in critically ill neurological patients. Neurologist 2003; 9(6):290–300.
46. Mayer SA, Solomon RA, Fink ME, et al. Effect of 5% albumin solution on sodium balance and blood volume after subarachnoid hemorrhage. Neurosurgery 1998; 42(4):759–767 (discussion 67–8).
47. Suarez JI, Qureshi AI, Parekh PD, et al. Administration of hypertonic (3%) sodium chloride/acetate in hyponatremic patients with symptomatic vasospasm following subarachnoid hemorrhage. J Neurosurg Anesthesiol 1999; 11(3):178–184.
48. Woo MH, Kale-Pradhan PB. Fludrocortisone in the treatment of subarachnoid hemorrhage-induced hyponatremia. Ann Pharmacother 1997; 31(5):637–639.
49. Wijdicks EF, Vermeulen M, van Brummelen P, et al. The effect of fludrocortisone acetate on plasma volume and natriuresis in patients with aneurysmal subarachnoid hemorrhage. Clin Neurol Neurosurg 1988; 90(3):209–214.
50. Knox FG, Burnett JC Jr., Kohan DE, et al. Escape from the sodium-retaining effects of mineralocorticoids. Kidney Int 1980; 17(3):263–276.
51. Forrest JN Jr., Cox M, Hong C, et al. Superiority of demeclocycline over lithium in the treatment of chronic syndrome of inappropriate secretion of antidiuretic hormone. N Engl J Med 1978; 298(4):173–177.
52. De Troyer A. Demeclocycline. Treatment for syndrome of inappropriate antidiuretic hormone secretion. JAMA 1977; 237(25):2723–2726.
53. Bhardwaj A. Neurological impact of vasopressin dysregulation and hyponatremia. Ann Neurol 2006; 59(2):229–236.
54. Verbalis JG. AVP receptor antagonists as aquaretics: review and assessment of clinical data. Cleve Clin J Med 2006; 73(suppl 3):S24–S33.
55. Verbalis JG. Vasopressin V2 receptor antagonists. J Mol Endocrinol 2002; 29(1):1–9.

56. Trandafir CC, Nishihashi T, Wang A, et al. Participation of vasopressin in the development of cerebral vasospasm in a rat model of subarachnoid haemorrhage. Clin Exp Pharmacol Physiol 2004; 31(4):261–266.
57. Fisher LA, Ko N, Miss J, et al. Hypernatremia predicts adverse cardiovascular and neurological outcomes after SAH. Neurocrit Care 2006; 5(3):180–185.
58. Adrogue HJ, Madias NE. Hypernatremia. N Engl J Med 2000; 342(20):1493–1499.
59. Claassen J, Vu A, Kreiter KT, et al. Effect of acute physiologic derangements on outcome after subarachnoid hemorrhage. Crit Care Med 2004; 32(3):832–838.
60. Sarrafzadeh A, Haux D, Kuchler I, et al. Poor-grade aneurysmal subarachnoid hemorrhage: relationship of cerebral metabolism to outcome. J Neurosurg 2004; 100(3):400–406.
61. Frontera JA, Fernandez A, Claassen J, et al. Hyperglycemia after SAH: predictors, associated complications, and impact on outcome. Stroke 2006; 37(1):199–203.
62. Charpentier C, Audibert G, Guillemin F, et al. Multivariate analysis of predictors of cerebral vasospasm occurrence after aneurysmal subarachnoid hemorrhage. Stroke 1999; 30(7):1402–1408.
63. De Georgia M. Hyperglycemia and subarachnoid hemorrhage: the critical care part of neurocritical care. Crit Care Med 2005; 33(7):1663–1664.
64. Badjatia N, Topcuoglu MA, Buonanno FS, et al. Relationship between hyperglycemia and symptomatic vasospasm after subarachnoid hemorrhage. Crit Care Med 2005; 33(7):1603–1609.
65. van den Berghe G, Wouters P, Weekers F, et al. Intensive insulin therapy in the critically ill patients. N Engl J Med 2001; 345(19):1359–1367.
66. Van den Berghe G, Schoonheydt K, Beex P, et al. Insulin therapy protects the central and peripheral nervous system of intensive care patients. Neurology 2005; 64(8): 1348–1353.
67. Finney SJ, Zekveld C, Elia A, et al. Glucose control and mortality in critically ill patients. JAMA 2003; 290(15):2041–2047.
68. Van den Berghe G, Wouters PJ, Bouillon R, et al. Outcome benefit of intensive insulin therapy in the critically ill: Insulin dose versus glycemic control. Crit Care Med 2003; 31(2):359–366.
69. Halperin ML, Kamel KS. Potassium. Lancet 1998; 352(9122):135–140.
70. Schaefer TJ, Wolford RW. Disorders of potassium. Emerg Med Clin North Am 2005; 23(3):723–747, viii–ix.
71. Sterns RH, Cox M, Feig PU, et al. Internal potassium balance and the control of the plasma potassium concentration. Medicine (Baltimore) 1981; 60(5):339–354.
72. Salem M, Munoz R, Chernow B. Hypomagnesemia in critical illness. A common and clinically important problem. Crit Care Clin 1991; 7(1):225–252.
73. Kruse JA, Carlson RW. Rapid correction of hypokalemia using concentrated intravenous potassium chloride infusions. Arch Intern Med 1990; 150(3):613–617.
74. Zivin JR, Gooley T, Zager RA, et al. Hypocalcemia: a pervasive metabolic abnormality in the critically ill. Am J Kidney Dis 2001; 37(4):689–698.
75. Zaloga GP. Hypocalcemia in critically ill patients. Crit Care Med 1992; 20(2):251–262.
76. Desai TK, Carlson RW, Geheb MA. Prevalence and clinical implications of hypocalcemia in acutely ill patients in a medical intensive care setting. Am J Med 1988; 84(2):209–214.
77. Wong ET, Rude RK, Singer FR, et al. A high prevalence of hypomagnesemia and hypermagnesemia in hospitalized patients. Am J Clin Pathol 1983; 79(3):348–352.

78. Rubeiz GJ, Thill-Baharozian M, Hardie D, et al. Association of hypomagnesemia and mortality in acutely ill medical patients. Crit Care Med 1993; 21(2):203–209.

79. Chernow B, Bamberger S, Stoiko M, et al. Hypomagnesemia in patients in postoperative intensive care. Chest 1989; 95(2):391–397.

80. van den Bergh WM, Algra A, van der Sprenkel JW, et al. Hypomagnesemia after aneurysmal subarachnoid hemorrhage. Neurosurgery 2003; 52(2):276–281 (discussion 81–2).

81. van den Bergh WM, Algra A, van Kooten F, et al. Magnesium sulfate in aneurysmal subarachnoid hemorrhage: a randomized controlled trial. Stroke 2005; 36(5): 1011–1015.

82. Dorhout Mees SM, van den Bergh WM, Algra A, et al. Achieved serum magnesium concentrations and occurrence of delayed cerebral ischaemia and poor outcome in aneurysmal subarachnoid haemorrhage. J Neurol Neurosurg Psychiatry 2007; 78(7): 729–731.

83. Agus ZS. Hypomagnesemia. J Am Soc Nephrol 1999; 10(7):1616–1622.

19

Management of Cardiopulmonary Dysfunction in Subarachnoid Hemorrhage

Thomas P. Bleck, MD, FCCM, Ruth Cain Ruggles Chairman[a], Vice Chairman[b], and Professor[c]

[a]Department of Neurology, Evanston Northwestern Healthcare,
[b]Department of Neurology, [c]Departments of Neurology, Neurosurgery, and Medicine, Northwestern University Feinberg School of Medicine, Chicago, Illinois, U.S.A.

Cardiac and pulmonary dysfunctions commonly accompany subarachnoid hemorrhage (SAH), particularly when it is due to aneurysmal rupture. The aggregate epidemiology of these problems has not been well studied, but some insight can be gained from a study of oxygenation abnormalities in which 80% of aneurysmal SAH patients had widened alveolar-arterial oxygen gradients ($AaDO_2$) during the first several days of illness (1). The vast majority of studies have focused on individual forms of heart or lung disorder in these patients. Because the pathogeneses of these problems vary, as do their treatment, they will be considered individually in this chapter. However, a given patient often suffers from more than one disorder simultaneously, and the tendency of these patients to have intravascular volume fluctuations due to cerebral salt wasting and its management, as well as volume expansion and vasopressor use for the treatment of cerebral vasospasm, further complicate any attempt to give simple therapeutic recommendations.

For clarity of exposition, these disorders are divided into those that primarily affect the lungs: neurogenic pulmonary edema (NPE), negative pressure pulmonary edema, and aspiration pneumonitis. Ventilator-associated pneumonia (VAP) is also common in SAH patients. The primarily cardiac disorders (contraction band necrosis, neurogenic stunned myocardium, tako-tsubo cardiomyopathy, repolarization

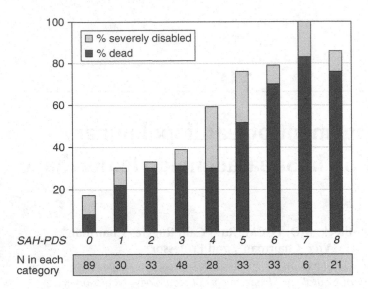

Figure 1   Effect of acute physiologic derangement score on outcome, SAH-PDS. *Abbreviation*: SAH-PDS, subarachnoid hemorrhage physiologic derangement score. *Source*: From Ref. 2.

Table 1   Components of the acute physiologic derangement score

Factor	Cutoff value	Points
AaDO$_2$	>125 mmHg	3
Serum bicarbonate concentration	<20 mmol/L	2
Serum glucose concentration	>180 mg/dL (10 mmol/L)	1
Mean arterial pressure	<70 or >130 mmHg	1

Source: From Ref. 2.

abnormalities and associated dysrhythmias) are probably all manifestations of the hypersympathetic state that accompanies aneurysmal rupture. They can produce varying degrees of left ventricular dysfunction, which leads to secondary pulmonary edema. To optimally manage these patients, one must determine the relative contributions of these problems to the patient's difficulties with oxygenation and hypotension. The effects of these problems on prognosis are apparent from their contributions to the acute physiologic derangement score developed by the Columbia group, which has a substantial predictive value for survival and functional outcome (Fig. 1), (Table 1) (2). The AaDO$_2$ had the strongest effect on outcome, and the mean arterial pressure (either depressed or elevated) was also important.

When a patient presents with pulmonary problems in the setting of acute SAH, it may not immediately be clear whether the primary dysfunction involves the lungs, the heart, or both. This chapter is divided into pulmonary and cardiac sections, but the physician will recognize that these systems are so intimately connected that, in practice, they must be treated as one. Furthermore, the principle of Occam's razor need not apply; a given patient may have more than one disorder in both systems. Thus, a major clinical challenge is sorting out what is at the root of the patient's problems. They must then be managed not only with reference to the heart and lungs but also with the primary view of protecting the brain from further damage as a result of hypoxemia, abnormal blood pressure, and inadequate cardiac output.

PRIMARILY PULMONARY DISORDERS

NPE

Acute pulmonary edema develops commonly in patients with acute SAH, but the genesis of this problem in a given patient may be difficult to determine. In a large Italian series of SAH patients, clinically apparent NPE was reported in 4% (3). NPE was the most common etiology in our series, in which 20% of SAH patients had symptomatic NPE (1). A similar percentage was reported in a multicentered trial (4). Other potential causes for pulmonary edema are discussed below. SAH is by far the most frequent etiology of NPE; head trauma, intracerebral hemorrhage, large ischemic stroke, and status epilepticus are the other commonly reported causes. A study of extravascular lung water in a mixed population of patients with SAH and intracerebral hemorrhage demonstrated an increase in $AaDO_2$ that was paralleled by an elevation of lung water content, as determined by a double-indicator dilution technique (5).

The pathogenesis of NPE in humans continues to be debated, but it is most likely a condition with more than one mechanism. While experimental models attempt to separate various possibilities in order to study them with clarity, patients may have a combination of disorders (e.g., simultaneous NPE and cardiac dysfunction). While it is tempting to assume that the causes of NPE share high circulating catecholamine levels (6), this remains to be demonstrated and is not in keeping with the mechanisms suggested by several experimental models. NPE following acute spinal cord injury and death by neurologic criteria suggests that neuronal outflow via the spinal cord is probably important.

The vast majority of reported NPE cases, as well as those not reported but encountered in clinical practice, are diagnosed within the first day or two of the onset of SAH. Investigators performed bronchoalveolar lavage in patients with NPE and concluded that seven of the patients had a hydrostatic disorder (low protein concentration in the bronchoalveolar lavage fluid) and that the remainder had evidence of a capillary leak (high protein concentration); five of the eight patients with SAH had low protein contents (7).

Experimental studies of NPE typically involve acute head injury, acute elevation of intracranial pressure, or cisternal injection of blood or other irritants. One group demonstrated that systemic hypertension was not necessary for the

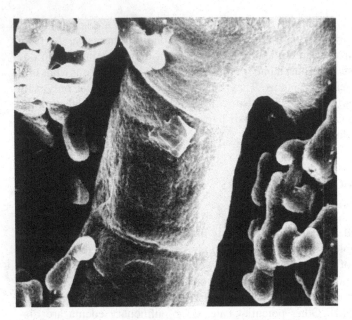

Figure 2 Scanning electron micrograph of sphincters on pulmonary venules. *Source*: From Ref. 11.

development of NPE (8) and further suggested that acute pulmonary hypertension was a prerequisite for its genesis (9). The reason for this pulmonary hypertension is uncertain but may be secondary to neurogenic constriction of post-capillary sphincters on pulmonary venules (10). These sphincters contract almost immediately after experimental head injury in rats (Fig. 2) (11). The neural origin of NPE is further suggested by work that indicated that transaction of nerves to one lung prevented it from developing edema when the other lung, exposed to the same hydrostatic pressure, became edematous (12). Output from the nucleus of the solitary tract via the vagi may be an important modulator (13). Many interrelated substances have been proposed as mediators of these effects, most prominently substance P (14), neuropeptide Y (15), nitric oxide (16), and most recently, neurokinins (17).

The diagnosis of NPE is usually suggested by an increasing $AaDO_2$, often manifested by a need for supplemental oxygen to maintain acceptable oxygen saturation. Many prefer to follow the ratio of partial pressure of oxygen to the fraction of inspired oxygen (PaO_2/FiO_2, or P/F ratio), which yields a similar trend with illness. The SAH patient who requires supplemental oxygen requires investigation for the cause of this problem and its management. At this time, the chest X ray may not yet show clear signs of pulmonary edema because the portable anteroposterior technique usually used is less sensitive to early markers (e.g., Kerley B-lines) than the formal posteroanterior projection used in the radiology suite. Later, the patient may develop interstitial, and eventually

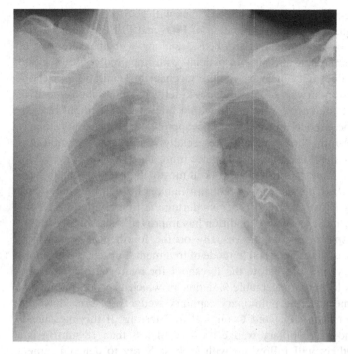

Figure 3 NPE in a 20-year-old patient with aneurysmal subarachnoid hemorrhage. Her pulmonary capillary wedge pressure was 12 mmHg, and her cardiac index was 4.2 L/min/m^2.

alveolar, edema that is visible on film (Fig. 3). Tachypnea is often present but may be overlooked among the numerous abnormalities that may be present on physical examination. Other signs of cardiac failure on examination should prompt consideration of neurogenic stunned myocardium (see below) as a cause of secondary pulmonary edema. An echocardiogram should be performed in the presence of any evidence that suggests cardiac dysfunction; some clinicians obtain this study in all cases of oxygenation abnormality in SAH patients.

In the absence of a clear understanding of pathophysiology, recommendations for management have been empiric (18). Supplemental oxygen is the mainstay of treatment. As the majority of SAH patients with NPE require mechanical ventilation, positive end-expiratory pressure (PEEP) is typically used to keep the FiO$_2$ below 50% if possible. Some of the applied PEEP will be transmitted from the alveoli to the pulmonary veins, thereby raising intrathoracic pressure and thus impairing jugular venous return and potentially increasing intracranial pressure. The diminished static pulmonary compliance associated with interstitial edema serves to limit this intrathoracic pressure transmission; measurement of the central venous pressure provides an estimate of the degree to which jugular venous return is affected. Diuresis to decrease lung water (see below) will decrease the need for PEEP but will also increase the transmitted pressure. Thus, the ideal combination of FiO_2 and PEEP cannot be prespecified but must be determined at the bedside, along with measurement of estimation of the intracranial pressure in patients with impaired consciousness.

If the patient does not otherwise require mechanical ventilation, or endotracheal intubation for airway protection, mask-delivered continuous positive airway pressure or noninvasive ventilation with a bilevel device might be considered. However, these modes of support are not appropriate for patients who may vomit into the tight-fitting mask required, especially if impaired consciousness makes it difficult for them to summon assistance immediately.

As hydrostatic forces are likely at work in most patients, attempts to keep the pulmonary capillary pressure low seem justifiable, and this is usually achieved with diuretics. Most severe NPE occurs during the first few days after the SAH occurs, and in most cases the condition has improved substantially before the period of vasospasm risk begins (usually on the fourth post–hemorrhage day); therefore, diuresis is an acceptable mode of treatment. Further, as the aim is to keep the capillary pressure below the threshold for hydrostatic edema production, this seems to be an acceptable situation in which to use a pulmonary artery catheter to measure the pulmonary capillary wedge pressure. However, this practice has not been subjected to clinical trial testing. If this measure is undertaken, a pulmonary capillary wedge pressure of less than 18 mmHg is a reasonable goal. Others will follow up with a chest X ray to detect incipient alveolar edema.

Cerebral salt wasting may also occur during this period and produce a diuresis of its own. However, when the patient is at risk for vasospasm between days 4 and 14, most physicians attempt to maintain the patient as close to euvolemia as possible (attempts at hypervolemia generally not being successful, unless cardiac or renal dysfunction supervene) in order to minimize cerebral damage as a result of vasospasm.

Lungs of patients who have suffered insults that lead to death by neurologic criteria often develop NPE. While this results in P/F ratios that are often thought to exclude the use of these lungs for transplantation, these organs often recover quickly when placed in the recipient. The recipient may require support with extracorporeal membrane oxygenation before adequate oxygen diffusion can be restored (19).

Negative-Pressure Pulmonary Edema

Negative-pressure pulmonary edema occurs when a patient, often young and in good physical condition, attempts to inspire vigorously against an obstructed airway. In neurocritical care, this typically develops after a seizure has produced upper airway compromise, as may occur when the patient's masseter contraction compresses an endotracheal tube. However, the condition may develop in conscious patients who struggle against an occluded airway for any cause. The edema appears to be a consequence of fluid transudation during a period of low alveolar pressure; a study of the protein content of the fluid supports this concept (20). Severe pressure gradients may cause alveolar hemorrhage (21). As these patients are by definition in very stressful circumstances, elevated catecholamine concentrations may also play a role in the genesis of the edema. The diagnosis is based on a compatible history, hypoxemia, and chest radiographic evidence of pulmonary edema. Less severe cases are probably underdiagnosed, especially because the time course of resolution is usually rapid, unless hemorrhage has supervened.

Because negative-pressure pulmonary edema is typically a relatively brief complication, supplemental oxygen and PEEP or continuous positive airway pressure for several hours to a few days is usually sufficient management (22). This condition usually occurs in patients who are otherwise healthy enough to develop very negative intrapleural pressures, and they seldom benefit from diuresis.

Aspiration Pneumonitis

Early in the course of acute SAH, patients with higher Hunt and Hess grades are often at risk for macroscopic aspiration because of impaired consciousness and vomiting. The diagnosis of aspiration is often apparent when the patient is intubated, or from the appearance of expectorated sputum. One group reported that 6% of their SAH patients developed aspiration (23). The chest X ray usually shows patchy infiltrates unless airway obstruction has occurred, resulting in segmental or lobar atelectasis. Patients often have a brief period of fever, typically in the absence of documentable infection.

Treatment for aspiration pneumonitis is supportive. Although many patients appear to have oxygenation problems related solely to either gastric acid injury or particulate matter in the airways, the question of antibiotic therapy is often raised. This is a contentious issue that is not likely to be resolved soon (24). If antibiotics are used, narrow-spectrum agents should be used for short courses, unless the patient develops evidence of a bacterial pneumonia. Antibiotic coverage for anaerobic organisms is often employed, but evidence for its benefit is lacking. If antibiotic therapy is deemed necessary, ceftriaxone is usually sufficient. Acid aspiration does not appear to benefit from anti-inflammatory drugs such as steroids.

Ventilator-Associated Pneumonia

Microscopic aspiration across the cuff of the endotracheal tube or tracheostomy tube is the putative cause of most cases of VAP. By definition, the patient must have received mechanical ventilation for three days or longer to be diagnosed with VAP; however, when patients are intubated for neurologic rather than pulmonary reasons, the real differential diagnosis of a new pneumonia is usually between macroscopic aspiration and VAP. Although a variety of measures to prevent VAP have been suggested (25), a full discussion of the choices is beyond the scope of this chapter. In general, they include elevation of the head of the bed to 30° or higher, use of endotracheal tubes to provide continuous aspiration of subglottic secretions, and meticulous attention to suctioning technique.

Treatment for VAP, an addition to improving oxygenation, depends on an adequate microbiologic diagnosis of the infecting organism. After obtaining blood and sputum cultures (the latter preferably with a quantitative technique), antibiotic therapy designed to cover the likely organisms, particularly resistant gram-negative rods such as *Pseudomonas aeruginosa*, should be initiated. After three days of treatment, the results of microbiologic studies should be used to "de-escalate" antibiotic therapy to cover the organism(s) isolated with the narrowest possible spectrum (26). Antianaerobic coverage is also debated in this setting but does not appear to improve clinical outcome measures.

PRIMARILY CARDIAC DISORDERS

The literature contains several descriptions of disorders of myocardial contractility in SAH patients. The terms *myocardial contraction band necrosis, neurogenic stunned myocardium,* and *tako-tsubo cardiomyopathy* most probably describe different manifestations of a unifying underlying disorder of excessive sympathetic nervous system activity. Some of this overactivity may reflect circulating catecholamine concentrations, while some is a manifestation of increased sympathetic nerve traffic in the cardiac nerves. As a consequence of myocardial dysfunction, the patient experiences diminished cardiac activity at a time when the cerebral circulation is at risk for vasospasm; as therapies for vasospasm involve attempts to raise arterial pressure and cardiac output, the patient is in a very precarious situation. Although β-adrenergic blockade may prevent or diminish these problems if instituted very early (27), adequately powered clinical trials are yet to be performed to determine whether, when, and how vigorously these agents should be used. Presently, we are only able to manage the manifestations of these problems.

Electrocardiographic abnormalities and elevated plasma concentrations of markers of myocardial damage are ubiquitous after SAH. They appear to be manifestations of the same problems underlying contractility disorders, but because they occasionally cause diagnostic confusion with coronary artery disease, they are discussed separately.

Myocardial Contraction Band Necrosis

Contraction band necrosis of the myocardium occurs in a number of settings that appear to share elevations of sympathetic tone as an underlying mechanism (28) (Fig. 4). It is likely the genesis of some of the electrocardiographic abnormalities as well as the leakage of muscle proteins into the circulation. The degree of

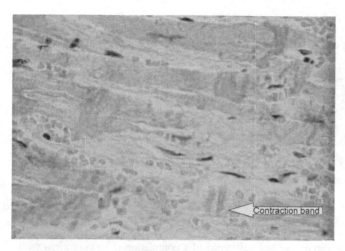

Figure 4 Light micrograph demonstrating myocardial contraction band necrosis. *Source*: From Ref. 28.

troponin elevation is probably a marker of the severity of SAH and, while correlated with functional outcome, is probably not an independent predictor of it (29).

No specific management for contraction band necrosis has been defined. If it is sufficiently extensive to produce symptomatic left ventricular failure, then the clinician is often in the difficult situation of needing to increase mean arterial pressure to treat vasospasm while wanting to decrease left ventricular overload. In such a situation, intra-aortic balloon pump counterpulsation may be the only therapeutic avenue. Similarly, the combination of cardiogenic and neurogenic pulmonary edema may occur, but here, the therapies are congruent.

Neurogenic Stunned Myocardium (Neurogenic Stress Cardiomyopathy)

Although the term neurogenic stunned myocardium has become more common in recent literature on SAH, it probably represents the macroscopic consequence of contraction band necrosis. It differs from tako-tsubo cardiomyopathy in that the depression of ventricular function is global rather than apical. The term *neurogenic stress cardiomyopathy* has been proposed as a more descriptive and inclusive alternative (30). Echocardiography reveals a poorly contracting myocardium, which can recover completely over time. More focal abnormalities of wall motion have also been reported (31), but in this circumstance, coincidental coronary disease with myocardial ischemia or infarction must be considered.

Inotropic therapy for patients with neurogenic stunned myocardium has been attempted with catecholamines and phosphodiesterase inhibition. It has been suggested that dobutamine may be a better choice in patients with impaired

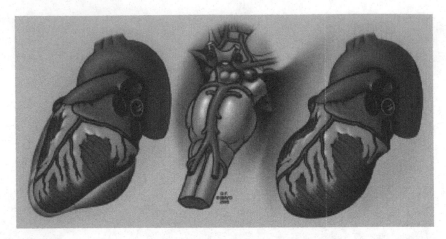

Figure 5 Artist's representation of normal ventricular contraction (*left*) contrasted with that seen in tako-tsubo cardiomyopathy. *Source*: From Ref. 29.

cardiac output (32). When these patients develop vasospasm, norepinephrine is probably preferable to phenylephrine because of the additional β agonism of the former. Often, a combination of norepinephrine and dobutamine may be required.

Tako-Tsubo Cardiomyopathy

Tako-tsubo cardiomyopathy is a descriptive term that reflects the echocardiographic appearance of the heart in patients with a variety of acute disorders. The apex of the left ventricle fails to contract normally, while the basal portion functions more normally, producing a shape resembling that of a Japanese octopus trap (33) (Fig. 5).

Cardiac Repolarization Disturbances and Dysrhythmias that Complicate Subarachnoid Hemorrhage

Prolongation of the (QTc) is the most common electrocardiographic disturbance in acute SAH patients, occurring in greater than 90% of patients (34). This finding is usually not clinically significant and has rarely been associated with deterioration into the polymorphic ventricular tachycardia known as torsade des pointes (35). However, torsade may also develop without premonitory QTc prolongation (36). Magnesium administration, which may be useful for vasospasm prevention as well, is often advocated for the prevention of torsade in other patient groups with prolonged QTc and seems reasonable. If episodes of torsade develop, magnesium should be administered, along with cardioversion or overdrive pacing.

The classic, although less common, electrocardiographic manifestations of acute SAH are deep, symmetric, inverted T waves, which may be seen across the precordium, inferiorly, laterally, or diffusely; they are commonly called "cerebral T waves." Although they resemble the inverted T waves suggestive of myocardial ischemia, their symmetric nature is unusual in ischemia, and they do not predict the discovery of coronary artery disease. They appear to be another manifestation of sympathetic overactivity and may be markers for contraction band necrosis. Less commonly, they are seen in other cerebrovascular diseases such as intracerebral hemorrhage without SAH or large ischemic strokes.

As patients with SAH are often hypertensive cigarette smokers, it is not surprising to realize that many of them also have coronary artery disease. The electrocardiogram should also be scrutinized to look for other dysrhythmias as well as evidence of ischemia or infarction.

CONCLUSION AND FUTURE DIRECTIONS

Cardiopulmonary dysfunction is commonly encountered in patients with SAH. The spectrum of these disorders is fairly broad and entails timely recognition, monitoring, and institution of appropriate therapy. Many of the pathophysiological mechanisms of these disorders are being unraveled that will bring forth appropriate management strategies and decrease mortality and morbidity in this subset of patients.

REFERENCES

1. Vespa PM, Bleck TP. Neurogenic pulmonary edema and other mechanisms of impaired oxygenation after aneurysmal subarachnoid hemorrhage. Neurocrit Care 2004; 1:157–170.
2. Claassen J, Vu A, Kreiter KT, et al. Effect of acute physiologic derangements on outcome after subarachnoid hemorrhage. Crit Care Med 2004; 32:832–838.
3. Citerio G, Gaini SM, Tomei G, et al. Management of 350 aneurysmal subarachnoid hemorrhages in 22 Italian neurosurgical centers. Intensive Care Med 2007; 33: 1580–1586.
4. Solenski NJ, Haley EC Jr, Kassell NF, et al. Medical complications of aneurysmal subarachnoid hemorrhage: a report of the multicenter, cooperative aneurysm study. Participants of the Multicenter Cooperative Aneurysm Study. Crit Care Med 1995; 23:1007–1017.
5. Touho H, Karasawa J, Shishido H, et al. Neurogenic pulmonary edema in the acute stage of hemorrhagic cerebrovascular disease. Neurosurgery 1989; 25:762–768.
6. Rassler B. The role of catecholamines in formation and resolution of pulmonary oedema. Cardiovasc Hematol Disord Drug Targets 2007; 7:27–35.
7. Smith WS, Matthay MA. Evidence for a hydrostatic mechanism in human neurogenic pulmonary edema. Chest 1997; 111:1326–1333.
8. Hoff JT, Nishimura M, Garcia-Uria J, et al. Experimental neurogenic pulmonary edema. Part 1: The role of systemic hypertension. J Neurosurg 1981; 54:627–631.

9. Garcia-Uria J, Hoff JT, Miranda S, et al. Experimental neurogenic pulmonary edema. Part 2: The role of cardiopulmonary pressure change. J Neurosurg 1981; 54:632–636.

10. Aharinejad S, Bock P, Lametschwandtner A, et al. Scanning and transmission electron microscopy of venous sphincters in the rat lung. Anat Rec 1992; 233:555–568.

11. Schraufnagel DE, Patel KR. Sphincters in pulmonary veins. An anatomic study in rats. Am Rev Respir Dis 1990; 141:721–726.

12. Grauer SE, Peterson BT, Kuenzig M, et al. Effect of lung denervation on development of pulmonary edema. Surgery 1981; 89:617–621.

13. Feng GG, Nishiwaki K, Kondo H, et al. Inhibition of fibrin-induced neurogenic pulmonary edema by previous unilateral left-vagotomy correlates with increased levels of brain nitric oxide synthase in the nucleus tractus solitarii of rats. Auton Neurosci 2002; 102:1–7.

14. Germonpre PR, Joos GF, Pauwels RA. Characterization of the neurogenic plasma extravasation in the airways. Arch Int Pharmacodyn Ther 1995; 329:185–203.

15. Hamdy O, Nishiwaki K, Yajima M, et al. Presence and quantification of neuropeptide Y in pulmonary edema fluids in rats. Exp Lung Res 2000; 26:137–147.

16. Hamdy O, Maekawa H, Shimada Y, et al. Role of central nervous system nitric oxide in the development of neurogenic pulmonary edema in rats. Crit Care Med 2001; 29:1222–1228.

17. Walsh DA, F McWilliams D. Tachykinins and the cardiovascular system. Curr Drug Targets 2006; 7:1031–1042.

18. Baumann A, Audibert G, McDonnell J, et al. Neurogenic pulmonary edema. Acta Anaesthesiol Scand 2007; 51:447–455.

19. Fiser SM, Kron IL, Long SM, et al. Donor lung salvage after neurogenic pulmonary edema with the use of post-transplant extracorporeal membrane oxygenation. J Thorac Cardiovasc Surg 2001; 122:1257–1258.

20. Fremont RD, Kallet RH, Matthay MA, et al. Postobstructive pulmonary edema: a case for hydrostatic mechanisms. Chest 2007; 131:1742–1746.

21. Patel AR, Bersten AD. Pulmonary haemorrhage associated with negative-pressure pulmonary oedema: a case report. Crit Care Resusc 2006; 8:115–116.

22. Chuang YC, Wang CH, Lin YS. Negative pressure pulmonary edema: report of three cases and review of the literature. Eur Arch Otorhinolaryngol 2007; 264:1113–1116.

23. Friedman JA, Pichelmann MA, Piepgras DG, et al. Pulmonary complications of aneurysmal subarachnoid hemorrhage. Neurosurgery 2003; 52:1025–1031.

24. Kane-Gill SL, Olsen KM, Rebuck JA, et al. Multicenter treatment and outcome evaluation of aspiration syndromes in critically ill patients. Ann Pharmacother 2007; 41:549–555.

25. Pieracci FM, Barie PS. Strategies in the prevention and management of ventilator-associated pneumonia. Am Surg 2007; 73:419–432.

26. Leone M, Garcin F, Bouvenot J. Ventilator-associated pneumonia: Breaking the vicious circle of antibiotic overuse. Crit Care Med 2007; 35:379–385.

27. Hamann G, Haass A, Schimrigk K. Beta-blockade in acute aneurysmal subarachnoid haemorrhage. Acta Neurochir (Wien) 1993; 121:119–122.

28. Samuels MA. The brain-heart connection. Circulation 2007 3; 116:77–84.

29. Pereira AR, Sanchez-Pena P, Biondi A, et al. Predictors of 1-year outcome after coiling for poor-grade subarachnoid aneurysmal hemorrhage. Neurocrit Care 2007; 7:18–26.

30. Lee VH, Oh JK, Mulvagh SL, et al. Mechanisms in neurogenic stress cardiomyopathy after aneurysmal subarachnoid hemorrhage. Neurocrit Care 2006; 5:243–249.
31. Khush K, Kopelnik A, Tung P, et al. Age and aneurysm position predict patterns of left ventricular dysfunction after subarachnoid hemorrhage. J Am Soc Echocardiogr 2005; 18:168–74.
32. Naidech A, Du Y, Kreiter KT, et al. Dobutamine versus milrinone after subarachnoid hemorrhage. Neurosurgery 2005; 56:21–27.
33. Lee VH, Connolly HM, Fulgham JR, et al. Tako-tsubo cardiomyopathy in aneurysmal subarachnoid hemorrhage: an underappreciated ventricular dysfunction. J Neurosurg 2006; 105:264–270.
34. Provencio JJ, Bleck TP. Cardiovascular Disorders Related to Neurologic and Neurosurgical Emergencies. In: Cruz J, ed. Neurologic and Neurosurgical Emergencies. Philadelphia: WB Saunders, 1998:39–50
35. Takenaka I, Aoyama K, Iwagaki T, et al. Development of torsade de pointes caused by exacerbation of QT prolongation during clipping of cerebral artery aneurysm in a patient with subarachnoid haemorrhage. Br J Anaesth 2006; 97:533–535.
36. Machado C, Baga JJ, Kawasaki R, et al. Torsade de pointes as a complication of subarachnoid hemorrhage: a critical reappraisal. J Electrocardiol 1997; 30:31–37.

20

Neuroradiologic Interventional Procedures for Cerebral Vasospasm

Pascal M. Jabbour, MD, Chief Resident[a]
Erol Veznedaroglu, MD, FACS, Associate Professor[a] and Director[b]
Robert H. Rosenwasser, MD, FACS, FAHA,
Professor and Chairman[a] and Professor[c]

[a]Department of Neurological Surgery, [b]Division of Neurovascular Surgery
and Endovascular Neurosurgery [c]Radiology, Neurovascular Surgery,
and Interventional Neuroradiology, Thomas Jefferson University,
Jefferson Hospital for Neuroscience, Philadelphia, Pennsylvania, U.S.A.

INTRODUCTION

Vasospasm affects 60% to 70% of patients after aneurysmal subarachnoid hemorrhage (aSAH), resulting in symptomatic ischemia in approximately half of these. Vasospasm reaches maximal severity in the second week after aSAH, typically resolving spontaneously in the third or fourth week. Vasospasm causes death or serious disability from infarction in up to one-third of patients with aSAH. Delayed neurologic deterioration after aSAH is presumed because of ischemic sequelae of vasospasm, unless proven otherwise and attributed to other causes. Although the pathogenesis is not clearly known, the risk of vasospasm is related to the amount of subarachnoid blood (1–3). The cause of cerebral vasospasm appears to be multifactorial, involving oxyhemoglobin, thromboxane, serotonin, and calcium (4). Calcium activates calmodulin, which activates the myosin light-chain kinase and interacts with actin filaments to cause vascular contractions (5). Vessel tone is a balance between both endothelium-derived constricting factors and endothelium-derived relaxation factors. Nitric oxide (NO) is the most prominent endothelium-derived relaxation factor. Studies have demonstrated that the vasospasm following aSAH is predominately a result of dysfunctional vasodilator

349

(e.g., NO) mechanisms (6,7). Histologic analysis has shown morphologic changes of the spastic vessel wall, with necrosis and fibrosis of the intima and media.

Numerous advances in neurosurgical critical care, such as rheologic manipulation of cerebral blood flow and the administration of calcium channel blockers, have reduced the ischemic and neurologic deficits associated with this devastating complication. Although the treatment protocol of intravascular volume expansion, hemodilution, induced hypertension, and cardiac performance enhancement [HHH therapy (8–11)] and the use of nimodipine (12) have had a substantial beneficial effect on the treatment of this condition, these therapies are not tolerated or are ineffective in some patients, who are subsequently susceptible to stroke, congestive heart failure, and death. Additional and alternative treatments for refractory vasospasm, particularly those that specifically target the dilation of cerebral vessels, are needed.

Vasospasm may be monitored noninvasively by insonating the circle of Willis vessels and its branches using transcranial-Doppler (TCD) techniques. This noninvasive bedside procedure has a high sensitivity and specificity for vasospasm but requires technical expertise and experience (13). The course of TCD-documented vasospasm correlates closely with the course and clinical sequelae of vasospasm detected on angiography, and its severity closely reflects clinical sequelae of brain ischemia. Angiography may be used to confirm vasospasm in clinical situations in which the cause of delayed neurologic deterioration is questionable, when TCD findings are nonconcordant with clinical progress, or when endovascular therapy for vasospasm is being contemplated.

ENDOVASCULAR OPTIONS

Cases of worsening vasospasm despite HHH therapy are considered for endovascular treatment (14–18). The precise threshold for endovascular interventions remains controversial, with some centers advocating early and frequent endovascular treatment of spasm and others reserving endovascular intervention solely for cases in which symptomatic vasospasm does not respond to HHH therapy. It is clear that not all cases of severe TCD spasm will require endovascular intervention, and such therapy introduces an added risk that must be considered and weighed. Conversely, endovascular treatment of spasm should not be delayed until actual infarction has developed.

Balloon Angioplasty

The first reported use of angioplasty for the treatment of vasospasm was published in 1984 (19), opening up a new modality of treatment for patients who were medically refractory to reversal of their ischemic neurologic syndrome (14,20,21). Despite successful improvement in the narrowing of the cerebral vessels with restored normal circulation time (as demonstrated angiographically), many cases of equivocal clinical improvement have been reported (14,16,22–24). It is possible that delayed treatment of patients may result in "end-organ failure," despite restoration of blood flow, which is analogous to the thrombolysis theme and to ischemic neural tissue after a thrombotic or embolic event.

Endovascular treatment of spasm has traditionally consisted of balloon angioplasty, mostly for large vessel spasm, and/or intra-arterial pharmacologic infusions for more distal branch vasospasm. Angioplasty is associated with greater risk of arterial rupture or dissection, especially if applied to more distal vessels, but its effect is more durable than intra-arterial pharmacologic infusions (25–28). For patients with delayed aSAH who have severe vasospasm proximal to the aneurysm site, a combined endovascular treatment with angioplasty and endovascular aneurysm coiling is safer than surgical clipping (29,30).

The clinical success rate of transluminal balloon angioplasty (TBA) is variable (18,23,24,31,32). The angiographic improvement with TBA seems to vary between 80% and 100% in most series. Clinical improvement ranges from 30% to 80%. Early treatment seems to be associated with better results. Randomized clinical studies that assess the effect of TBA on outcome are few, and little is known of the long-term effects of TBA. The effect of angioplasty in the setting of cerebral vasospasm has been found to be lasting. Furthermore, the angioplastied vessels normalize in luminal diameter over time on the basis of follow-up angiography. Risks, including vessel perforation, unprotected aneurysm rerupture, branch occlusion, hemorrhagic infarction, and arterial dissection, are associated with this procedure. Vessel rupture is reported in 4% of patients, usually with catastrophic outcome, and rebleeding from unclipped aneurysms is found in roughly 5% of patients (21,23,24,33).

Timing of the Angioplasty

In a study of the importance of the timing of the angioplasty, between July 1993 and December 1997, a total of 466 patients were admitted to Thomas Jefferson University Hospital-Wills Neurosensory Institute with the diagnosis of "acute" aSAH. In the intensive care unit, all patients were treated prophylactically with HHH when, as shown by TCD imaging, their velocities were consistent with vasospasm, elevated, or showed a trend toward elevation with increasing ratios (25,34,35). If the patients developed a new focal deficit or a change in their mental status, a CT scan was performed to eliminate a diagnosis of hydrocephalus or subsequent bleeding (Fig. 1). HHH therapy would then be maximized to the point of elevating the mean arterial pressure to 130–140 mmHg. If the patients did not demonstrate neurologic reversal within 60 minutes, they were transferred to the endovascular suite for angiography and possible angioplasty. All patients who required angioplasty received a ventriculostomy, if one was not already in place.

Of the entire group of 466 patients, 93 (22%) underwent endovascular management of medically refractory cerebral vasospasm, with 84 available for a minimum of six months of follow-up. The breakdown of these 84 patients by grade was as follows: Grade I, 2 of 33 patients (6%); Grade II, 9 of 84 patients (10%); Grade III, 57 of 260 patients (22%); and Grade IV, 16 of 42 patients (38%).

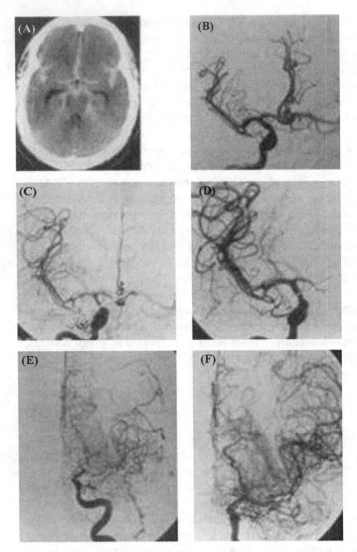

Figure 1   (**A**) Noncontrast CT scan, showing diffuse subarachnoid hemorrhage, Fisher's Grade 3, with early hydrocephalus, as evidenced by enlarged temporal horns. (**B**) Right internal carotid angiogram, demonstrating no spasm and a small anterior communicating artery aneurysm. (**C**) Right internal carotid angiogram, one week postoperatively, demonstrating severe spasm of the right internal carotid system. (**D**) Angiogram, posttreatment. (**E**) Left internal carotid angiogram, demonstrating severe spasm of the supraclinoid carotid and middle cerebral artery, pretreatment. (**F**) Left internal carotid angiogram, posttreatment.

Fifty-one patients (61%) underwent endovascular management within a two-hour window because of the inability to reverse the patients' neurologic deficits with medical measures. In this group, 90% of patients demonstrated improvement angiographically, and 70% sustained clinical improvement. Thirty-three patients (39%) failed to improve with the best medical therapy available; they were treated in more than a two-hour window (range, 2 hr, 15 min–17 hr) and had 88% angiographic improvement, but only 40% sustained clinical improvement. Clinical improvement was noted as early as 60 minutes after the procedure, when gross motor movement could be evaluated. However, global improvement (as assessed by Glasgow Coma Scale) continued for up to 48 hours.

Technique

The protocol for TBA involves angiography with placement of an 8F femoral sheath. Full heparinization is performed to achieve an activated clotting time of twice baseline to prevent thromboembolic complications. TBA is conducted on patients under general anesthesia and with neurophysiologic monitoring. Endovascular management is performed using an Endeavor silicone balloon with thumb pressure inflations for periods of one to five seconds or a stealth system (Target Therapeutics/Boston Scientific, Boston, Massachusetts). Vessels amenable to angioplasty include all of the intracranial proximal vessels (e.g., internal carotid artery, proximal branches of the middle cerebral or anterior cerebral artery). For more distal vasospasm, intra-arterial pharmacologic (vasodilator) infusion should be considered because trying to perform an angioplasty on more distal vessels carries a higher risk of rupturing the vessel.

Intra-Arterial Infusion

A variety of calcium channel antagonists and other vasodilators have been studied via intrathecal and intra-arterial delivery. Intrathecal nitroprusside has been proven safe, but efficacy is still controversial (36–38). The use of intra-arterial calcium channel blockers, such as nicardipine, verapamil, and nimodipine, has been shown to significantly reduce TCD velocities, to provide clinical improvement in up to 72% of patients, and to increase vessel caliber by 44% (39–41). The application of nicardipine prolonged release implants in the basal cistern of Fisher Grade III aSAH patients has shown promising results (42). Future therapies for vasospasm will be aimed at improved delivery systems and developing biologic agents that target the numerous cellular substrates responsible for vasospasm. Many animal research studies are being conducted on intrathecal immunotherapy, which is also a vast field open to exploration (43–45).

CONCLUSION

Neurosurgical critical care has made dramatic improvements in the perioperative management of the patient suffering from aSAH. Calcium channel blockers and HHH therapy continue to be a cornerstone in the management of this problem and are effective in approximately 80% of patients. In patients who are refractory to medical therapy, timely application of angioplasty in the affected blood vessels may be of benefit in improving both the angiographic appearance and the ultimate outcome. Anecdotal experience indicates that a two-hour window may exist for the restoration of blood flow, which is analogous to a patient who presents with a vascular-related event from either an embolic or thrombotic occlusion. Although early reports of improved neurologic recovery resulting from the use of TBA in aSAH vasospasm are encouraging, prospective randomized controlled trials are necessary to determine the true efficacy of angioplasty in the treatment of vasospasm and whether it influences ultimate outcome.

REFERENCES

1. Fisher M, Cameron DG. Concerning cerebral vasospasm. Neurology 1953; 3(6): 468–473.
2. Friedman JA, Goerss SJ, Meyer FB, et al. Volumetric quantification of Fisher Grade 3 aneurysmal subarachnoid hemorrhage: a novel method to predict symptomatic vasospasm on admission computerized tomography scans. J Neurosurg 2002; 97(2): 401–407.
3. Suzuki H, Muramatsu M, Kojima T, et al. Intracranial heme metabolism and cerebral vasospasm after aneurysmal subarachnoid hemorrhage. Stroke 2003; 34(12): 2796–2800.
4. Sonobe M, Suzuki J. Vasospasmogenic substance produced following subarachnoid haemorrhage, and its fate. Acta Neurochir (Wien) 1978; 44(1–2):97–106.
5. Winder SJ, Allen BG, Clement-Chomienne O, et al. Regulation of smooth muscle actin-myosin interaction and force by calponin. Acta Physiol Scand Dec 1998; 164(4):415–426.
6. Sobey CG. Cerebrovascular dysfunction after subarachnoid haemorrhage: novel mechanisms and directions for therapy. Clin Exp Pharmacol Physiol 2001; 28(11): 926–929.
7. Inagawa T. Cerebral vasospasm in elderly patients treated by early operation for ruptured intracranial aneurysms. Acta Neurochir (Wien) 1992; 115(3–4):79–85.
8. Kosnik EJ, Hunt WE. Postoperative hypertension in the management of patients with intracranial arterial aneurysms. J Neurosurg 1976; 45(2):148–154.
9. Pritz MB, Giannotta SL, Kindt GW, et al. Treatment of patients with neurological deficits associated with cerebral vasospasm by intravascular volume expansion. Neurosurgery 1978; 3(3):364–368.
10. Kassell NF, Peerless SJ, Durward QJ, et al. Treatment of ischemic deficits from vasospasm with intravascular volume expansion and induced arterial hypertension. Neurosurgery 1982; 11(3):337–343.
11. Wood JH, Simeone FA, Fink EA, et al. Hypervolemic hemodilution in experimental focal cerebral ischemia. Elevation of cardiac output, regional cortical blood flow, and ICP after intravascular volume expansion with low molecular weight dextran. J Neurosurg 1983; 59(3):500–509.

12. Allen GS, Ahn HS, Preziosi TJ, et al. Cerebral arterial spasm—a controlled trial of nimodipine in patients with subarachnoid hemorrhage. N Engl J Med 17 1983; 308(11):619–624.

13. Kim P, Schini VB, Sundt TM, Jr., et al. Reduced production of cGMP underlies the loss of endothelium-dependent relaxations in the canine basilar artery after subarachnoid hemorrhage. Circ Res 1992; 70(2):248–256.

14. Eskridge JM, McAuliffe W, Song JK, et al. Balloon angioplasty for the treatment of vasospasm: results of first 50 cases. Neurosurgery 1998; 42(3):510–516 (discussion 516–517).

15. Eskridge JM, Newell DW, Pendleton GA. Transluminal angioplasty for treatment of vasospasm. Neurosurg Clin N Am 1990; 1(2):387–399.

16. Higashida RT, Halbach VV, Cahan LD, et al. Transluminal angioplasty for treatment of intracranial arterial vasospasm. J Neurosurg 1989; 71(5 Pt 1):648–653.

17. Rosenwasser RH. Endovascular tools for the neurosurgeon. Clin Neurosurg 2002; 49:115–135.

18. Rosenwasser RH, Armonda RA, Thomas JE, et al. Therapeutic modalities for the management of cerebral vasospasm: timing of endovascular options. Neurosurgery 1999; 44(5):975–979 (discussion 979–980).

19. Zubkov YN, Nikiforov BM, Shustin VA. Balloon catheter technique for dilatation of constricted cerebral arteries after aneurysmal ASAH. Acta Neurochir (Wien) 1984; 70(1–2):65–79.

20. Eskridge JM. Interventional neuroradiology. Radiology 1989; 172(3 Pt 2):991–1006.

21. Eskridge JM, Song JK. A practical approach to the treatment of vasospasm. AJNR Am J Neuroradiol 1997; 18(9):1653–1660.

22. Yamamoto Y, Smith RR, Bernanke DH. Mechanism of action of balloon angioplasty in cerebral vasospasm. Neurosurgery 1992; 30(1):1–5 (discussion 5–6).

23. Polin RS, Coenen VA, Hansen CA, et al. Efficacy of transluminal angioplasty for the management of symptomatic cerebral vasospasm following aneurysmal subarachnoid hemorrhage. J Neurosurg 2000; 92(2):284–290.

24. Bejjani GK, Bank WO, Olan WJ, et al. The efficacy and safety of angioplasty for cerebral vasospasm after subarachnoid hemorrhage. Neurosurgery 1998; 42(5):979–986 (discussion 986–977).

25. Newell DW, Eskridge JM, Mayberg MR, et al. Angioplasty for the treatment of symptomatic vasospasm following subarachnoid hemorrhage. J Neurosurg 1989; 71(5 pt 1):654–660.

26. Linskey ME, Horton JA, Rao GR, et al. Fatal rupture of the intracranial carotid artery during transluminal angioplasty for vasospasm induced by subarachnoid hemorrhage. Case report. J Neurosurg 1991; 74(6):985–990.

27. Kassell NF, Helm G, Simmons N, et al. Treatment of cerebral vasospasm with intra-arterial papaverine. J Neurosurg 1992; 77(6):848–852.

28. Elliott JP, Newell DW, Lam DJ, et al. Comparison of balloon angioplasty and papaverine infusion for the treatment of vasospasm following aneurysmal subarachnoid hemorrhage. J Neurosurg 1998; 88(2):277–284.

29. Murayama Y, Song JK, Uda K, et al. Combined endovascular treatment for both intracranial aneurysm and symptomatic vasospasm. AJNR Am J Neuroradiol 2003; 24(1):133–139.

30. Brisman JL, Roonprapunt C, Song JK, et al. Intentional partial coil occlusion followed by delayed clip application to wide-necked middle cerebral artery aneurysms in

patients presenting with severe vasospasm. Report of two cases. J Neurosurg 2004; 101(1):154–158.

31. Higashida RT, Halbach VV, Dowd CF, et al. Intravascular balloon dilatation therapy for intracranial arterial vasospasm: patient selection, technique, and clinical results. Neurosurg Rev 1992; 15(2):89–95.

32. Newell DW, Eskridge JM, Aaslid R. Current indications and results of cerebral angioplasty. Acta Neurochir Suppl 2001; 77:181–183.

33. Eskridge JM, Newell DW, Winn HR. Endovascular treatment of vasospasm. Neurosurg Clin N Am 1994; 5(3):437–447.

34. Grosset DG, Straiton J, du Trevou M, et al. Prediction of symptomatic vasospasm after subarachnoid hemorrhage by rapidly increasing transcranial Doppler velocity and cerebral blood flow changes. Stroke 1992; 23(5):674–679.

35. Newell DW, Winn HR. Transcranial Doppler in cerebral vasospasm. Neurosurg Clin N Am 1990; 1(2):319–328.

36. Rosenwasser RH. Re: Safety of intraventricular sodium nitroprusside and thiosulfate for the treatment of cerebral vasospasm in the intensive care unit setting. Stroke 2002; 33(4):1165–1166 (author reply 1165–1166).

37. Thomas JE, Rosenwasser RH. Reversal of severe cerebral vasospasm in three patients after aneurysmal subarachnoid hemorrhage: Initial observations regarding the use of intraventricular sodium nitroprusside in humans. Neurosurgery 1999; 44(1):48–57 (discussion 57–48).

38. Thomas JE, Rosenwasser RH, Armonda RA, et al. Safety of intrathecal sodium nitroprusside for the treatment and prevention of refractory cerebral vasospasm and ischemia in humans. Stroke 1999; 30(7):1409–1416.

39. Badjatia N, Topcuoglu MA, Pryor JC, et al. Preliminary experience with intra-arterial nicardipine as a treatment for cerebral vasospasm. AJNR Am J Neuroradiol 2004; 25(5):819–826.

40. Biondi A, Ricciardi GK, Puybasset L, et al. Intra-arterial nimodipine for the treatment of symptomatic cerebral vasospasm after aneurysmal subarachnoid hemorrhage: preliminary results. AJNR Am J Neuroradiol 2004; 25(6):1067–1076.

41. Feng L, Fitzsimmons BF, Young WL, et al. Intra-arterially administered verapamil as adjunct therapy for cerebral vasospasm: Safety and 2-year experience. AJNR Am J Neuroradiol 2002; 23(8):1284–1290.

42. Kasuya H, Onda H, Sasahara A, et al. Application of nicardipine prolonged-release implants: analysis of 97 consecutive patients with acute subarachnoid hemorrhage. Neurosurgery 2005; 56(5):895–902 (discussion 895–902).

43. Cirak B, Kiymaz N, Ari HH, et al. The effects of endothelin antagonist BQ-610 on cerebral vascular wall following experimental subarachnoid hemorrhage and cerebral vasospasm. Clin Auton Res 2004; 14(3):197–201.

44. Frazier JL, Pradilla G, Wang PP, et al. Inhibition of cerebral vasospasm by intra-cranial delivery of ibuprofen from a controlled-release polymer in a rabbit model of subarachnoid hemorrhage. J Neurosurg 2004; 101(1):93–98.

45. Pradilla G, Wang PP, Legnani FG, et al. Prevention of vasospasm by anti-CD11/CD18 monoclonal antibody therapy following subarachnoid hemorrhage in rabbits. J Neurosurg 2004; 101(1):88–92.

21

Intraoperative Management of Spinal Cord Injury

Dawn Dillman, MD, Assistant Professor
Ansgar Brambrink, MD, PhD, Professor
Department of Anesthesiology & Peri-Operative Medicine,
Oregon Health & Science University, Portland, Oregon, U.S.A.

Spinal cord injury (SCI) has an incidence in the United States of approximately 2 cases per 100,000 in both children and adults. The most common mechanisms of injury for both groups are motor vehicle collision, falls, violence, and sports in descending order—notably, all traumatic (1,2). Regions where motor vehicle collisions are more commonly associated with alcohol use and low rates of seatbelt use have higher rates of injury (3). Given the current U.S. population, this translates to approximately 11,000 new cases of SCI each year. Some of the controversies currently surrounding intraoperative management of acute SCI will be discussed in this chapter, and suggestions for practice based on evidence will be provided when possible.

PATHOPHYSIOLOGY

The spinal cord extends from the foramen magnum to approximately the second lumbar vertebra (L2) in adults. Its blood supply is through the anterior spinal artery and two posterior spinal arteries, which are fed by paired radicular arteries at each level of the spine. One large radicular artery at the level of the diaphragm (the artery of Adamkiewicz) may be responsible for much of the blood flow to the lower two-thirds of the cord. Similar to the brain, the spinal cord has a blood-spinal cord barrier. Also similar to the brain, under normal circumstances, spinal cord blood flow (SCBF) is autoregulated to prevent changes in blood flow in the setting of changes in blood pressure. Similar to traumatic brain injury, SCI results in a disruption of both the blood-spinal cord barrier and autoregulation of SCBF (4,5).

Injuries to the spinal cord can occur through several mechanisms. Direct force applied to one area of the spine in a rapid manner that causes hyper-extension and translocation of one vertebral body over another can lead to cord compression, such as with the face hitting the windshield during a motor vehicle collision. Rotational force applied to the spine can result in contusion or tearing injury to the cord, such as may occur in ejection from a motor vehicle collision. Direct axial loading may cause a burst disruption of the vertebrae, which may lead to a compression injury of the cord. Less common are distraction injuries, such as with hanging. Penetrating trauma, such as with gunshots or stabbing, may cause direct partial or complete disruption to the cord as well. The relative flexibility of the cervical spine makes it a susceptible location for injury, so that, the majority of acute SCIs are in the cervical spine (2). The stabilizing force of the thoracic cage make mid-thoracic spine injuries less common, and their presence should prompt the practitioner into looking for additional injuries that may be related to a high-force impact. Complete disruptions or transsections, in which all sensation and function below an injured level are lost, have poor prognosis. However, incomplete lesions with some preserved function may indicate continuity of the underlying cord. Spinal shock, a transient sensorimotor deficit, may present this way and has a much better prognosis. Spinal shock may or may not be accompanied by neurogenic shock, a cardiovascular phenomenon characterized by hypotension and bradycardia secondary to loss of sympathetic tone.

In all cases, the SCI will go though several phases. The primary anatomic injury to the cord will be a result of the physical mechanism of injury. However, several mechanisms of secondary injury can threaten the cord over the next hours to days. One that is intuitively easy to understand—and relatively correctable—is ischemia related to decreased SCBF. It may be related to systemic hypotension, but hypoxemia and anemia may also contribute to an ischemic state in the acute SCI setting. Venodilation may increase the blood volume in the cord, increase the cord pressure, and contribute to ischemia as well (by decreasing perfusion pressure, the difference between arterial and venous or spinal cord pressure). Preservation of SCBF may become particularly problematic in the setting of multisystem trauma, in which hemorrhage coupled with neurogenic shock can rapidly lead to a reduction in perfusion to the cord and a worsening of the cord injury. Secondary injury may also be related to the initiation of an inflammatory cascade that results in the release of inflammatory mediators, including but not limited to, tumor necrosis factor-α, IL-1β, and inducible nitric oxide synthase. This inflammation can result in the disruption of normal regulation of SCBF and in an increased permeability of the blood-spinal cord barrier that leads to edema formation in the cord (6). Several therapeutic agents have been investigated toward interfering with these mechanisms of secondary injury and improving long-term outcome, with the most commonly used example being high-dose steroids (e.g., methylprednisolone) (7–9). Finally, the inflammatory responses associated with ischemia may lead to tertiary injury from apoptosis, which may manifest even up to weeks later. Death of interneurons may lead to retrograde and anterograde neuronal degeneration over weeks to months. Interestingly, high-dose steroid administration may also help to prevent these mechanisms of tertiary injury (10,11).

PREOPERATIVE EVALUATION

Understanding the mechanism and extent of injury is critical prior to undertaking surgical correction. As alluded to earlier, a high potential exists for associated injuries with the SCI acquired in a traumatic setting. For example, the hypovolemia that could develop from occult abdominal bleeding secondary to liver laceration may be difficult to diagnose intraoperatively but may have a profound effect on the spinal cord perfusion and secondary injury. Timing of surgery has been an area of controversy. A recent review suggested an improvement in outcomes with early (<8 hours) decompression compared to delayed or nonoperative treatment, particularly for those with incomplete injury, and it is a safe treatment option (12). However, decompressive surgery is only emergent in the setting of bilateral locked facets with incomplete quadriplegia or in the setting of neurologic deterioration (13). Therefore, most patients have time to have a complete evaluation and preparation for surgery.

History and physical examination should be performed to evaluate both the extent of SCI and coexisting medical diseases. Complete sensory and motor neurologic examination should be documented preoperatively. Particular attention should also be paid to the cardiovascular system, especially in the high thoracic or cervical cord injury. The spinal cord sends sympathetic afferents to the heart from T1–T4, to the vascular bed from T1–L2, and to the adrenal medulla from T3–L3. Therefore, it is common for the patient with a cervical or high thoracic cord injury to experience bradycardia and hypotension, manifesting as neurogenic shock. The more severe the injury, the more likely the autonomic system will be involved.

Pulmonary involvement may manifest (*i*) as respiratory compromise in patients with any thoracic spine injury because of dysfunction of intercostal muscles or (*ii*) as respiratory failure in an injury above C5, which affects the phrenic nerves and thereby the diaphragmatic respiration. Acute pulmonary edema may also occur and impair respiration from overaggressive hydration in the setting of neurogenic shock. Coexisting injuries, such as aspiration, pneumothorax, or pulmonary contusion, may all occur in the setting of trauma as well.

Laboratory analysis should at least include a complete blood count to evaluate for anemia, as anemia has been correlated with the presence and severity of acute SCI (14). Electrolyte and clotting analysis, as well as blood typing and cross matching, may also be beneficial, particularly for multilevel or large procedures in which significant blood loss may be expected. An electrocardiogram is indicated for baseline evaluation. Benign elevation of the ST segments consistent with early repolarization is common, particularly in injuries above T5, most likely secondary to high vagal tone (15). Cardiac contusions in the setting of trauma may also be suggested by electrocardiogram. Patients with multisystem injury should have a chest X ray and may benefit from spiral CT scanning to evaluate for associated traumatic injuries, such as pneumothorax, pulmonary contusion, or splenic or liver lacerations.

OPERATIVE MANAGEMENT

Premedication

The choice of appropriate premedication will be dependent on the preoperative state and comorbidities of the patient. If the patient with an isolated SCI is completely alert and oriented and expresses anxiety about the impeding procedure, judicious anxiolysis with midazolam may be indicated. In the setting of multi-system trauma or decreased levels of consciousness related to intoxication or traumatic brain injury, benzodiazepines may best be avoided to prevent both respiratory depression and confusing the neurologic examination postoperatively. Premedication with gastric antacids (sodium citrate), histamine blockers (ranitidine), and promotility agents (metoclopramide) may be indicated, as gastric motility will be impaired with cervical and high thoracic cord lesions (16).

Communication about preoperative antibiotics and neuroprotectants should occur between the surgical and anesthesia teams. Preoperative antibiotics should be administered less than an hour prior to skin incision. High-dose steroid (methylprednisolone) therapy should be continued if started. If not yet started, the preoperative period can be considered a time to reconsider whether steroids or other potentially neuroprotective agents should be initiated. However, sub-stantial controversy surrounds the use of high-dose steroids in the setting of SCI. Methylprednisolone given for acute SCI has been demonstrated to lead to significant neurologic improvement up to one year after injury if given within eight hours after injury (9,17). On the other hand, positive studies have been significantly criticized, and concerns have been raised regarding the increased risk for infectious complications or myopathy (18). A survey of spine surgeons revealed that, although 90% use a steroid protocol for acute SCI, only 24% believe that it will improve outcomes (19).

Premedication with a vagolytic, either atropine or glycopyrrolate, should be considered for patients with high thoracic or cervical injury. Lesions above the level of T4 will cause a loss of sympathetic innervation to the heart, and the remaining autonomic input will be parasympathetic. Thus, this stimulus that would result in vagal stimulation, such as placement of an endotracheal tube, may result in profound bradycardia or asystole (20). The incidence of life-threatening bradycardia with vagal stimulation is greatest during the first two weeks after injury (21). If a patient has been experiencing bradycardic episodes preoperatively, preparation for transvenous pacing should be considered, as transcutaneous pacing can be unreliable (22).

Airway Management

Considerable controversy certainly surrounds the optimal methods of securing the airway in the setting of SCI (23). Many patients with SCI who present for surgical procedures will have already been intubated as part of their prehospital or emergency department care. However, when faced with the necessity of achieving intubation, the primary concerns relate to the emergency of intubation, maintaining stability of unstable cervical spine segments, and operator skill.

First and foremost, airway patency and respiratory drive are necessary to maintain oxygenation, and their compromise may lead to cardiac arrest and/or brain death. Secondarily, the development of hypoxemia can contribute to furthering the secondary injury of the at-risk spinal cord. Therefore, if it appears that the patient is in danger of becoming hypoxic, either from respiratory distress from the SCI or from other injuries sustained concurrently, the airway should be controlled as soon as possible. If airway management is not otherwise anticipated to be difficult (e.g., no micrognathia, no retropharyngeal or neck hematomas, normal mouth opening), the most expeditious means of securing the airway is preferred. Rapid-sequence induction followed by direct laryngoscopy is one option available. Manual in-line immobilization (MILI) has been found to be effective at limiting the motion indicative of instability in a model of complete ligamentous injury during orotracheal intubation with direct laryngoscopy and superior to traction because of the potential for distraction injury with traction (24). MILI in the setting of severe ligamentous injury and direct laryngoscopy is also superior to collar immobilization, as there is less cervical displacement and improved laryngeal view (25). Several retrospective case series have documented success with the direct laryngoscopic technique after induction in the setting of cervical spine injury, without progression of SCI attributed to intubation (23,26–32). It is also worth noting that cricoid pressure was utilized as part of the rapid-sequence induction for these series without evidence of complication.

In contrast, the patient who presents to the operating room with an isolated SCI for nonemergent surgery may benefit from an awake intubation, with the goal being to exclude intubation as a potential source of injury by allowing examination of neurologic status before and after intubation and allowing examination after positioning for surgery. In a survey of anesthesiologists given the situation of intubating a patient with an unstable cervical spine injury, 78% reported that they would perform an awake intubation (33). Awake intubation may be accomplished using several approaches (blind nasal, nasal, or oral fiberoptic being the most common). If awake intubation is chosen, local anesthetics should be used to improve patient tolerance, as coughing or gagging can result in movement of an unstable spine. Topicalization can be accomplished via many routes: nebulizer, atomizer, direct application via applicators or through the bronchoscope, or injection for nerve block. Sedation and systemic analgesics should be given judiciously, as they may contribute to hypoxemia. Awake intubation is not without risk. Laryngospasm with loss of airway has been reported in patients with unstable cervical spine fractures who undergo awake fiberoptic intubation (FOI) (34). One controlled study on awake FOI (not on SCI patients) reported an 8% failure rate, with 11% of patients desaturating to less than 90% during the attempt (35).

If induction is chosen, FOI may still be a useful option, as less neck movement is associated with nasal FOI, compared to direct laryngoscopy, esophageal combitube, intubating laryngeal mask airway, and conventional laryngeal mask airway placement, even with MILI (36). Of note, mask ventilation produces a significant amount of neck motion in and of itself in the setting of cervical spine injury (36,37). Operator skill is probably the most under-considered factor. A survey of 1000 anesthesiologists demonstrated that only 59% reported they had skill with FOI, while 78% felt skilled at blind intubation (38). Certainly, the argument is convincing for using a technique that the practitioner feels comfortable accomplishing quickly and safely. At this time, no series of cases in the setting of unstable cervical spine injury have been published that demonstrate a convincing benefit of choosing an awake intubation over induction and tracheal intubation using MILI.

Induction

The goal of the provider should be to maintain oxygen delivery and SCBF, which can be a challenge in the setting of acute SCI. In a study of the response of SCI patients to induction and intubation (39), it was found that catecholamine levels and heart rate were lower in acute quadriplegic patients than in control patients (no SCI) at baseline, after induction, and postintubation. In contrast, acute paraplegic patients had higher baseline norepinephrine levels compared with controls and comparable increases in heart rate and systolic arterial pressure to controls. Furthermore, the norepinephrine and systolic arterial pressure increases seen in response to intubation in both the controls and acute paraplegics were abolished in acute quadriplegics. Hypotension (systemic arterial pressure < 70% of baseline, or < 90 mmHg) occurred in 35% of acute quadriplegics, whereas hypertension (systemic arterial pressure > 130% of baseline, or > 160 mmHg) occurred in 83% of acute paraplegics. Therefore, induction agents should be cautiously dosed in patients with acute cervical SCI.

The optimal neuromuscular blocker to use with induction, if any, is not clear. Extrajunctional nicotinic receptors begin to proliferate within hours of denervation injury. However, in a study that examined denervations of a single limb, hyperkalemia in response to succinylcholine did not occur until four days after injury (40). No reports of fatal hyperkalemia in response to succinylcholine have been reported in exposures prior to four days after an acquired injury. Therefore, if neuromuscular blockers are to be used, succinylcholine may likely be used safely up to 72 hours post-SCI (41). Rocuronium is an alternative to succinylcholine for rapid sequence induction without potential for development of hyperkalemia; however, the intubating conditions may be inferior (42). Avoidance of neuromuscular blockers should be considered another advantage of awake intubation. Induction and intubation may also be performed without any neuromuscular blockers. The practitioner should be cognizant of the potential for hypotension with large doses of induction agents that may be necessary when intubating without muscle relaxants.

Monitoring

Hemodynamic Monitoring and Management

As maintaining perfusion is critical in the acute SCI patient, a low threshold for invasive monitoring should be considered. For the cervical SCI patient at risk for neurogenic shock, an arterial line placed prior to sedation or induction can help to identify the onset of hypotension more quickly and definitively intraoperatively and may be used to guide management in the postoperative period as well. Central venous pressure monitoring may be helpful in guiding fluid replacement therapy, as well as providing access for administration of vasopressors. Some authors have advocated goal-directed therapy (mean arterial pressure > 85 90 mmHg) guided by pulmonary artery catheters to target whether fluids or vasopressors are needed, and they suggest that outcomes may be improved by this technique (43,44). The main benefit of this technique is the avoidance of overvolume resuscitation and potential prevention of pulmonary edema, while providing maximal cord perfusion. In addition, a pulmonary artery catheter can help to distinguish between (*i*) the need for a vasopressor such as phenylephrine or norepinephrine to increase systemic vascular resistance secondary to lack of sympathetic tone, and (*ii*) the need for an inotrope such as dopamine or dobutamine from the lack of sympathetic tone to the heart. However, numerous large studies on critically ill patients (not in the setting of SCI) have failed to demonstrate any benefit of pulmonary artery catheterization on outcomes, and they have demonstrated potentially more complications (45–47). Therefore, routine pulmonary artery catheterization should be considered controversial and cannot be recommended as a standard at this time. In the setting of a lower thoracic or lumbar injury, with which less sympatholysis is seen, central venous access may still be useful for guiding fluid therapy if an extensive procedure is to be performed that has the potential for significant blood loss.

Hemodynamic goal targeting is one area in which intraoperative management of acute SCI is dramatically different from other types of spinal surgery. Controlled hypotension using antihypertensive agents has for decades been a successful technique for limiting blood loss during elective spine surgery. However, in the setting of SCI and a loss of autoregulation of SCBF, as well as potential ischemia, controlled hypotension is not recommended as a standard practice. As discussed above, mean arterial pressures should be targeted to at least normal levels, based on preoperative blood pressure monitoring, in order to ensure perfusion to the cord.

As of writing this chapter, little data exist regarding fluid management in the setting of SCI, and the best strategy for replacement remains unknown. Transfusion in the perioperative period is currently an area of controversy, as it has the inherent risks of infection and transfusion reaction, as well as immunomodulatory effects, the significance of which is still unclear. Although severe anemia (hemoglobin of <6 g/dL) has been shown not to change evoked potential transmission in healthy volunteers (48), the patient with SCI and inflammation may be different. This level of anemia has been shown to increase the level of cerebral cortical nitric oxide synthase, presumably as an attempt to vasodilate and increase cerebral blood flow (49). If the injured spinal cord is unable to autoregulate SCBF, it may have lost this compensatory mechanism of maintaining oxygen delivery. Although no data support any specific recommendation, rheologic properties maximize oxygen delivery at a hemoglobin level of approximately 10 g/dL, and transfusion may be indicated to maintain this level.

In animal studies, hypertonic saline administered after SCI reduces spinal cord vascular resistance and preserves evoked potentials, compared to isotonic saline (50,51). Although the use of hypertonic saline for SCI has not been studied in humans, it may be an attractive choice for maintaining intravascular volume in contrast to isotonic crystalloids. This is particularly true for the patient at risk for pulmonary edema from overvigorous hydration in the setting of neurogenic shock. One concern regarding use of hypertonic saline is the potential for development of a hyperchloremic metabolic acidosis (52). Although it appears that the acidosis is transient, the hypertonic saline may be prepared and delivered as a 50% sodium chloride and 50% sodium acetate mix to reduce the total chloride load and prevent development of hyperchloremic metabolic acidosis.

Neurologic Monitoring and Maintenance

Neuromonitoring of spinal cord integrity intraoperatively may be useful, particularly for those patients with incomplete injury who would be at risk for injury progression. Monitoring may include somatosensory-evoked potentials (SSEPs) and/or motor-evoked potentials (MEPs). As the sensory tracts are carried in the posterior cord and motor tracts are carried in the anterior cord, both are often monitored to assess cord integrity. As transcortical MEPs are very sensitive to many of the commonly used anesthetics, consideration of neuromonitoring must be anticipated when formulating an anesthetic plan.

Neuromuscular-blocking agents are incompatible with monitoring MEPs. If neuromuscular blockers are used during induction on a patient who will have MEP monitoring, they should not be redosed. If SSEPs alone are monitored, neuromuscular blockers may be helpful to reduce movement artifact and background noise in the signal.

The ideal maintenance agent for neuromonitoring is an area of continued discussion. Potent inhalational agents (isoflurane, sevoflurane, desflurane) all depress amplitude and increase latency of SSEPs and MEPs in a dose-dependent fashion (53–55). Levels of more than 1 minimum alveolar concentration (MAC) are likely to significantly impair the detection of MEPs. Although nitrous oxide (N_2O) seems to have little effect on latency (56), it also depresses amplitude of SSEPs and MEPs and does so more effectively than isoflurane at equipotent doses (57,58). Because of the potential interference with evoked-potential monitoring, it may seem reasonable to try to minimize the amount of inhaled agents used and utilize IV anesthetics instead. However, IV agents may also affect SSEPs and MEPs. Propofol, in particular, increases latency and reduces amplitude in a dose-dependent manner (59,60). Ketamine, etomidate, benzo-diazepines, and opiates have less effect on evoked potentials (60). Even with these effects, an anesthetic with either one-half MAC desflurane and two-thirds MAC N_2O or a propofol anesthetic is consistent with monitoring MEPs for scoliosis surgery (61). If MEPs are consistently obtainable at the beginning of surgery, it is not likely to matter which technique is used—inhalational or intravenous—but the goal should be to minimize the usage of any particular anesthetic agent. However, if MEPs are marginal at the start, the anesthetic technique should be converted to intravenous, with consideration of using etomidate and/or ketamine to minimize the influence on neuromonitoring.

Degradation of MEP or SSEP signals may be because of several causes, and not all are correlated with new neurologic deficits. Gradual decreases in amplitude and increases in latency may be from cumulative effects of anesthesia (62) or from the development of facial or scalp edema that reduces conductivity of electrodes. This condition can usually be compensated for by changes in monitoring parameters. However, in the presence of acute changes in amplitude and latency, cord injury must be assumed to be the cause. Table 1 outlines steps that may be taken if this situation is encountered.

Table 1 Interventions for the Acute Change in Somatosensory-evoked Potentials/ Motor-evoked Potentials

1. Ensure that surgical, anesthesia and neuromonitoring teams are all aware of the change.
2. Pursue reversible anatomic causes, such as a surgical intervention, which may have placed tension on the cord.
3. Adjust the positioning to relieve any pressure on the brachial plexus or ulnar nerve if the change is limited to an upper extremity.
4. Adjust the FiO_2 to 1.0.
5. Deliver vasopressors as needed to ensure that the mean arterial pressure is > 90–100 mmHg to improve cord perfusion.
6. Transfuse packed red blood cells if the hemoglobin is < 10 g/dL.

Positioning

Several risks may be attributed to positioning. First, positioning may exacerbate injury to the cord by movement of the unstable spine. If an awake intubation is performed, positioning may take place with the patient's assistance to avoid movements that may induce cord injury. This ensures that no additional damage to the cord occurs with positioning. Alternatively, baseline SSEPs and MEPs may be taken after induction and prior to positioning to confirm that no change in signals has occurred with positioning.

Second, prone positioning has the potential to cause neuropraxia secondary to pressure on point of the brachial plexus. The chest supports should be low enough on the pectoral region to avoid direct pressure on the infraclavicular or axillary fossa, which will also prevent the chest roll from being high enough to put pressure on the neck and reduce venous outflow from the head. The shoulders should be at less than 90°, and forearms should be positioned slightly lower than the chest to avoid tension on the brachial plexus. SSEPs can help to diagnose impeding brachial plexus injury from prone positioning, and if changes in amplitude of the SSEPs are noted, repositioning often corrects the conduction deficit (63).

Third, prone positioning during spinal surgery have been associated with perioperative vision loss (64). The American Society of Anesthesiologists issued a practice advisory in 2006; their recommendations are summarized in Table 2 (65). Positioning of the face should be done carefully, as pressure directly on the eye can reduce blood flow and places the eye at risk for central retinal artery occlusion. However, hypotension and anemia may place the eye at risk for ischemic optic neuropathy, regardless of pressure on the eye. Risk is likely greater with coexisting vascular disease, predisposing to lower flows (66).

Table 2 Recommendations from the ASA Practice Advisory on Perioperative Vision Loss in Spine Surgery

---

1. Prolonged procedures and high blood loss procedures should be considered risk factors, with the combination of the two being considered high risk.
2. Provide informed consent to patients about the small but real risk of perioperative vision loss.
3. Colloids should be used to reduce the formation of facial edema in high blood loss surgeries.
4. No specific transfusion threshold is supported by current data for preventing vision loss.
5. Attention should be given to positioning, including keeping the head at or above the level of the heart to reduce venous pressure in the eyes and maintaining neutral neck and head position.

Source: From Ref. 65.

Temperature

Hypothermia has long been used as a prophylactic measure to reduce ischemic neuroinjury in cardiac and vascular surgery, but little evidence supports the use of hypothermia in patients following SCI. A recent review identified 15 publications that investigated the potential role of hypothermia in traumatic SCI (67). All studies reviewed were based on experimental injury models, as no human studies have been done on the effects of either systemic or local hypothermia in SCI. Neurologic injury may be partially mitigated by hypothermia in experimental models of mild-to-moderate SCI; however, hypothermia has no benefit for severe SCI. As always, caution should be applied when trying to transfer evidence from experimental studies directly to the clinical setting. It is also noteworthy that hypothermia will reduce amplitude, increase latency of SSEPs, and, therefore, potentially mask a significant injury (68). In addition, intraoperative hypothermia is known to contribute to the development of surgical-site infection (69). Currently, hypothermia cannot be recommended as a standard practice intraoperatively. However, hyperthermia has the potential to increase metabolic demand and impair neurologic injury following ischemia, and as it has no known intraoperative benefits, it should be avoided rigorously.

POSTOPERATIVE CONSIDERATIONS

Postoperative extubation may be considered for those patients who come to the operating room extubated. However, several issues must be considered. First, a cervical SCI that was below the level of C3–C5 preoperatively may have edema formation and cranial progression of the injury significant enough to cause respiratory compromise postoperatively. Second, cervical surgery may be accompanied by soft tissue swelling so that even if a posterior approach is used, anterior tracking of edema can cause some element of tracheal or upper airway compromise. Third, prolonged prone positioning can lead to facial and upper airway swelling even in thoracic or lumbar surgeries. Fourth, if the patient had any element of difficult airway management preoperatively, this is only likely to be enhanced postoperatively. In addition, fusion or fixation of the occiput-C1 and/or C1–C2 is likely to make reintubation extremely difficult. A cuff-leak test may be performed to evaluate the extent of upper airway edema; however, if there is significant concern, the conservative approach is to leave the patient's trachea intubated postoperatively and allow for controlled extubation in the intensive care unit. Extubation of the presumed difficult airway should be performed only with all necessary equipment for reintubation prepared. A useful technique is to extubate over an airway-exchange catheter, leaving the catheter in place. If reintubation is then required, it can be accomplished over the catheter.

Postoperative pain in the setting of SCI may be multifactorial, as the pain will have both nociceptive and neuropathic components. Opiates are a mainstay of treatment for nociceptive pain. Treatments aimed at neuropathic pain, such as gabapentin or pregabalin, may be effective in treating a component of pain in the setting of SCI (70). Early consultation of an acute pain service may be beneficial.

CONCLUSION

The intraoperative management of patients with acute SCI aims to prevent secondary injury to the injured spinal cord. Maintenance of adequate perfusion, sufficient oxygen-carrying capacity, and normoxia are of paramount importance for preventing spinal ischemia. Neurogenic shock and the reduction in sympathetic tone are particularly concerning in the perioperative period, as they can contribute to or cause significant morbidity. Prospective controlled research in the perioperative setting is sparse, and more is necessary to delineate the optimal hemodynamic goals, fluid management choices, and anesthetic and intraoperative neuroprotective strategies. Until more scientific evidence is available, empiric physiology and knowledge from experimental research may be carefully translated to guide intraoperative decisions.

REFERENCES

1. Vitale MG, Goss JM, Matsumoto H, et al. Epidemiology of pediatric spinal cord injury in the United States: years 1997 and 2000. J Pediatr Orthop 2006; 26(6):745–749.
2. Jackson AB, Dijkers M, Devivo MJ, et al. A demographic profile of new traumatic spinal cord injuries: Change and stability over 30 years. Arch Phys Med Rehabil 2004; 85(11):1740–1748.
3. Burke DA, Linden RD, Zhang YP, et al. Incidence rates and populations at risk for spinal cord injury: a regional study. Spinal Cord 2001; 39(5):274–278.
4. Popovich PG, Horner PJ, Mullin BB, et al. A quantitative spatial analysis of the blood-spinal cord barrier. I. Permeability changes after experimental spinal contusion injury. Exp Neurol 1996; 142(2):258–275.
5. Guha A, Tator CH, Rochon J. Spinal cord blood flow and systemic blood pressure after experimental spinal cord injury in rats. Stroke 1989; 20(3):372–377.
6. Pannu R, Christie DK, Barbosa E, et al. Post-trauma Lipitor treatment prevents endothelial dysfunction, facilitates neuroprotection, and promotes locomotor recovery following spinal cord injury. J Neurochem 2007; 101(1):182–200.
7. Bracken MB, Collins WF, Freeman DF, et al. Efficacy of methlprednisolone in acute spinal cord injury. JAMA 1984; 251(1):45–52.
8. Bracken MB, Shepard MJ, Collins WF, et al. A randomized, controlled trial of methylprednisolone or naloxone in the treatment of acute spinal-cord injury. Results of the Second National Acute Spinal Cord Injury Study. N Engl J Med 1990; 322(20): 1405–1411.
9. Bracken MB, Shepard MJ, Holford TR, et al. Administration of methylprednisolone for 24 or 48 hours or tirilazad mesylate for 48 hours in the treatment of acute spinal cord injury. Results of the Third National Acute Spinal Cord Injury Randomized Controlled Trial. National Acute Spinal Cord Injury Study. JAMA 1997; 277(20):1597–1604.
10. Oudega M, Vargas CG, Weber AB, et al. Long-term effects of methylprednisolone following transection of adult rat spinal cord. Eur J Neurosci 1999; 11(7), 2453–2464.

11. Vaquero J, Zurita M, Oya S, et al. Early administration of methylprednisolone decreases apoptotic cell death after spinal cord injury. Histol Histopathol 2006; 21(10): 1091–1102.

12. La Rosa G, Conti A, Cardali S, et al. Does early decompression improve neurological outcome of spinal cord injured patients? Appraisal of the literature using a meta-analytical approach. Spinal Cord 2004; 42(9):503–512.

13. Fehlings MG, Perrin RG. The timing of surgical intervention in the treatment of spinal cord injury: a systematic review of recent clinical evidence. Spine 2006; 31(11 suppl):S28–S35.

14. Furlan JC, Krassioukov AV, Fehlings MG. Hematologic abnormalities within the first week after acute isolated traumatic cervical spinal cord injury: a case-control cohort study. Spine 2006; 31(23):2674–2683.

15. Marcus RR, Kalisetti D, Raxwal V, et al. Early repolarization in patients with spinal cord injury: prevalence and clinical significance. J Spinal Cord Med 2002; 25(1):33–38.

16. Segal JL, Milne N, Brunnemann SR, et al. Metoclopramide-induced normalization of impaired gastric emptying in spinal cord injury. Am J Gastroenterol 1987; 82(11): 1143–1148.

17. Bracken MB. Steroids for acute spinal cord injury. Cochrane Database Syst Rev 2002; (3):CD001046.

18. Sayer FT, Kronvall E, Nilsson OG. Methylprednisolone treatment in acute spinal cord injury: the myth challenged through a structured analysis of published literature. Spine J 2006; 6(3):335–343.

19. Eck JC, Nachtigall D, Humphreys SC, et al. Questionnaire survey of spine surgeons on the use of methylprednisolone for acute spinal cord injury. Spine 2006 Apr 20; 31(9): E250–E253.

20. Frankel HL, Mathias CJ, Spalding JM. Mechanisms of reflex cardiac arrest in tetraplegic patients. Lancet 1975; 2(7946):1183–1185.

21. Lehmann KG, Lane JG, Piepmeier JM, et al. Cardiovascular abnormalities accompanying acute spinal cord injury in humans: incidence, time course and severity. J Am Coll Cardiol 1987; 10(1):46–52.

22. Ruiz-Arango AF, Robinson VJ, Sharma GK. Characteristics of patients with cervical spinal injury requiring permanent pacemaker implantation. Cardiol Rev 2006; 14(4): E8–E11.

23. Lord SA, Boswell WC, Williams JS. Airway control in trauma patients with cervical spine fractures. Prehospital Disaster Med 1994; 9(1):44–49.

24. Lennarson, PJ, Smith DW, Sawin PD, et al. Cervical spinal motion during intubation: efficacy of stabilization maneuvers in the setting of complete segmental instability. J Neurosurg 2001; 94(2 suppl):265–270.

25. Gerling MC, Davis DP, Hamilton RS, et al. Effects of cervical spine immobilization technique and laryngoscope blade selection on an unstable cervical spine in a cadaver model of intubation. Ann Emerg Med 2000; 36(4):293–300.

26. Holley J, Jordan R. Airway management in patients with unstable cervical spine fractures. Ann Emerg Med 1989; 18(11):1237–1239.

27. Shatney CH, Brunner RD, Nguyen TQ. The safety of orotracheal intubation in patients with unstable cervical spine fracture or high spinal cord injury. Am J Surg 1995; 170(6):676–679.

28. Patterson H. Emergency department intubation of trauma patients with undiagnosed cervical spine injury. Emerg Med J 2004; 21(3):302–305.

29. Criswell JC, Parr MJ, Nolan JP. Emergency airway management in patients with cervical spine injuries. Anaesthesia 1994; 49(10):900–903.
30. Suderman VS, Crosby ET, Lui A. Elective oral tracheal intubation in cervical spine-injured adults. Can J Anaesth 1991; 38(6):785–789.
31. McCrory C, Blunnie WP, Moriarty DC. Elective tracheal intubation in cervical spine injuries. Ir Med J 1997; 90(6):234–235.
32. Scannell G, Waxman K, Tominaga G, et al. Orotracheal intubation in trauma patients with cervical fractures. Arch Surg 1993; 128(8):903–905.
33. Rosenblatt WH, Wagner PJ, Ovassapian A, et al. Practice patterns in managing the difficult airway by anesthesiologists in the United States. Anesth Analg 1998: 87: 153–157.
34. McGuire G, el-Beheiry H. Complete upper airway obstruction during awake fibreoptic intubation in patients with unstable cervical spine fractures. Can J Anaesth 1999; 46(2):176–178.
35. Langeron O, Semjen F, Bourgain JL, et al. Comparison of the intubating laryngeal mask airway with the fiberoptic intubation in anticipated difficult airway management. Anesthesiology 2001; 94(6):968–972.
36. Brimbacombe J, Keller C, Kunzel KH, et al. Cervical spine motion during airway management: a cinefluoroscopic study of the posteriorly destabilized third cervical vertebrae in human cadavers. Anesth Analg 2000; 91(5):1274–8.
37. Hauswald M, Sklar DP, Tandberg D, et al. Cervical spine movement during airway management: cinefluoroscopic appraisal in human cadavers. Am J Emerg Med 1991; 9(6):535–538.
38. Ezri T, Szmuk P, Warters RD, et al. Difficult airway management practice patterns among anesthesiologists practicing in the United States: have we made any progress? J Clin Anesth 2003; 15(6):418–422
39. Yoo KY, Jeong SW, Kim SJ, et al. Cardiovascular responses to endotracheal intubation in patients with acute and chronic spinal cord injuries. Anesth Analg 2003; 97:1162–1167.
40. John DA, Tobey RE, Homer LD, et al. Onset of succinylcholine-induced hyperkalemia following denervation. Anesthesiology 1976; 45:294–299.
41. Martyn JA, Richtsfeld M. Succinylcholine-induced hyperkalemia in acquired pathologic states: etiologic factors and molecular mechanisms. Anesthesiology 2006; 104(1):158–169.
42. Perry J, Lee J, Wells G. Rocuronium versus succinylcholine for rapid sequence induction intubation. Cochrane Database Syst Rev 2003; (1):CD002788.
43. Vale FL, Burns J, Jackson AB, et al. Combined medical and surgical treatment after acute spinal cord injury: results of a prospective pilot study to assess the merits of aggressive medical resuscitation and blood pressure management. J Neurosurg 1997; 87(2):239–246.
44. Levi L, Wolf A, Belzberg H. Hemodynamic parameters in patients with acute cervical cord trauma: description, intervention, and prediction of outcome. Neurosurgery 1993; 33(6):1007–1016.
45. Richard C, Warszawski J, Anguel N, et al. Early use of the pulmonary artery catheter and outcomes in patients with shock and acute respiratory distress syndrome: a randomized controlled trial. JAMA 2003; 290(20):2713–2720.

46. Sandham JD, Hull RD, Brant RF, et al. A randomized, controlled trial of the use of pulmonary-artery catheters in high-risk surgical patients. N Engl J Med 2003; 348(1): 5–14.

47. Wheeler AP, Bernard GR, Thompson BT, et al. Pulmonary-artery versus central venous catheter to guide treatment of acute lung injury. National Heart, Lung, and Blood Institute Acute Respiratory Distress Syndrome (ARDS) Clinical Trials Network. N Engl J Med 2006; 354(21):2213–2224.

48. Weiskopf RB, Aminoff MJ, Hopf HW, et al. Acute isovolemic anemia does not impair peripheral or central nerve conduction. Anesthesiology 2003; 99(3):546–551.

49. Hare GM, Mazer CD, Mak W, et al. Hemodilutional anemia is associated with increased cerebral neuronal nitric oxide synthase gene expression. J Appl Physiol 2003; 94:2058–2067.

50. Young WF, Rosenwasser RH, Vasthare US, et al. Preservation of post-compression spinal cord function by infusion of hypertonic saline. J Neurosurg Anesthesiol 1994; 6(2):122–127.

51. Spera PA, Vasthare US, Tuma RF, et al. The effects of hypertonic saline on spinal cord blood flow following compression injury. Acta Neurochir (Wien) 2000; 142(7): 811–817.

52. Moon PF, Kramer GC. Hypertonic saline-dextran resuscitation from hemorrhagic shock induces transient mixed acidosis. Crit Care Med 1995; 23(2):323–331.

53. Freye E, Bruckner J, Latasch L. No difference in electroencephalographic power spectra or sensory-evoked potentials in patients anaesthetized with desflurane or sevoflurane. Eur J Anaesthesiol 2004; 21(5):373–378.

54. Sekimoto K, Nishikawa K, Ishizeki J, et al. The effects of volatile anesthetics on intraoperative monitoring of myogenic motor evoked potentials to transcranial electrical stimulation and on partial neuromuscular blockade during propofol/fentanyl/nitrous oxide anesthesia in humans. J Neurosurg Anesthesiol 2006; 18(2): 106–111.

55. Haghighi SS, Sirintrapun SJ, Keller BP, et al. Effect of desflurane anesthesia on transcortical motor evoked potentials. J Neurosurg Anesthesiol 1996; 8(1):47–51.

56. Kunisawa T, Nagata O, Nomura M, et al. A comparison of the absolute amplitude of motor evoked potentials among groups of patients with various concentrations of nitrous oxide. J Anesth 2004; 18(3):181–184.

57. Thornton C, Creagh-Barry P, Jordan C, et al. Somatosensory and auditory evoked responses recorded simultaneously: differential effects of nitrous oxide and isoflurane. Br J Anaesth 1992; 68(5):508–514.

58. Lam AM, Sharar SR, Mayberg TS, et al. Isoflurane compared with nitrous oxide anaesthesia for intraoperative monitoring of somatosensory-evoked potentials. Can J Anaesth 1994; 41(4):295–300.

59. Nathan N, Tabaraud F, Lacroix F, et al. Influence of propofol concentrations on multipulse transcranial motor evoked potentials. Br J Anaesth 2003; 91(4):493–497.

60. Sihle-Wissel M, Scholz M, Cunitz G. Transcranial magnetic-evoked potentials under total intravenous anaesthesia and nitrous oxide. Br J Anaesth 2000; 85(3):465–467.

61. Lo YL, Dan YF, Tan YE, et al. Intraoperative motor-evoked potential monitoring in scoliosis surgery: comparison of desflurane/nitrous oxide with propofol total intravenous anesthetic regimens. J Neurosurg Anesthesiol 2006; 18(3):211–214.

62. Lyon R, Feiner J, Lieberman JA. Progressive suppression of motor evoked potentials during general anesthesia: the phenomenon of "anesthetic fade". J Neurosurg Anesthesiol 2005; 17(1):13–19.
63. Schwartz DM, Drummond DS, Hahn M, et al. Prevention of positional brachial plexopathy during surgical correction of scoliosis. J Spinal Disord 2000; 13(2):178–182.
64. Lee LA, Roth S, Posner KL, et al. The American Society of Anesthesiologists Postoperative Visual Loss Registry: analysis of 93 spine surgery cases with postoperative visual loss. Anesthesiology 2006; 105(4):652–659.
65. American Society of Anesthesiologists Task Force on Perioperative Blindness. Practice advisory for perioperative visual loss associated with spine surgery: a report by the American Society of Anesthesiologists Task Force on Perioperative Blindness. Anesthesiology 2006; 104(6):1319–1328.
66. Rupp-Montpetit K, Moody ML. Visual loss as a complication of non-ophthalmic surgery: A review of the literature. Insight 2005; 30(1):10–17.
67. Inamasu J, Nakamura Y, Ichikizaki K. Induced hypothermia in experimental traumatic spinal cord injury: an update. J Neurol Sci 2003; 209(1–2):55–60.
68. Jou IM. Effects of core body temperature on changes in spinal somatosensory-evoked potential in acute spinal cord compression injury: an experimental study in the rat. Spine 2000; 25(15):1878–1885.
69. Kurz A, Sessler DI, Lenhardt R. Perioperative normothermia to reduce the incidence of surgical-wound infection and shorten hospitalization. Study of Wound Infection and Temperature Group. N Engl J Med 1996; 334(19):1209–1215.
70. Levendoglu F, Ogun CO, Ozerbil O, et al. Gabapentin is a first line drug for the treatment of neuropathic pain in spinal cord injury. Spine 2004; 29(7):743–751.

22

Medical Management of Acute Spinal Cord Injury

Steven Casha, MD, PhD, FRCSC, Assistant Professor
R. John Hurlbert, MD, PhD, FRCSC, FACS, Associate Professor

*Department of Clinical Neurosciences, Division of Neurosurgery
and University of Calgary Spine Program, Foothills Hospital
and Medical Centre, Calgary, Alberta, Canada*

INTRODUCTION

The field of spinal cord injury (SCI) has benefited from significant attention in both the preclinical and clinical research arenas. The pathophysiology of this condition has been extensively studied, and strategies aimed at neuroprotection, neuroregeneration, and neuroaugmentation or rehabilitation have shown significant promise and efficacy in animal models. The largest challenge, perhaps, has been the translation of these results into human application. While several agents (discussed below) have been subject to rigorous testing in human trials, none have shown enough evidence to become standards of care. In the 2002 Guidelines for the Management of Acute Cervical Spine and Spinal Cord Injury (1) published by the American Association of Neurological Surgeons and Congress of Neurological Surgeons Joint Section on Disorders of the Spine and Peripheral Nerves, two agents were commented on specifically: methylprednisolone and GM-1 ganglioside. Both were recommended as options for treatment in patients with acute SCI "without demonstrated clinical benefit," in the case of GM-1 ganglioside and with the caveat that "the evidence suggesting harmful side effects is more consistent than any suggestion of clinical benefit" in the case of methylprednisolone. Two other agents, tirilazad and naloxone, were felt to have been studied less extensively and inadequately to warrant consideration in the guidelines.

Several possible reasons exist for the failure to translate promising animal strategies to human therapies. Some strategies are difficult to apply in the human without significant toxicity or morbidity and have not reached human studies because of the lack of an adequate pharmacologic agent. Animal models are generally very reproducible and consistent in the neurologic deficit produced and in the extent of recovery seen. However, human SCI is characterized by significant heterogeneity in mechanism of injury, level of injury, clinical syndrome, and extent of recovery. This added variability significantly hinders the ability to detect a beneficial effect of treatment. Furthermore, many models do not duplicate human pathology and, thus, likely human pathophysiology adequately. For instance, while mouse models have several advantages (including the relative ease of genetic manipulation), they lack the cavitation that is typically seen after human SCI (2). Mechanisms identified in such models may not be as significant in human SCI. Other models are desirable for studying specific strategies; however, they do not represent common mechanisms of human SCI. For example, transection models allow less ambiguous identification of regenerated axons, but spinal transection or even laceration is rarely seen in humans. Most strategies can be expected to achieve only a modest improvement in neurologic outcome, and almost certainly a multipronged therapeutic approach will be necessary in the future in order to have significant functional impact. This, together with the inherent variability in human SCI, necessitates large trials to achieve adequate power to detect an effect. Such multicentered trials are difficult and expensive to conduct. The outcome measures used in animals are different from those used in humans, and those applicable in humans may lack sensitivity in some patients (e.g., improvement of a few spinal segments in thoracic SCI will not be apparent in lower extremity motor recovery, often a key component of outcome instruments). Finally, the window of opportunity for application of an intervention almost certainly differs between human and other species. Adequate biomarkers to correlate the timing of pathologic events between species and to guide the selection of a comparable therapeutic window are generally lacking.

In spite of these and other such challenges, several pharmacologic agents have been evaluated in controlled human studies and will be reviewed in this chapter. All of the human randomized controlled trials of pharmacotherapy are summarized in Table 1, with other studies included in the discussion. The wealth of animal studies that have not reached clinical investigation are beyond the scope of this discussion. Likewise, treatment strategies aimed at neuroaugmentation and neuroregeneration in the chronic phase of SCI will not be discussed.

METHYLPREDNISOLONE AND OTHER CORTICOSTEROIDS

Steroids, in various forms, have been used in the treatment of SCI for many years; however, their role became more rigorously considered following publication of the National Acute Spinal Cord Injury Study (NASCIS) II. Initial

Table 1 Human Clinical Trials in Spinal Cord Injury

Author	Year	Design	Agent	Reported result
Methylprednisolone and other corticosteroids				
Bracken et al. (NASCIS I)	1984	Prospective, randomized, double-blinded	Methylprednisolone	Negative
Bracken et al. (NASCIS II)	1990 1992	Prospective, randomized, double-blinded	Methylprednisolone	Positive
Bracken et al. (NASCIS III)	1997 1998	Prospective, randomized, double-blinded	Methylprednisolone	Positive
Otani et al.	1994	Prospective, randomized, no blinding	Methylprednisolone	Positive
Pointillart et al.	2000	Prospective, randomized, blinded	Methylprednisolone	Negative
Kiwerski	1993	Retrospective, concurrent case controlled	Dexamethasone	Positive
Gangliosides				
Geisler et al.	1991	Prospective, randomized, double-blinded	GM-1 Gangliocyde	Positive
Geisler et al.	2001	Prospective, randomized, double-blinded	GM-1 Gangliocyde	Negative
Opiod antagonists				
Bracken et al. (NASCIS II)	1990 1992	Prospective, randomized, double-blinded	Naloxone	Negative
Flamm et al.	1985	Prospective feasibility/ safety study	Naloxone	N/A
Pitts et al.	1995	Prospective, randomized, double-blinded	Thyrotropin-releasing hormone	Positive
Excitatory amino acid antagonists				
Tadie et al.	1999	Prospective, randomized, double-blinded	Gacyclidine	Negative
Calcium channel blockers				
Pointillart et al.	2000	Prospective, randomized, double-blinded	Nimodipine	Negative
Antioxidants and free radical scavengers				
Bracken et al. (NASCIS III)	1997 1998	Prospective, randomized, double-blinded	Tirilazad	Positive

enthusiasm for an apparent positive effect of methylprednisolone in SCI has not stood up to the extensive scrutiny that ensued (3–6). In spite of significant criticism, this medication continues to be used by many, and a 2002 study suggested that most practitioners prescribe it because of peer pressure or fear of litigation rather than a firm belief that it is indeed efficacious (7).

The first NASCIS study which compared low- and high-dose methyl-prednisolone did not include a placebo group and failed to demonstrate a difference between the doses tested (8). It was followed by a randomized controlled trial that compared a 24-hour protocol to placebo in NASCIS II (9,10). The dose selected in NASCIS II was higher than that of the original study because of further animal work that suggested a therapeutic threshold of 30 mg/kg (10). NASCIS II concluded that improved neurologic recovery was seen when the methylprednisolone treatment protocol was initiated within 8 hours of injury. That study was followed by NASCIS III, which compared patients who were randomized to the 24-hour NASCIS II protocol to those randomized to a 48-hour protocol (11,12). That study concluded that patients in whom therapy is initiated within three hours do not gain any benefit from extending treatment to 48 hours, while those in whom therapy is initiated between three hours and eight hours do benefit further. No benefit had been shown in NASCIS II if therapy was initiated beyond eight hours.

Both the NASCIS II and NASCIS III trials were well designed and executed. However, closer scrutiny reveals that the primary analyses of methylprednisolone treatment effect were negative in both studies. The stated conclusions were based on post hoc analyses, which suggested minor treatment effects on motor scores at one year and when therapy was initiated in the eight- and three to eight-hour windows identified in NASCIS II and III, respectively. Statistical probability was slightly greater than 0.05 for one-year motor scores in the NASCIS III 48-hour steroid group. None of the sensory scores were different between treatment groups in either study. Several concerns have arisen regarding the post hoc analyses of NASCIS II and III. The left-sided motor scores were not published but were reported to be "similar" to right-sided scores. Thus, half of the available data was excluded. The statistical analyses failed to correct for multiple statistical comparisons, and it is unclear if the repeated measures design was considered. More than 65 methylprednisolone-related t-tests were performed in NASCIS II, and more than 100 were performed in NASCIS III representing a high likelihood of type I error (erroneously detecting a statistical difference that does not exist) through random chance. The rationale for an 8-hour subanalysis (NASCIS II) is unclear. It has been claimed that this subgroup was selected on the basis of median time to treatment. However, by definition, 50% of patients should have initiated treatment before the median time of treatment initiation. In fact, only 38% of patients (183 of 487) were included in this post hoc analysis. The justification for the three- and eight-hour windows in NASCIS III is similarly obscure. Finally, the outcomes lacked an assessment of function recovery meaningful to the patient's expected activities.

In addition to the NASCIS studies, a prospective randomized trial was published that investigated the NASCIS II methylprednisolone dosing protocol (13). The investigators were not blinded to treatment, and the control group was allowed to receive alternate steroids at the physicians' discretion. Of 158 patients entered, 117 were analyzed. The primary outcome measures [American Spinal

Injury Association (ASIA) motor and sensory scores] were not different between treatment groups. Post hoc analyses suggested that more patients improved on the NASCIS II steroid regimen compared to controls. However, for a greater number of steroid-treated patients to improve, the fewer control patients who also improved must have demonstrated a larger magnitude of recovery (as overall ASIA motor and sensory scores were no different between groups). Thus, such post hoc analyses become difficult to interpret in the face of a negative overall effect.

A retrospective study with concurrent case controls also suggested a benefit with corticosteroid administration (14). This study investigated the use of dexamethasone initiated within 24 hours of injury, with the specific dose left to the discretion of the attending physicians. Length of follow-up was not specified, and a new but unvalidated neurologic grading system was used for outcome assessment. This study reported that the percentage of patients improved was significantly higher in the methylprednisolone-treated group. However, a much higher mortality rate was found within the control group, suggesting a selection bias to more severely injured patients in the control arm. The magnitude of the mortality rate is also a concern and suggests that the study population may not be representative and that the results are not generalizable.

A randomized controlled trial designed to examine the potential therapeutic benefit of nimodipine (a calcium channel antagonist, discussed below) included an NASCIS II methylprednisolone regimen as well as a placebo group (15). This study, which included approximately 25 patients in each group, failed to show any difference between any of the four groups (placebo, nimodipine, and methylprednisolone plus nimodipine) using ASIA scores and ASIA grade outcomes. However, this study was remarkable for an increase in infectious complications in the methylprednisolone group.

In summary, while well-designed and well-executed studies have been performed, they have failed to convincingly demonstrate a beneficial effect of methylprednisolone or other corticosteroids in the management of SCI. Post hoc analyses have been used to argue a small effect on motor function in three randomized trials. However, all these analyses contain significant flaws, rendering conclusions of efficacy dubious. These observations have led two national organizations to publish guidelines that recommend methylprednisolone administration as a treatment option rather than as a standard of care or recommended treatment (1,16). It must also be recognized that corticosteroid administration comes with increased risk of several adverse events, including pneumonia, sepsis, and steroid-induced myopathy, all of which may negatively impact outcome in SCI patients, potentially overshadowing any unproven beneficial effect (17). In addition, the Corticosteroid Randomisation After Significant Head Injury (CRASH) trial, which investigated the use of a corticosteroid regimen similar to that used in NASCIS III in the setting of closed-head injury demonstrated increased mortality with steroid use in that population (18). The possibility of an elevated mortality risk in SCI patients must also be recognized.

GANGLIOSIDES

Gangliosides are sialic acid-containing glycosphingolipids that are found in high concentration in the outer cell membranes of central nervous system cells, especially in the vicinity of synapses. Although their exact function is unknown, they appear to play a role in neural development and plasticity. The proposed mechanisms of action of exogenously administered gangliosides include anti-excitotoxic activities, prevention of apoptosis, augmentation of neurite outgrowth, and induction of neuronal sprouting and regeneration (19–22).

GM-1 ganglioside has been the subject of two human studies. The first study was a randomized placebo-controlled trial of 37 patients (23). Patients were administered 100 mg of IV GM-1 ganglioside or placebo daily for 18 to 32 days, starting within 72 hours of injury. In addition, all patients received methylprednisolone for 72 hours. A significant difference was seen between groups, as analyzed using change in Frankel grades and mean ASIA motor score from baseline at one year. Furthermore, the improved recovery in the GM-1-treated group was attributed to recovery of useful strength in the initially paralyzed muscle groups, rather than to strengthening of paretic muscles. No adverse events attributable to the study drug were reported.

Based on the encouraging results of the first trial, a larger prospective, multicentered, double-blinded, randomized trial of GM-1 ganglioside in SCI patients was initiated (24). All the 797 patients enrolled received NASCIS II protocol methylprednisolone and were randomized to placebo, low-dose GM-1 (300 mg loading dose, then 100 mg/day for 56 days), and high-dose GM-1 (600 mg loading dose, then 200 mg/day for 56 days), starting at completion of the 23-hour methylprednisolone infusion. The primary outcome assessed was the proportion of patients who improved two or more grades from baseline using the modified Benzel score at 26 weeks. Secondary outcomes included timing of recovery, ASIA motor and sensory evaluations, relative and absolute sensory levels of impairment, and assessments of bladder and bowel function. The high-dose regimen was discontinued after 180 patients when an interim assessment revealed a trend toward increased mortality. At the end of the study, in 760 patients, the authors found no significant difference in mortality between the groups and no significant difference in the primary outcome. However, the authors also reported a large, consistent, and at some points, significant effect in the primary outcome in the subgroup of nonoperated patients. The ASIA motor, light touch, and pinprick scores showed a consistent trend in favor of GM-1, as did bladder function, bowel function sacral sensation, and anal contraction.

In summary, these studies provide suggestive but not conclusive evidence of a positive effect on neurologic recovery after SCI with administration of GM-1 ganglioside.

OPIATE ANTAGONISTS

Vasospasm, posttraumatic ischemia, and infarction are known contributors to the pathophysiology of SCI (25). In addition, human SCI may occur in the setting of polytrauma and spinal shock syndromes, which contribute to the ischemic pathophysiology. Opiate receptor antagonists and physiologic opiate antagonists improve blood pressure and survival following traumatic shock (26). In addition, endogenous opioid peptides are released in the spinal cord after SCI (27,28). Dynorphin decreases microcirculatory blood flow in the spinal cord and may contribute directly to neurotoxicity, possibly through the NMDA receptor (29–31). Opiate antagonists may thus be useful in maintaining circulation and in preventing some neurotoxicity. Of these, nalmefene, naloxone, and thyrotropin-releasing hormone (TRH) are neuroprotective in animal models (27,32–42). The latter two have been studied in humans.

Naloxone was administered as one of the treatment arms in NASCIS II (10) and was therefore compared to methylprednisolone and placebo treatment. Comparison of naloxone (5.4 mg/kg bolus, followed by a 23-hour, 4.0-mg/kg/hr infusion) and placebo failed to demonstrate a therapeutic benefit (9,10). Post hoc analysis suggested an effect on long tract recovery when naloxone was started within eight hours of injury, which may warrant further study (43).

In a dose escalation phase 1 study of naloxone in SCI, 20 patients received a 0.14- to 1.43-mg/kg loading dose, followed by 20% of loading, 47 hour infusion (low dose), and 9 patients received a 2.7- to 5.4-mg/kg loading dose, followed by 75% of loading, 23-hour infusion (high dose) (44). More patients in the low-dose group had complete injuries (85% vs. 44%) and initiated their treatment later (average 12.9 hours vs. 6.6 hours). No improvement in neurologic exam or somatosensory-evoked potentials was seen with the low-dose regimen, but in the high-dose group, a small number of patients demonstrated sustained improvement of both. The observed improvements were encouraging, but this study was not designed to examine efficacy. The authors were able to show that the high doses of naloxone that were required to achieve consistency with animal data in SCI were tolerated clinically with minimal side effects.

In one human study of TRH, 20 SCI patients were administered a 0.2-mg/kg bolus followed by a 0.2-mg/kg/hr, 6-hour infusion or placebo within 12 hours of injury (45). No discernible treatment effect was found in 6 patients with complete injuries, while in 11 incompletely injured patients, TRH treatment was associated with significantly higher motor, sensory recovery, and Sunnybrook cord injury scale scores at four months. While this is a small study and should be interpreted cautiously, it was nonetheless positive. Unfortunately, it has not as yet been replicated (17).

In summary, to date, three human studies have provided positive evidence that likely deserves further study. Definitive efficacy studies remain lacking, although one small randomized trial was positive.

EXCITATORY AMINO ACID RECEPTOR ANTAGONISTS

Receptor-mediated excitotoxicity of neurons and glia is a well-recognized secondary injury mechanism following neural injury (46–52). Inhibition of excitotoxicity in animal models of SCI results in improved behavioral and histologic outcomes (48,53,54). However, the rise in excitatory amino acids after SCI occurs early and is transient (likely complete within 2 hours), suggesting that the therapeutic window is small (46).

To date, one human SCI study has been performed using the NMDA (N-methyl-D-aspartate) ionotropic glutamate receptor antagonist gacyclidine (55). The 272 enrolled patients were randomized into four groups (0.005 mg/kg, 0.01 mg/kg, or 0.02 mg/kg gacyclidine or placebo). The doses selected were similar to those used in a safety and efficacy trial in patients with traumatic brain injury (56). Gacyclidine was administered twice, first within two hours of injury, followed by another administration four hours later. While the one-month data showed a nonsignificant trend to better outcome in the high-dose group, no significant differences in ASIA or FIM scores were observed at one year (17,55).

Thus, strong animal data suggest that inhibition of posttraumatic excitotoxicity is likely to be efficacious in the treatment of SCI; however, the therapeutic window may be very short. A single human study to date did not show efficacy.

CALCIUM CHANNEL BLOCKERS

Dysregulation of calcium homeostasis and cytoplasmic calcium-mediated events are common to many pathways leading to cell death (57). Calcium channel blockers may ameliorate calcium fluxes, decreasing cell death. They may also affect vascular smooth muscle and decrease vasospasm. In animal SCI models, calcium channel blockade is neuroprotective (58–61) and increases posttraumatic spinal blood flow (62,63). In a single, human, randomized placebo-controlled trial of the calcium-channel blocker nimodipine, 106 SCI patients were administered methylprednisolone (NASCIS II protocol), nimodipine (0.015 mg/kg/hr for 2 hours, followed by 0.03 mg/kg/hr for 7 days), both agents, or placebo (15,64). No difference in blinded neurologic recovery (ASIA score and grade) was found among these groups at one year.

Thus, cellular calcium fluxes are thought to be key regulators of cell death after neural trauma, and calcium channel inhibition in animal studies has proven neuroprotective. However, to date, a single study failed to reproduce this finding in humans.

ANTIOXIDANTS AND FREE RADICAL SCAVENGERS

Following neural trauma, free radical-mediated macromolecule peroxidation may lead to cell death (65). Several conditions following SCI promote increased formation of free radicals, and ample animal evidence suggests that this is a significant targetable secondary injury event after SCI (66–73).

Tirilazad mesylate is thought to act through inhibition of iron-dependent lipid peroxidation. The NASCIS III study included a 166-patient tirilazad group (2.5 mg/kg bolus infusion every six hours for 48 hours, administered after a 30-mg/kg methylprednisolone bolus) (74). This study showed no difference in motor recovery compared to 24-hour methylprednisolone treatment (11,12). Given the lack of convincing evidence regarding the role of methylprednisolone (as discussed above), this study does not provide evidence that tirilazad is effective in human SCI. In addition, while the predominant mechanism of action of methylprednisone is unclear, it is thought to include inhibition of peroxidation reactions (methylprednisolone is discussed in detail above).

In summary, the human data on methylprednisolone and tirilazad mesylate, which are believed to decrease peroxidation, do not support their use in the treatment of SCI.

CONCLUSION

A wealth of interest in the pathophysiology of SCI has identified many potential therapeutic targets in animal models. Of these, several have come to high-quality human investigations. Unfortunately, none have been proven effective in humans. Several challenges exist when translating successful strategies from animal models to human studies. However, several groups have now demonstrated an ability to coordinate and execute large trials that are well designed.

Currently, several human trials are ongoing that will add to an already interesting, although largely disappointing, human literature in SCI, which to date, has not established any clearly effective therapeutic options. These trials include investigations of minocycline (a tetracycline derivative that may affect several secondary injury mechanisms, including apoptotic cell death and inflammation), cethrin (75) (an Rho antagonist that is believed to promote axonal regeneration), anti-Nogo-A antiserum (17) (Nogo A is a myelin-associated inhibitor of central nervous system axonal regeneration), and autologous activated macrophages (76) (thought to act through elaboration of growth factors and modulation of the inflammatory response). In addition, interest is significant in stem cell, Schwann cell, and olfactory unsheathing glia transplantation therapies, all of which are involved in ongoing human investigations (17).

REFERENCES

1. Hadley MN, Walters BC, Grabb PA, et al. Guidelines for the management of acute cervical spine and spinal cord injuries: pharmacological therapy after acute cervical spinal cord injury. Neurosurgery 2002; 50(suppl 3):S63–S72.
2. Joshi M, Fehlings MG. Development and characterization of a novel, graded model of clip compressive spinal cord injury in the mouse: Part 1. Clip design, behavioral outcomes, and histopathology. J Neurotrauma 2002; 19(2):175–190.
3. Nesathurai S. Steroids and spinal cord injury: revisiting the NASCIS 2 and NASCIS 3 trials. J Trauma 1998; 45(6):1088–1093.

4. Coleman WP, Benzel D, Cahill DW, et al. A critical appraisal of the reporting of the National Acute Spinal Cord Injury Studies (II and III) of methylprednisolone in acute spinal cord injury. J Spinal Disord 2000; 13(3):185–199.

5. Hurlbert RJ. Methylprednisolone for acute spinal cord injury: an inappropriate standard of care. J Neurosurg 2000; 93(suppl 1):1–7.

6. Short DJ, El Masry WS, Jones PW. High dose methylprednisolone in the management of acute spinal cord injury—a systematic review from a clinical perspective. Spinal Cord 2000; 38(5):273–286.

7. Hurlbert RJ, Moulton R. Why do you prescribe methylprednisolone for acute spinal cord injury? A Canadian perspective and a position statement. Can J Neurol Sci 2002; 29(3):236–239.

8. Bracken MB, Collins WF, Freeman DF, et al. Efficacy of methylprednisolone in acute spinal cord injury. JAMA 1984; 251(1):45–52.

9. Bracken MB, Shepard MJ, Collins WF Jr., et al. Methylprednisolone or naloxone treatment after acute spinal cord injury: 1-year follow-up data. Results of the second National Acute Spinal Cord Injury Study. J Neurosurg 1992; 76(1):23–31.

10. Bracken MB, Shepard MJ, Collins WF, et al. A randomized, controlled trial of methylprednisolone or naloxone in the treatment of acute spinal-cord injury. Results of the Second National Acute Spinal Cord Injury Study. N Engl J Med 1990; 322(20): 1405–1411.

11. Bracken MB, Shepard MJ, Holford TR, et al. Administration of methylprednisolone for 24 or 48 hours or tirilazad mesylate for 48 hours in the treatment of acute spinal cord injury. Results of the Third National Acute Spinal Cord Injury Randomized Controlled Trial. National Acute Spinal Cord Injury Study. JAMA 1997; 277(20): 1597–1604.

12. Bracken MB, Shepard MJ, Holford TR, et al. Methylprednisolone or tirilazad mesylate administration after acute spinal cord injury: 1-year follow up. Results of the third National Acute Spinal Cord Injury randomized controlled trial. J Neurosurg 1998; 89(5):699–706.

13. Otani K, Abe H, Kadoya S. Beneficial effect of methylprednisolone sodium succinate in the treatment of acute spinal cord injury. Sekitsui Sekizui J 1994; 7:633–647.

14. Kiwerski JE. Application of dexamethasone in the treatment of acute spinal cord injury. Injury 1993; 24(7):457–460.

15. Pointillart V, Petitjean ME, Wiart L, et al. Pharmacological therapy of spinal cord injury during the acute phase. Spinal Cord 2000; 38(2):71–76.

16. Hugenholtz H, Cass DE, Dvorak MF, et al. High-dose methylprednisolone for acute closed spinal cord injury—only a treatment option. Can J Neurol Sci 2002; 29(3): 227–235.

17. Tator CH. Review of treatment trials in human spinal cord injury: issues, difficulties, and recommendations. Neurosurgery 2006; 59(5):957–982 (discussion 982–957).

18. Roberts I, Yates D, Sandercock P, et al. Effect of intravenous corticosteroids on death within 14 days in 10008 adults with clinically significant head injury (MRC CRASH trial): randomised placebo-controlled trial. Lancet 2004; 364(9442): 1321–1328.

19. Zeller CB, Marchase RB. Gangliosides as modulators of cell function. Am J Physiol 1992; 262(6 pt 1):C1341–C1355.

20. Rahmann H. Brain gangliosides and memory formation. Behav Brain Res 1995; 66(1–2):105–116.

21. Sabel BA, Stein DG. Pharmacological treatment of central nervous system injury. Nature 1986; 323(6088):493.

22. Gorio A. Gangliosides as a possible treatment affecting neuronal repair processes. Adv Neurol 1988; 47:523–530.

23. Geisler FH, Dorsey FC, Coleman WP. Recovery of motor function after spinal-cord injury—a randomized, placebo-controlled trial with GM-1 ganglioside. N Engl J Med 1991; 324(26):1829–1838.

24. Geisler FH, Coleman WP, Grieco G, et al. The Sygen multicenter acute spinal cord injury study. Spine 2001; 26(suppl 24):S87–S98.

25. Tator CH, Fehlings MG. Review of the secondary injury theory of acute spinal cord trauma with emphasis on vascular mechanisms. J Neurosurg 1991; 75(1):15–26.

26. McIntosh TK, Faden AI. Opiate antagonist in traumatic shock. Ann Emerg Med 1986; 15(12):1462–1465.

27. Faden AI, Jacobs TP, Mougey E, et al. Endorphins in experimental spinal injury: therapeutic effect of naloxone. Ann Neurol 1981; 10(4):326–332.

28. Faden AI, Holaday JW. A role for endorphins in the pathophysiology of spinal cord injury. Adv Biochem Psychopharmacol 1981; 28:435–446.

29. Winkler T, Sharma HS, Gordh T, et al. Topical application of dynorphin A (1–17) antiserum attenuates trauma induced alterations in spinal cord evoked potentials, microvascular permeability disturbances, edema formation and cell injury. An experimental study in the rat using electrophysiological and morphological approaches. Amino Acids 2002; 23(1–3):273–281.

30. Hauser KF, Knapp PE, Turbek CS. Structure-activity analysis of dynorphin A toxicity in spinal cord neurons; intrinsic neurotoxicity of dynorphin A and its carboxyl-terminal, nonopioid metabolites. Exp Neurol 2001; 168(1):78–87.

31. Hu WH, Lee FC, Wan XS, et al. Dynorphin neurotoxicity induced nitric oxide synthase expression in ventral horn cells of rat spinal cord. Neurosci Lett 1996; 203(1):13–16.

32. Behrmann DL, Bresnahan JC, Beattie MS. A comparison of YM-14673, U-50488H, and nalmefene after spinal cord injury in the rat. Exp Neurol 1993; 119(2):258–267.

33. Benzel EC, Khare V, Fowler MR. Effects of naloxone and nalmefene in rat spinal cord injury induced by the ventral compression technique. J Spinal Disord 1992; 5(1):75–77.

34. Akdemir H, Pasaoglu A, Ozturk F, et al. Histopathology of experimental spinal cord trauma. Comparison of treatment with TRH, naloxone, and dexamethasone. Res Exp Med (Berl) 1992; 192(3):177–183.

35. Hashimoto T, Fukuda N. Effect of thyrotropin-releasing hormone on the neurologic impairment in rats with spinal cord injury: treatment starting 24 h and 7 days after injury. Eur J Pharmacol 1991; 203(1):25–32.

36. Benzel EC, Hoffpauir GM, Thomas MM, et al. Dose-dependent effects of naloxone and methylprednisolone in the ventral compression model of spinal cord injury. J Spinal Disord 1990; 3(4):339–344.

37. Faden AI, Sacksen I, Noble LJ. Opiate-receptor antagonist nalmefene improves neurological recovery after traumatic spinal cord injury in rats through a central mechanism. J Pharmacol Exp Ther 1988; 245(2):742–748.

38. Arias MJ. Treatment of experimental spinal cord injury with TRH, naloxone, and dexamethasone. Surg Neurol 1987; 28(5):335–338.

39. Arias MJ. Effect of naloxone on functional recovery after experimental spinal cord injury in the rat. Surg Neurol 1985; 23(4):440–442.

40. Flamm ES, Young W, Demopoulos HB, et al. Experimental spinal cord injury: treatment with naloxone. Neurosurgery 1982; 10(2):227–231.

41. Faden AI, Jacobs TP, Holaday JW. Opiate antagonist improves neurologic recovery after spinal injury. Science 1981; 211(4481):493–494.

42. Faden AI, Jacobs TP, Holaday JW. Thyrotropin-releasing hormone improves neurologic recovery after spinal trauma in cats. N Engl J Med 1981; 305(18):1063–1067.

43. Bracken MB, Holford TR. Effects of timing of methylprednisolone or naloxone administration on recovery of segmental and long-tract neurological function in NASCIS 2. J Neurosurg 1993; 79(4):500–507.

44. Flamm ES, Young W, Collins WF, et al. A phase I trial of naloxone treatment in acute spinal cord injury. J Neurosurg 1985; 63(3):390–397.

45. Pitts LH, Ross A, Chase GA, et al. Treatment with thyrotropin-releasing hormone (TRH) in patients with traumatic spinal cord injuries. J Neurotrauma 1995; 12(3):235–243.

46. Farooque M, Hillered L, Holtz A, et al. Changes of extracellular levels of amino acids after graded compression trauma to the spinal cord: an experimental study in the rat using microdialysis. J Neurotrauma 1996; 13(9):537–548.

47. Panter SS, Yum SW, Faden AI. Alteration in extracellular amino acids after traumatic spinal cord injury. Ann Neurol 1990; 27(1):96–99.

48. Mills CD, Johnson KM, Hulsebosch CE. Group I metabotropic glutamate receptors in spinal cord injury: roles in neuroprotection and the development of chronic central pain. J Neurotrauma 2002; 19(1):23–42.

49. Liu D, Xu GY, Pan E, et al. Neurotoxicity of glutamate at the concentration released upon spinal cord injury. Neuroscience 1999; 93(4):1383–1389.

50. Liu D. An experimental model combining microdialysis with electrophysiology, histology, and neurochemistry for studying excitotoxicity in spinal cord injury. Effect of NMDA and kainate. Mol Chem Neuropathol 1994; 23(2–3):77–92.

51. Agrawal SK, Fehlings MG. Role of NMDA and non-NMDA ionotropic glutamate receptors in traumatic spinal cord axonal injury. J Neurosci 1997; 17(3):1055–1063.

52. Agrawal SK, Theriault E, Fehlings MG. Role of group I metabotropic glutamate receptors in traumatic spinal cord white matter injury. J Neurotrauma. 1998; 15(11):929–941.

53. Lang-Lazdunski L, Heurteaux C, Vaillant N, et al. Riluzole prevents ischemic spinal cord injury caused by aortic crossclamping. J Thorac Cardiovasc Surg 1999; 117(5):881–889.

54. Wrathall JR, Choiniere D, Teng YD. Dose-dependent reduction of tissue loss and functional impairment after spinal cord trauma with the AMPA/kainate antagonist NBQX. J Neurosci 1994; 14(11 pt 1):6598–6607.

55. Tadie M, Gaviria M, Mathe JF, et al. Early care and treatment with a neuroprotective drug, Gacyclidine, in patients with acute spinal cord injury. Rachis 2003; 15:363–376.

56. Lepeintre JF, D'Arbigny P, Mathe JF, et al. Neuroprotective effect of gacyclidine. A multicenter double-blind pilot trial in patients with acute traumatic brain injury. Neurochirurgie 2004; 50(2–3 pt 1):83–95.

57. Tymianski M, Tator CH. Normal and abnormal calcium homeostasis in neurons: a basis for the pathophysiology of traumatic and ischemic central nervous system injury. Neurosurgery 1996; 38(6):1176–1195.

58. Ross IB, Tator CH, Theriault E. Effect of nimodipine or methylprednisolone on recovery from acute experimental spinal cord injury in rats. Surg Neurol 1993; 40(6): 461–470.

59. Agrawal SK, Nashmi R, Fehlings MG. Role of L- and N-type calcium channels in the pathophysiology of traumatic spinal cord white matter injury. Neuroscience 2000; 99(1):179–188.

60. Pointillart V, Gense D, Gross C, et al. Effects of nimodipine on posttraumatic spinal cord ischemia in baboons. J Neurotrauma 1993; 10(2):201–213.

61. De Ley G, Leybaert L. Effect of flunarizine and methylprednisolone on functional recovery after experimental spinal injury. J Neurotrauma 1993; 10(1):25–35.

62. Ross IB, Tator CH. Spinal cord blood flow and evoked potential responses after treatment with nimodipine or methylprednisolone in spinal cord-injured rats. Neurosurgery 1993; 33(3):470–476.

63. Guha A, Tator CH, Piper I. Effect of a calcium-channel blocker on posttraumatic spinal cord blood flow. J Neurosurg 1987; 66(3):423–430.

64. Petitjean ME, Pointillart V, Dixmerias F, et al. Medical treatment of spinal cord injury in the acute stage. Ann Fr Anesth Reanim 1998; 17(2):114–122.

65. Gardner AM, Xu FH, Fady C, et al. Apoptotic vs. nonapoptotic cytotoxicity induced by hydrogen peroxide. Free Radic Biol Med 1997; 22(1–2):73–83.

66. Kowaltowski AJ, Castilho RF, Vercesi AE. Ca(2+)-induced mitochondrial membrane permeabilization: role of coenzyme Q redox state. Am J Physiol 1995; 269(1 Pt 1): C141–C147.

67. Lewen A, Matz P, Chan PH. Free radical pathways in CNS injury. J Neurotrauma 2000; 17(10):871–890.

68. Kaptanoglu E, Sen S, Beskonakli E, et al. Antioxidant actions and early ultra-structural findings of thiopental and propofol in experimental spinal cord injury. J Neurosurg Anesthesiol 2002; 14(2):114–122.

69. Liu D, Li L, Augustus L. Prostaglandin release by spinal cord injury mediates production of hydroxyl radical, malondialdehyde and cell death: a site of the neuroprotective action of methylprednisolone. J Neurochem 2001; 77(4):1036–1047.

70. Farooque M, Isaksson J, Olsson Y. Improved recovery after spinal cord injury in neuronal nitric oxide synthase-deficient mice but not in TNF-alpha-deficient mice. J Neurotrauma 2001; 18(1):105–114.

71. Fujimoto T, Nakamura T, Ikeda T, et al. Effects of EPC-K1 on lipid peroxidation in experimental spinal cord injury. Spine 2000; 25(1):24–29.

72. Katoh D, Ikata T, Katoh S, et al. Effect of dietary vitamin C on compression injury of the spinal cord in a rat mutant unable to synthesize ascorbic acid and its correlation with that of vitamin E. Spinal Cord 1996; 34(4):234–238.

73. Naftchi NE. Treatment of mammalian spinal cord injury with antioxidants. Int J Dev Neurosci 1991; 9(2):113–126.

74. Kavanagh RJ, Kam PC. Lazaroids: efficacy and mechanism of action of the 21-aminosteroids in neuroprotection. Br J Anaesth 2001; 86(1):110–119.

75. Baptiste DC, Fehlings MG. Pharmacological approaches to repair the injured spinal cord. J Neurotrauma 2006; 23(3–4):318–334.

76. Kigerl K, Popovich P. Drug evaluation: ProCord—a potential cell-based therapy for spinal cord injury. IDrugs 2006; 9(5):354–360.

23

Pediatric Spine Injury

Brian Jankowitz, MD, Resident
David O. Okonkwo, MD, PhD, Assistant Professor
Department of Neurosurgery, University of Pittsburgh
School of Medicine, Pittsburgh, Pennsylvania, U.S.A.

Christopher Shaffrey, MD, Professor
Department of Neurological Surgery, University of Virginia,
Charlottesville, Virginia, U.S.A.

INTRODUCTION

Pediatric spine injury is a preventable epidemic with an incidence of 10–50 cases per million children annually (1–3). Children represent less than 10% of spinal injuries seen in emergency departments, while spine fractures represent 1% to 2% of all pediatric fractures (4,5). Over the span of a year, a large medical center can expect to see approximately 57 pediatric spine injuries (6). The cost to society, both financially and physically, is substantial. Children form a cohort of victims with unique anatomy, pathogenesis, and recovery. Insight into these aspects should facilitate prevention, care, and rehabilitation.

The most commonly reported data regarding pediatric spinal cord injury (SCI) quotes an incidence of 18 per million children per year, resulting in approximately 1300 cases annually (7). The most recent data, reported in 2006, substantiate these numbers, stating that 20 of every million children will experience SCI (8). The data may be misleading, as an estimated 50% of children who suffer from SCI in association with multisystem trauma die prior to hospitalization. An additional 20% die after admission to a hospital (9). The expense of

Table 1 Mechanism of Injury Among Age Groups, Total = 137 Patients

Injury	0–9 y	10–14 y	15–17 y	Total
MVA	18(13%)	25(18%)	36(26%)	79(58%)
Fall	8(6%)	8(6%)	4(3%)	20(15%)
Sports	0	5(4%)	5(4%)	10(7%)
Pedestrian	5(4%)	4(3%)	3(2%)	12(9%)
Diving	0	2(1%)	2(1%)	4(3%)
Gunshot	2(1%)	2(1%)	0	4(3%)
Other	3(2%)	3(2%)	2(1%)	8(6%)

Abbreviation: MVA, motor vehicle accident.
Source: From Ref. 89.

caring for these children is estimated to reach $300,000 in the acute setting, with a subsequent annual expense of approximately $50,000 (10). Considering that these figures were derived in 1985, the current cost likely greatly exceeds these sums.

The mechanism of injury varies by age group (Table 1). Younger children (aged 0–8 years) are most often injured by falls or as pedestrians involved in vehicular trauma. Older children (ages > 8 years) are often injured as passengers in motor vehicle crashes or during sports and recreational activities (4). Cervical injuries predominate, followed by lumbar and thoracic injuries with near equivalent incidence (4,5). In particular, injuries of C_1–C_2 and the cranioverte-bral junction predominate in younger children, while subaxial injuries comprise the most common location in older children (11). Younger children more commonly suffer spinal column injury without fracture (12). Approximately half of children will present without evidence of SCI, with younger children more likely to incur neurologic deficit (5). Males have a greater incidence of spinal injury, a statistic that is skewed by adolescent males taking part in more aggressive sports and activities.

PEDIATRIC SPINE ANATOMY

An understanding of pediatric spinal anatomy is essential to grasp the unique injuries and age distribution. The more horizontal orientation of pediatric facet joints (Fig. 1) allows translational motion in the anteroposterior plane and facilitates excessive flexion, extension, and rotation. Greater elasticity of the interspinous ligaments, facet joint capsules, and cartilaginous end plates allows hypermobility. While predisposing to injury, this laxity also allows the recoil of dislocated anatomy back into anatomic alignment. Weaker paraspinal muscles and the larger inertial mass of the head in relation to the body, with a fulcrum of movement at C_2–C_3 rather than at C_5–C_6 contribute to an increased risk of upper cervical spine, and particularly atlantoaxial, injury (13). The uncinate process, which normally restricts lateral and rotational movement between adjacent vertebral bodies, is usually absent in children younger than 10 years. In addition,

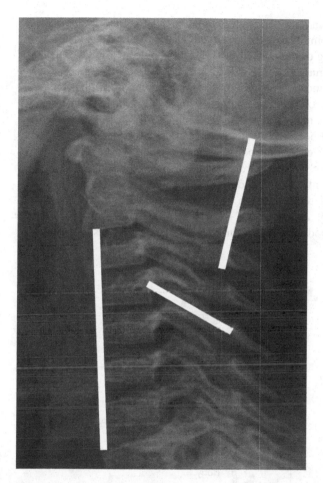

Figure 1 Lateral cervical x-ray of a 3-year-old child. The anterior vertebral body line is drawn to highlight the pseudosubluxation of C_2 on C_3. The line of Swischuk has been drawn to show normal alignment of the C_1–C_3 spinous processes. Also note the relatively horizontal orientation of the facet joint and the rounded corners of the vertebral bodies consistent with anterior wedging.

incomplete ossification of the superior vertebral body end plates creates anterior wedging that facilitates spondylolisthesis, often referred to as pseudosubluxation when occurring in a normal pediatric spine (Fig. 1).

The complexity of pediatric anatomy can lead to misinterpretation of radiography. In particular, the preossified skeleton and joint laxity allow a significant incidence of false-positive interpretations. Careful review of films read by a radiologist have shown error rates of 24% and 15% for children younger than 9 years and older than 8 years, respectively (14). Predisposing factors to misinterpretations include unfamiliarity of pediatric spine anatomy, the inability to recognize normal spine variants, and suboptimal imaging. The craniovertebral junction was the most common site of misinterpretation. One typical variant is known as pseudospreading or the normal lateral overriding of C_1 on C_2. The sum of the bilateral overhang may be up to 6 mm in children up to age 7 years (15). Pseudosubluxation is the most common false-positive finding on pediatric lateral films (Fig. 1). Up to 40% of children younger than 8 years will display anterior spondylolisthesis occurring at C_2–C_3, with 14% exhibiting C_3–C_4 subluxation (16). Pseudosubluxation should not be present after age 14 years. Anterior wedging of the C_3–C_5 vertebrae, which can mimic compression fractures, is normal in children up to age 14 years because of the encircling ring apophysis (Fig. 1).

The ossification centers of the developing spine may be mistaken for fractures. Knowledge of their location is integral to avoid misdiagnosis of traumatic pathology (Fig. 2). C_1 and C_3–C_7 share three common ossification centers that connect the body and two neural arches. The arches fuse to the body

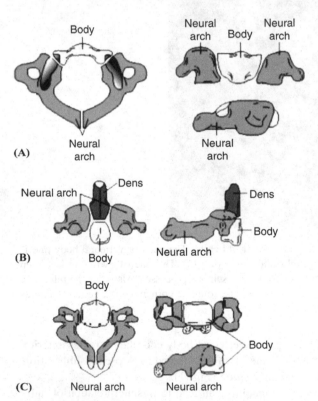

Figure 2 Schematic representation of the developmental ossification centers in the pediatric cervical spine. (A) C_1 has three synchondroses connecting the two lateral arches with the central body. (B) C_2 has four synchondroses connecting two lateral arches with the body and dens. (C) C_3–C_7 has three synchondroses, similar to C_1. *Source*: From Ref. 17.

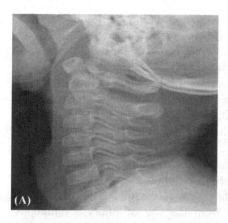 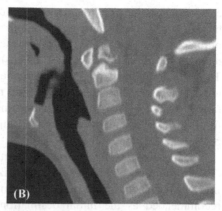

Figure 3 Os odontoideum. Also note the radiolucent basal odontoid synchondrosis. (**A**) Lateral cervical x-ray. (**B**) Cervical CT with sagittal reconstruction.

by age 6 years, and the posterior arch fuses by age 3 years. The C_2 vertebra develops from four ossification centers, incorporating a body, odontoid, and two neural arches. The most commonly misinterpreted ossification center, the neurocentral synchondrosis between the dens and body, remains radiolucent in all children up to age 4 years and in half of children up to age 11 years (Fig. 3). Fusion of the posterior C2 synchondrosis occurs between ages 2 and 3 years, while the arch-body synchondroses fuse by age 6 years (15). The atlanto-dens interval (ADI), which acts as a surrogate measure of C_1–C_2 stability, relies on the transverse and alar ligament to maintain a distance of 3 mm or less in adults. This interval can be up to 5 mm in children (17). Overriding of the anterior arch of the atlas on the dens can be seen in 20% of normal children (18). Finally, loss of lordosis can be normal in children up to age 16 years when the neck is in a neutral position.

The pediatric spine is a dynamic entity, continuously evolving. The infant spine (ages 0–2 years) can display all of the above characteristics. Between the ages of 2 and 14 years, the musculature develops, the head:body ratio reduces, the torso elongates and matures, and the bones ossify. The upper cervical spine reaches its maturity around ages 8 to 10 years, while the subaxial spine development is usually completed by age 14 years (19). The entire spinal column reaches physiologic maturity by ages 15 to 16 years, at which time injury patterns begin to mimic those of adults.

DIAGNOSIS AND TRIAGE

A low threshold of suspicion for pediatric spine injury will enable early diagnosis and facilitate appropriate triage and immobilization on the scene. Of note, the greater head:body ratio in children younger than 8 years will force the cervical spine into flexion when a child is placed supine on a uniformly flat board (20). This position may compromise the airway, exacerbate injury, or mimic a loss of lordosis in an otherwise normal cervical spine. This condition requires elevation of the body ($\sim$ 2.5 cm) in relation to the head during transport. The goal should be to align the external auditory meatus with the shoulders. One must remember that the incidence of multiple, noncontiguous spine injuries range from 11% to 16% (4,12). Concomitant systemic injury has been reported in up to 37% of patients, while head injury has been noted in 30% to 66% of patients with spine injury (21).

Management of pediatric SCI begins with early recognition and immobilization followed by appropriate specialized care to prevent secondary insults or injury. Specialized pediatric trauma centers with access to SCI specialists are recommended as the initial destination from the site of injury. Continuous monitoring and a high suspicion for associated injuries are paramount to avoid exacerbation of noted or occult injuries. Spinal injury may facilitate hypoventilation and hypoxemia because of the loss of motor and sympathetic tone. The clinician should have a low threshold for early intubation and even tracheotomy. Fiberoptic intubation to prevent excessive cervical extension is recommended when clinically feasible (22).

Initial Imaging

The guidelines for the management of acute cervical spine and SCI state that in children who have suffered trauma and have a distracting injury or pain an anteroposterior and lateral x-ray of the cervical spine should be obtained. Conspicuously absent is the mention of open-mouthodontoid views. Considering the difficulty in obtaining these views in children younger than 9 years combined with the low sensitivity of these images in detecting injury from the occiput to C_3, some experts recommend eliminating their routine use (23,24). However, one might reconsider foregoing the standard three-view series, as the false-negative value for a single cross-table lateral x-ray at ruling out fracture is 21% to 26% (25). A compromise voiced by Swischuk recommends abandoning the open-mouth view after one or two attempts if the lateral film is normal (26). Anteroposterior and lateral x-rays of the thoracolumbar spine should be obtained on the basis of injury, exam, and the clinician's judgment.

Routine x-rays must often be supplemented with a fine-cut CT to evaluate the occiput-to-C_2 region. Furthermore, a CT should be obtained in all instances of suspected injury on plain films or to supplement questionable or inadequate x-rays at any level. Flexion-extension views may be necessary to rule out ligamentous instability in a patient with neck pain and no evidence of osseous injury. Muscle spasm and pain may limit adequate movement, necessitating placement in a cervical collar, with repeat flexion-extension views in the following weeks. These dynamic studies can be performed with the aid of fluoroscopy and neurophysiologic monitoring in patients who cannot limit their movement on the basis of pain, such as very young, uncooperative, distracted, or comatose children (27). A greater reliance on MRI has burgeoned from the superior diagnostic capability regarding ligamentous or neural injury, absence of ionizing radiation, and avoidance of passive flexion or extension of the cervical spine that is necessary under fluoroscopy. In particular, for the pediatric population, diffusion-weighted imaging may be more sensitive for the diagnosis and prognosis of SCI without radiographic evidence of abnormality (SCIWORA), as hyperintensity of diffusion-weighted imaging may be observed in the absence of T2 signal change within the spinal cord (28). However, even MRI lacks the sensitivity to detect all SCIs. Up to 35% of patients with a persistent neurologic deficit can have a normal MRI. Electrophysiologic studies or somatosensory-evoked potentials are other diagnostic tests that can detect SCI, with a sensitivity of 88%. It is essential to note that 12% to 15% of children with definitive signs and symptoms of SCI can present with no evidence of SCI by imaging or electrophysiologic criteria, highlighting the continued importance of a meticulous neurologic examination.

Of note, certain congenital diseases may predispose children to inherently unstable spinal anatomy because of a combination of joint laxity and bony abnormalities. Down syndrome confers a 10% to 40% incidence of atlantoaxial and occipitocervical instability (29). The Klippel-Feil syndrome, basilar invagination, and Chiari malformation are but a few disease entities with well known accompanying spine pathology. The presence of these syndromes should raise the suspicion of injury in patients who suffer even minor trauma. These syndromes may also affect decisions regarding surgery, given the likelihood of incipient instability.

Excluding Cervical Instability

A protocol for the clearance of the pediatric cervical spine after trauma was developed and prospectively validated in 3065 children (30). By implementing these National Emergency X Radiography Utilization Study (NEXUS) criteria in communicating children who were aged 3 years or more, two or three plain-view films +/– flexion-extension views were used to successfully clear 68% of 746 pediatric cervical spines with no late or missed injuries (Fig. 4) (31). Certain accepted radiographic standards can be used to exclude cervical instability. Intervertebral angulation greater than $7°$ at all ages, C_2–C_4 anterior subluxation greater than 4.5 mm in children younger than 8 years, and anterior subluxation greater than 3.5 mm in children older than 8 years are all considered signs of ligamentous injury (32). A line can also be drawn that connects the anterior aspect of the posterior arch of C_1 and C_3, referred to as the line of Swischuk (Fig. 1). This line should touch or lie within 1 mm of the C_2 posterior arch. In the presence of anterior wedge compression fractures, greater than $15°$ of vertebral body angulation is considered unstable.

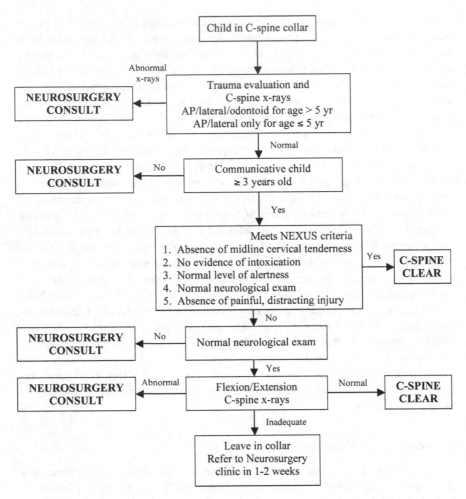

Figure 4 Algorithm for clearing the pediatric cervical spine after trauma. Neurosurgery consult denotes triage based on the clinicians judgment. *Source*: From Ref. 31.

SPINAL COLUMN INJURY

Cervical spine injuries predominate in the pediatric age group, comprising well over half of all spine trauma. A review of more than 75,000 injured children over a 10-year period revealed a 1.5% incidence of cervical spine injury (33). Upper cervical spine injury (C1–4) was almost twice as common, overall, although lower cervical spine injury predominated in children who were older than 8 years, comprising 85% of the injured levels in this age group (Tables 2 and 3) (34). The 83% of patients who presented with bony injury exhibited fractures (67%), dislocations (27%), or both (6%).

Table 2 Injury to Vertebral Column or Spinal Cord

Injury Level	O-C4	C5-7	T1-10	T11-L1	L2-S	Total
Infant	7(63.6%)	2(18.2%)	1(9.1%)	1(9.1%)	0	11(7.6%)
Toddler	15(48.4%)	5(16.1%)	3(9.7%)	2(6.5%)	6(19.4%)	31(21.4%)
School	18(60.0%)	5(16.7%)	1(3.3%)	2(6.7%)	4(13.3%)	30(20.7%)
Adolescent	27(37.0%)	10(13.7%)	9(12.3%)	4(5.5%)	23(31.5%)	73(50.3%)
Total (%)	67(46.2%)	22(15.2%)	14(9.7%)	9(6.2%)	33(22.9%)	145(100%)

Abbreviations: O, occipital; C, cervical; T, thoracic; L, lumbar; S, sacral.
Source: From Ref. 34.

Table 3 Summary of Clinical Data in 102 Pediatric Patients with Cervical Injuries at Admission

Age Range: Years	Cervical Level		Neurological Status at Admission			Type of Injury			
	Upper	Lower	Intact	Incomplete SCI	Complete SCI	Fx	Sub	Fx & Sub	No Fx or Sub
birth–9 (38 patients)	31	7	16	16	6	7	15	4	12
10–16 (64 patients)	22	42	26	30	8	27	7	24	6

Abbreviation: Fx, fracture; Sub; subluxation.
Source: From Ref. 21.

Craniovertebral Junction

Atlanto-occipital dislocation constitutes an avulsion of the ligamentous attachments between the occiput and atlas (Fig. 5). The infantile craniovertebral junction may be particularly susceptible to this injury because of an inherently unstable atlanto-occipital joint. Predisposing anatomic factors include a relatively small C_1 arch in relation to the larger foramen magnum, a lax condylar capsule with flat articulating surfaces, and redundant atlanto-occipital ligaments (35). Imaging findings include a powers ratio (the distance from the basion to the posterior arch of C_1 divided by the distance from the opisthion to the anterior arch of C_1) greater than 1, greater than 10 mm between the dens and basion, or subarachnoid hemorrhage at the level of the cervicomedullary junction (36). Quadriparesis and apnea should alert physicians to this diagnosis. Halo immobilization or occipital-cervical fusion should be performed as soon as medically feasible, usually spanning from the occiput to C_2 or C_3. Atlanto-occipital dislocation was classically considered a fatal injury, with the highest mortality rate (48%) of all cervical spine injuries (33). With the advent of rapid triage and transport, early immobilization, and aggressive resuscitation, increasing numbers of case reports have shown survivability after

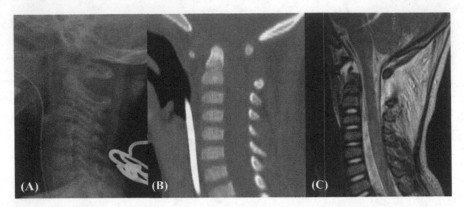

Figure 5 Craniovertebral junction injury involving both atlanto-occipital and atlantoaxial dislocation. (**A**) Lateral cervical x-ray showing C_1 distracted from C_2 with the entire C_1 ring lying above the dens. (**B**) Cervical CT with sagittal reconstruction, again showing distraction between the occiput-C_1 and C_1–C_2. The basion-dens interval was 13 mm. (**C**) Sagittal T2-weighted MRI showing anterior and posterior hyperintensity at the craniovertebral junction consistent with extensive ligamentous disruption.

atlanto-occipital dislocation in some patients with incomplete spinal cord injury, resulting in a good outcome (37,38).

Atlantoaxial injuries compromise the next subset of osseous injuries to the pediatric spine. Fractures of C_1 are a rare entity in children, as the cartilaginous ring can absorb and dissipate loads without fracturing. C_1 fractures in children may present without the classic dual-ring Jefferson fracture seen in adults, instead revealing a unilateral hinge at the synchondrosis (39). The mainstay of treatment involves immobilization in a rigid cervical collar or halo vest. Fractures of C_2 are the most common site of fracture, usually occurring at the odontoid basal synchondrosis. In young children, incomplete ossification allows this neurocentral synchondrosis to be distracted (11,40). A true type II odontoid fracture at the odontoid-body junction can be distinguished from a synchondrosis separation, as the latter occurs below the level of the superior facets within the C_2 body. Reduction requires gentle extension and posterior translation, rarely necessitating traction. The treatment of choice is rigid cervical immobilization, usually with a halo orthosis, for 10 weeks. Success rates approach 80%. Surgery is rarely necessary, although odontoid screws, transarticular screws, and posterior sublaminar wiring have all been described in the pediatric population (24,41).

Os odontoideum represents a cryptic entity, which is defined as an ossicle with smooth circumferential cortical margins, representing the odontoid process that has no osseous continuity with the body of C_2 (Fig. 3). While the etiology remains uncertain, with the debate vacillating between acquired and congenital, treatment depends upon presentation. Patients without neurologic signs or symptoms may be followed conservatively, even in the presence of radiographic instability. Symptomatic patients with instability require fixation, with good results reported from both transarticular screw fixation and posterior C_1–C_2 wire fixation combined with halo immobilization (24).

Atlantoaxial rotatory subluxation is a specific variant of C_1–C_2 injury. Trauma, including minor injuries, is one cause, although spontaneous displacement, infection (Grisel syndrome), and tumors more commonly induce the subluxation. These scenarios allow the anterior facet of C_1 to become locked or "sticky" to the facet of C_2, creating a spectrum of cervical rotation inhibition. Children tend to exhibit a cock-robin appearance, with the chin rotated in one direction and the head flexed toward the contralateral side. Displacement may occur, whereupon there is anterior translation of the lateral mass of C_1 in relation to C_2. Fielding and Hawkins classified this spectrum into types 1 through 4 (Fig. 6), ranging from no displacement of C_1, 3–5 mm displacement of C_1 on C_2, greater than 5 mm anterior displacement, or posterior displacement, respectively (42). Pang et al. created a new diagnostic, classification, and treatment algorithm on the basis of dynamic CT in three positions, which compares the orientation of C_1 to C_2 with the head in the presenting "cocked" position, neutral nose-up position, and maximal rotation in the opposite direction (43–45). For all patients,

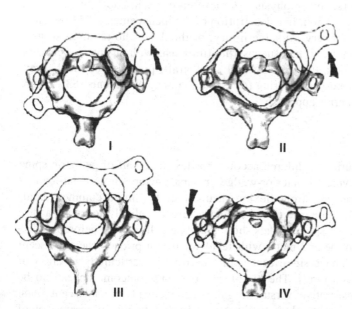

Figure 6 These drawings illustrate the Fielding classification scheme for atlantoaxial rotatory fixation. Type I demonstrates no displacement of C_1, type II demonstrates 3–5 mm of anterior displacement and is associated with abnormality of the transverse ligament, type III demonstrates over 5 mm of anterior displacement of C_1 on C_2 and is associated with deficiency of the transverse and alar ligament, and type IV demonstrates C_1 displacement posteriorly. Arrows indicate direction of movement. *Source*: From Ref. 15.

immediate closed reduction with traction is recommended, followed by a cervicothoracic brace. Nonreducible subluxation or repeated, failed attempts at closed reduction with halo immobilization require posterior C_1–C_2 fusion. The severity and, more importantly, the chronicity of C_1–C_2 fixation led to poorer outcomes, with 6 of 29 patients requiring surgery. In another review, 6 of 20 patients ultimately required posterior cervical fusion after recurrence of the subluxation or unsuccessful reduction, with a 100% success rate (46).

Subaxial Cervical Spine

Subaxial spine injuries tend to occur in older children and at higher levels compared with adults because of a more rostral moment arm, located at C_2–C_3, C_3–C_4, C_4–C_5, and C_5–C_6 at ages 0, 5, 10, and 15, years respectively (47). Common injury patterns include vertebral body compression or facet fractures from hyperextension or physical end plate fractures from hyperextension. Physical fractures are unique to the pediatric population and involve separation of the vertebral end plate from the body through the epiphysis. Fractures in which the epiphysis is intact and separated from the metaphysis, often seen in infants and younger children, are highly unstable and require surgical stabilization (48). Fractures that traverse the epiphysis, which often occur in adolescents, can be treated with immobilization. In a description of the management of 51 pediatric patients with subaxial cervical spine injury, of the 36% who required surgery (age range, 8–16 years), all had successful arthrodesis with an anterior cervical discectomy and fusion, corpectomy and strut graft, posterior cervical screw and rod fixation, or posterior wiring (49). The majority of patients (83%) were managed via an anterior approach.

Thoracolumbar Spine

Thoracolumbar injuries in children account for less than half of pediatric spine injuries. They are typically anterior-wedge or burst fractures from axial-loading or three-column fractures from flexion distraction. The more common axial-loading injury with resultant compression fracture is unlikely to cause a disc herniation as immature spine models show the bone will fracture before the disc fails (50). Injury to the end plate, with resultant fusion prior to the adolescent growth spurt, can induce significant spinal deformity, particularly in areas of multiple contiguous injuries. The long-term functional outcome appears to be equivalent for conservative versus surgical management in adolescent burst fracture, although nonsurgical treatment is associated with greater progression of posttraumatic kyphosis during the first year (51).

Flexion-distraction injuries often produce Chance fractures, or transverse fractures, through the vertebral body extending into the pedicle, typically caused by lap belt restraint in a motor vehicle crash (Fig. 7). Standard adult management applies, with the application of reduction, bracing in a thoracolumbar-sacral

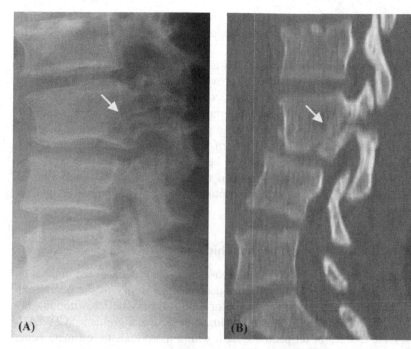

Figure 7 L₃ flexion distruction injury with fracture extending from vertebral body into pedicle, consistent with a Chance fracture. (**A**) Lateral x-ray of lumbar spine. (**B**) CT with sagittal reconstruction of lumbar spine.

orthosis for two to three months, and surgery utilized as necessary in the presence of neurologic deficit or significant ligamentous injury. To aid in the prognosis of successful bracing, one small series defined less than 20° kyphosis as the cutoff for reliable bracing and avoidance of surgical fusion (52). Surgical stabilization is also recommended for greater than 50% loss of vertebral body height or lateral compression of greater than 15° (53).

Shear injuries comprise another rare subset of spinal column traumas that often occur in the thoracic spine but may occur in the cervical or lumbar spine as well. Violent shearing can fracture the thick, cartilaginous end plate, resulting in a limbus or apophysial fracture. Typically seen in adolescents or young adults, patients may present with radiculopathy consistent with a herniated nucleus pulposus. Surgery is often required to extract the compressive fragment.

SPINAL CORD INJURY

Half of pediatric spine injuries present with evidence of SCI upon examination (4). Much like spinal column injury, age often determines location of injury in pediatric SCI. Most of the injuries in the younger age group involve the upper cervical spine. One group reported that 79% of SCI in children younger than 9 years involved the cervical spine, as opposed to 53% of children aged 9 to 16 years (40).

The anatomic predisposition for SCI in children involves a spine that is lax enough to be stressed without fracture, providing excessive stretch, shearing, or transient concussion to the encased spinal cord. This hypermobility often allows the deformed but unfractured spinal column to return to its normal anatomic alignment. This scenario is typified by the physiologic normal variant of pseudosubluxation, which allows up to 4 mm of translational gliding between C_2–C_3 and C_3–C_4 in younger children (54). It has also been shown that while the neonatal spinal column can withstand up to 2 in of stretch without signs of structural disruption, the spinal cord ruptures after only one-quarter inch of stretch (55).

Spinal Cord Injury Without Radiographic Abnormality

First defined in 1982, SCIWORA is a disease entity that predated the innovation of MRI technology (56). The syndrome described an injury to the neural elements of the spinal column, causing a motor and/or sensory deficit without x-ray or CT evidence of vertebral fracture, subluxation, or misalignment. SCIWORA comprises 1% to 62% of all pediatric SCI, with a more realistic estimate being 30% to 40% (4,5,21,57). SCIWORA is seen in all age groups; however, the unique anatomy of children younger than 8 years predisposes to more severe injury, a greater incidence, and a threefold increase in abnormal imaging by MRI, compared with children older than 8 years (58,59). In fact, two-thirds of SCIWORA injuries occur in children younger than 8 years (12,56). In one large review, of those aged 0 to 9 years with spine trauma, the frequency of SCIWORA was 42%, compared with 8% in those aged 15 to 17 years (4).

Various theories regarding the etiology of SCIWORA have been proposed. Possible explanations include transient vascular injury or forcible extension that results in buckling of the ligamentum flavum, axial distraction, and stretch of the spinal cord (55,56,60).

Five consistent patterns of cord injury may be noted on MRI after SCIWORA, consisting of complete disruption, major hemorrhage (hemorrhage in > 50% of the cross-sectional area of the cord), minor hemorrhage, edema only, and normal (58). All classification schemata have attempted to correlate imaging findings with neurologic outcome; however, no large-scale prospective classifications have been validated. In retrospective reviews, complete disruption and major hemorrhage are always associated with a poor outcome (61), minor hemorrhage or edema is associated with moderate-to-good recovery (62–64), and absence of MR findings predicts complete recovery (65). Forty percent of patients with minor hemorrhage will ultimately improve to a mild deficit, compared with 100% improvement to mild deficit or normal in those with edema only. Approximately 35% of patients with clinical or electrophysiologic evidence of SCI do not have an MRI abnormality of their cord.

Repeat imaging is recommended, as resolution of signal change predicts a better return of function and persistence of MR abnormality is a poor prognostic indicator (66,67). Also, early imaging may miss edema, which can take three to four hours to manifest.

The inability to alter the outcome of patients suffering from SCIWORA once the incipient injury took place led Pang to publish three recommendations to improve outcome once injury had occurred. These recommendations include ruling out overt spinal instability, identifying and inhibiting delayed neurologic deterioration, and preventing recurrent injury (59). Prevention of delayed SCIWORA and recurrence is of the utmost importance and may be possible with early diagnosis and immobilization to prevent excessive spine motion. Recurrent SCIWORA may result from noncompliance with spine immobilization or inadequate treatment and often results in more severe deficits than the initial injury (66,68,69). One group described a 19% recurrence during the initial two months of follow-up, which included recommendations of rigid cervical immobilization and avoidance of contact sports (70). Clearly defined trauma preceded seven of the eight recurrences, and five of the seven had removed their cervical collar. Most of the traumatic episodes were relatively trivial. These results prompted the recommendation of strict adherence to a rigid cervical collar for three months followed by repeat dynamic imaging, with avoidance of all sporting activity for six months. An algorithm for the care of possible SCI-WORA is presented in Figure 8.

Delayed presentation of SCIWORA has been noted up to four days after injury in 22% to 27% of patients (4,5,59). These children reported transient symptoms, including subjective paralysis, distal paresthesias, and the Lhermitte phenomenon; these symptoms may indicate an incipiently unstable spinal column, prompting some clinicians to recommend six weeks of rigid cervical collar bracing, even with normal imaging studies (59). The greater sensitivity of somatosensory-evoked potentials to detect occult SCI may be helpful in this situation, allowing cautious consideration of one to two weeks in a cervical collar, with follow-up as espoused by Pang in the setting of fleeting symptoms with normal imaging and somatosensory-evoked potentials. Such significant numbers of delayed presentations have not been reproduced in other, more recent retrospective reviews (11,12,21,56,59). The reduced incidence may be because of more rigorous early detection and immobilization for all children with neck pain and transient neurologic symptoms. In the guidelines for the management of acute cervical and spinal cord injury, it currently remains an option to treat SCIWORA with 12 weeks of immobilization, as no documented neurologic deterioration has been reported after this rigid management (71). Conversely, no child with SCIWORA and a normal, adequate flexion-extension x-ray, regardless of MRI findings, has developed spinal instability.

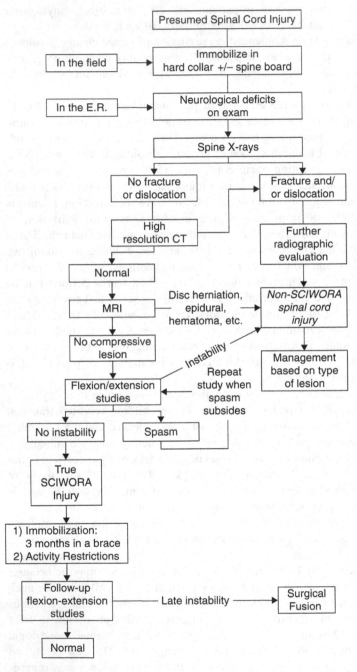

Figure 8 Management algorithm for the evaluation and treatment of children with SCI. *Source*: From Ref. 69 with permission.

Injury patterns from SCIWORA include complete cord transaction and partial cord, Brown Sequard, or central cord syndromes. Complete injuries tend to predominate with thoracic injuries, and younger children consistently sustain the most severe deficits (11,12,56).

Birth-Related Injuries

Patients with birth-related spine trauma comprise an often-overlooked group, representing up to 4% of all SCIs (11). With an incidence of 1 of every 60,000 births, SCI is estimated to cause 10% of perinatal deaths (72,73). The affected level is usually the upper cervical spine or cervicothoracic junction, resulting in apnea, loss of deep tendon reflexes, and flaccid quadriparesis. High cervical cord injuries are usually associated with shoulder dystocia and/or complicated vertex deliveries necessitating forceps for rotational maneuvers (74). In utero hyperextension of the fetal head is another proposed mechanism of SCI, usually associated with breech and persistent transverse lie positioning (75). Vaginal delivery under these conditions may induce longitudinal traction of the spine with subsequent rupture of the cord (76). In a review of the methods of delivery for neonates with persistent hyperextension in utero, delivery via cesarean section produced no deficits, while 21% of those delivered vaginally suffered an SCI, leading the investigators to recommend cesarean section for all fetuses with persistent hyperextension noted on imaging (77). One must also remember that 20% to 25% of injuries occur during uncomplicated deliveries (78). Outcome is universally poor. No reports in the literature support a specific management; however, spinal immobilization in suspected patients who survive is reasonable.

Child Abuse

Infants who suffer child abuse or the shaken-baby syndrome comprise a rare subset of injured patients that may develop cord injury from the rapid oscillation between hyperextension and hyperflexion. Most patients will present with associated systemic injury such as traumatic brain injury or rib fractures. The injury pattern often mimics a central cord syndrome and is considered a type of SCIWORA, with the same treatment goals (56).

TREATMENT

Treatment of pediatric SCI is based upon immobilization to prevent secondary injury. Cervical and thoracolumbar spine precautions include maintaining a rigid cervical collar at all times, log rolling when mobilization is necessary, and maintaining spinal alignment.

The only therapy that has been shown to reduce secondary injury in clinical trials is the administration of methylprednisolone if started within eight hours of injury. This protocol involves an initial bolus of 30 mg/kg within

15 minutes of injury, followed by infusion of 5.4 mg/kg/hr over the following 23 hours if started within three hours of injury, or 48 hours if started after three hours (79). While often employed, this protocol does not represent the standard of care and has not been rigorously evaluated in the pediatric population, as children younger than 13 years were excluded from the initial studies.

Secondary insults, including gastric ulcers, aspiration, hypovolemia, urinary retention, and deep vein thrombosis/pulmonary embolism, can be reduced with simple interventions such as H_2-receptor blockers, early intubation and tracheotomy, early and aggressive volume resuscitation with or without a central venous catheter, Foley catheter, and early serial compression devices, respectively.

Most cervical injuries can be managed with a rigid cervical collar or halo vest. Children as young as 1-year old can be managed in a halo vest by maximizing the number of pins to distribute cranial compression; however, complication rates are high. Pin site infections, pin loosening, calvarial penetration, and supraorbital nerve injury were noted in 68% of young children (80). The most conservative application requires 8 to 10 pins to allow as little as 1 to 2 lb of torque at each site. Injuries of the lower cervical and cervicothoracic spine can be managed in customized multicomponent braces such as the Minerva, SOMI, or Guilford brace. Thoracic or lumbar spine injuries can be managed in custom-molded, acrylic, clamshell-style braces. Traction may be necessary to reduce dislocations or fractures. One pound per cervical level in children younger than 4 years and 2 lb per cervical level for children older than 4 years is often adequate (48). As few as 5% of children will fail nonoperative therapy even though it may be initially deemed appropriate (5).

Surgical treatment should be pursued to decompress neural structures or in the presence of gross instability, irreducible dislocations, incomplete injury with progressive neurologic deficit, or progressive spinal deformity. Specific indications include greater than15° kyphosis, significant vertebral compression, or ligamentous injury with facet dislocation. Approximately one-third of pediatric spine injuries will require surgery (5,21). Surgical fusion should be confined to the unstable segments to allow normal physiologic maturation and bone growth. The surgical technique depends on the maturity of the spine (48). The size of the spine in children younger than 5 years routinely disallows invasive instrumented fusion. Posterior cervical wiring with graft onlay and rigid external immobilization is often sufficient. By age 5 years, anterior cervical discectomy and fusion is another alternative. As most cervical spine growth and elongation occurs in the epiphysis of the end plate, complete discectomy and decortication allows symmetric anterior and posterior growth. By age 10 years, near-adult spine physiology has been reached, allowing anterior or posterior spine instrumentation, including screw, rod, and plate fixation, with a low risk of progressive deformity. Surgeons should minimize exposure and manipulation of the periosteum in adjacent segments because the highly osteogenic pediatric bone is prone to fuse across areas of exposed periosteum; however, this provides for excellent fusion rates. In a review of the treatment for pediatric cervical spine trauma, it was noted that the entire surgical cohort of 30 patients showed evidence of solid arthrodesis within six months (21).

OUTCOMES

Outcome of SCI greatly depends on the extent of the initial insult and neurologic status upon presentation (Table 4). Injury type does not predict outcome, only extent of neurologic deficit. In a review of 174 pediatric patients, 77% of patients with only a fracture were neurologically intact compared with 20% of those patients with fracture and subluxation. Complete injury occurred in 68% of the fracture- and-subluxation groups, compared with 27% in the fracture-only group. SCIWORA tended to result in more severe injuries, particularly for the youngest age group. Complete injury following SCIWORA was noted in 50% of those aged 0 to 9 years versus 11% in those aged 15 to 17 years (4).

Complete versus incomplete injury provides a reliable predictor of recovery. Mortality rates range from 4% to 35% overall, with an approximate threefold increase in complete (53%) versus incomplete (16%) injury (5,21,33,81,82). The cause of death is most often related to complications from associated injuries (such as closed-head injury) or secondary insults (such as pneumonia and hypoventilation). Patients who suffer complete injuries rarely improve or have good outcomes, even with early stabilization and surgery. In general, surgery has not been shown to influence neurological outcome (5). In one series, it was reported that only one-quarter of complete patients showed any improvement (12). Conversely, the majority of incomplete patients experience some level of improvement. Investigators reported 89% of the incomplete injury cohort experienced measurable recovery, with most mild-to-moderate injuries regaining near complete neurologic function (12). A follow-up to this review during the subsequent decade reported that 83% of incomplete injuries recovered completely (21). Another study reported similar results, with only 1 of 42 patients who suffered complete injury regaining useful motor recovery and 1 of 26 patients with severe injury regaining independent motor function. The most recent large review of severe SCI provides more optimistic data. A 2004 review reported that 5 of 20 children who presented with complete injuries eventually became ambulatory, with functional improvement occurring as late as 50 weeks postinjury (83). Children may show improvement up to two years postinjury (12).

Although the level of injury does not consistently correlate with outcome, it does influence the rehabilitation potential. High cervical injuries understandably have worse outcomes, with one report that none of 67 patients experienced a good outcome after presenting with quadriplegia (2). The few patients with functional outcomes had injuries below T 12 (84).

Close follow-up is also necessary to monitor for progressive spinal deformity or syrinx formation. Cadaveric studies have shown that fractures in

Table 4 Outcome in 908 Children with Bony Spine Injury

| Leval | Type of Bony Injury | | | Outcome | | | | |
	Fracture	Dislocation	Both	Nonsurvivors: Dead	Mortality Rate (%)	Survivors: Complete SCI	Incomplete SCI	No Deficits
Single level								
C1	52	54	4	36	32.73%	0	1	73
C2	100	29	2	6	4.58%	0	0	125
C3	16	11	1	4	14.29%	3	2	19
C4	8	12	2	3	13.64%	2	1	16
C5	42	2	1	1	2.22%	0	0	44
C6	25	8	3	1	2.78%	1	2	32
C7	71	6	3	2	2.50%	1	2	75
Multiple levels								
Upper[a]	128	47	19	64	32.99%	9	46	75
Lower[b]	73	15	8	8	8.33%	8	33	47
Both[c]	42	10	12	7	10.94%	4	11	42
UNSP[d]	53	47	2	29	28.43%	0	2	71
TOTAL	610	241	57	161	17.73%	28	100	619

[a]Upper cervical spine injury (C_1–C_4), multiple levels.
[b]Lower cervical spine injury (C_5–C_7), multiple levels.
[c]Both upper and lower cervical spine.
[d]Unspecified level of cervical spine injury.
Abbreviation: SCI, spinal cord injury.
Source: From Ref. 33.

young children tend to occur through the cartilaginous vertebral end plates, thus injuring the active growth zones (85). Destruction of these growth plates can lead to stunted and asymmetric vertebral growth, with delayed spinal deformity involving scoliosis, kyphosis, and exaggerated lordosis (86). Ischemic necrosis of epiphyseal growth plates, asymmetric bone destruction, fusion between adjacent injured segments, and imbalance of the paraspinous muscles can also contribute to growth imbalance. Studies from the 1970s reported progressive posttraumatic spinal deformity in 50% to 90% of patients (75,87,88). After the advent of early stabilization and fusion, recent studies have shown that 8% to 12% of patients with severe SCI will go on to develop kyphoscoliosis (5,89). As further proof of deformity stemming from bone disruption, SCIWORA rarely results in progressive deformity (56).

PREVENTION

Prevention has become an important focus of pediatric spine injury. Local and federal government-sponsored legislation and the efforts of private groups such as ThinkFirst (a service mark of the American Association of Neurological Surgeons and Congress of Neurological Surgeons, The ThinkFirst Foundation) are integral to disseminating information regarding injury avoidance and child safety. The use of seat belts, age- and weight-appropriate child seats, and protective sporting gear are but a few areas worthy of further intervention and improvement. In a review of pediatric cervical spine injury, 81% of the injuries caused by a motor vehicle crash involved children who were either unrestrained or inappropriately restrained (90). In the older subset of this group, 87% were totally unrestrained. These findings have been substantiated in the literature, whereby adherence to age-appropriate motor vehicle restraints resulted in a decreased incidence of cervical spine injury (91).

Future Perspectives and Evolving Paradigms

The recent past has seen a significant change in the management of pediatric spine injury. Surgeons are gaining comfort with the use of instrumentation in this population, with pedicle screws utilized in children as young as 8-months old (92). Gaining considerable popularity is the use of percutaneous instrumentation without arthrodesis as an internal, temporary brace. An example of this is percutaneous pedicle screw instrumentation for a potentially unstable Chance fracture. By avoiding decortication and bone grafting, children may have time to heal by themselves and avoid the adverse effects of premature fusion or cumbersome external orthosis. The instrumentation can even be removed at a later date to allow normal physiologic growth.

Another technique to avoid permanent instrumentation involves the use of bioresorbable hardware. The first large-scale reviews involving resorbable cervical plating systems are in publication, with MRI studies showing no evidence of local irritation or swelling following degradation at two years (93,94). As evidence accrues that these systems provide equivalent fusion or stabilization rates, their use in children will likely grow.

Pharmacologic therapy with bisphosphonates can increase bone mineral density and reduce fracture rates in children as young as 1-month old, providing a possible therapeutic augmentation of bone healing or fusion in the very young who sustain spine injury (95,96). Perhaps the greatest pharmacologic benefit lies in the potential application of stem cell therapy or granulocyte-colony stimulating factor to directly repopulate or induce neuronal repair and growth following SCI. Both of these have been shown to improve motor outcome in animal models following SCI (97,98). The plasticity of the pediatric immune system may translate into safer utility of stem cell transplantation.

CONCLUSION

The pediatric spine is not simply a miniature adult spine. It is a unique dynamic entity that requires specialized attention and treatment. The clinician must avoid the pitfalls of misdiagnosis. Familiarization with pediatric anatomy and imaging is essential. Treatment relies on early stabilization and immobilization. Surgical options will continue to improve toward accommodating the smaller immature spine. Overall, pediatric spinal trauma patients fare better than their adult counterparts.

Currently, outcomes remain most closely associated with the severity of the initial injury. An ounce of prevention is far superior to a pound of care in pediatric SCI. Future interventions tailored to the pediatric central nervous system, with the aim of diminishing secondary injury combined with neuro-augmentation to facilitate the repair or replacement of damaged neuronal tissue, are eagerly awaited. Unfortunately, widespread application of these initiatives remains in the distant future.

REFERENCES

1. Griffin MR, Opitz JL, Kurland LT, et al. Traumatic spinal cord injury in Olmsted County, Minnesota, 1935–1981. Am J Epidemiol 1985; 121:884–895.
2. Kewalramani LS, Kraus JF, Sterling HM. Acute spinal-cord lesions in a pediatric population: epidemiological and clinical features. Paraplegia 1980; 18(3):206–219.
3. McGrory BJ, Klassen RA, Chao EY, et al. Acute fractures and dislocations of the cervical spine in children and adolescents. J Bone Joint Surg Am 1993; 75(7):988–995.
4. Hamilton MG, Myles ST. Pediatric spinal injury: review of 174 hospital admissions. J Neurosurg 1992; 77(5):700–704.
5. Osenbach RK, Menezes AH. Pediatric spinal cord and vertebral column injury. Neurosurgery 1992; 30(3):385–390.
6. Stulik J, Pesl T, Kryl J, et al. [Spinal injuries in children and adolescents]. Acta Chir Orthop Traumatol Cech 2006; 73(5):313–320.
7. Kokoska ER, Keller MS, Rallo MC, et al. Characteristics of pediatric cervical spine injuries. J Pediatr Surg 2001; 36(1):100–105.

8. Vitale MG, Goss JM, Roye BD. The epidemiology of pediatric spinal cord injury in the Unites States. #183. Presented at the American Academy of Orthopaedic Surgeons 73rd Annual Meeting, March 22–26, 2006.

9. Adelson PD, Resnick DK. Spinal Cord Injury in Children. Principles and Practice of Pediatric Neurosurgery. Ed. Albright AL, Pollack IF, Adelson PD. New York: Thieme, 1999:955–969.

10. Wilberger JE Jr. Spinal Cord Injuries in Children. Mount Kisco, NY: Futura Publishing Co., 1986:7–11.

11. Ruge JR, Sinson GP, McLone DG, et al. Pediatric spinal injury: the very young. J Neurosurg 1988; 68(1):25–30.

12. Hadley MN, Zabramski JM, Browner CM, et al. Pediatric spinal trauma. Review of 122 cases of spinal cord and vertebral column injuries. J Neurosurg 1988; 68(1):18–24.

13. Bailey DK. The normal cervical spine in infants and children. Radiology 1952; 59 (5):712–719.

14. Avellino AM, Mann FA, Grady MS, et al. The misdiagnosis of acute cervical spine injuries and fractures in infants and children: the 12-year experience of a level I pediatric and adult trauma center. Childs Nerv Syst 2005; 21(2):122–127.

15. Lustrin ES, Karakas SP, Ortiz AO, et al. Pediatric cervical spine: normal anatomy, variants, and trauma. Radiographics 2003; 23(3):539–560.

16. Cattell HS, Filtzer DL. Pseudosubluxation and other normal variations in the cervical spine in children. A study of one hundred and sixty children. J Bone Joint Surg Am 1965; 47(7):1295–1309.

17. Sullivan J. Fractures of the Spine in Children. Skeletal Trauma in Children. 2nd ed. Philadelphia: WB Saunders, 1998:343–368.

18. Swischuk LE. Emergency Imaging of the Acutely Ill or Injured Child. In: The Spine and the Spinal Cord, 4th ed. Philadelphia: Lippincott Williams and Wilkins, 2000;532–587.

19. Brockmeyer D. Pediatric Spinal Cord and Spinal Column Trauma. AANS/CNS Section on Pediatric Neurological Surgery, 2006.

20. Nypaver M, Treloar D. Neutral cervical spine positioning in children. Ann Emerg Med 1994; 23(2):208–211.

21. Eleraky MA, Theodore N, Adams M, et al. Pediatric cervical spine injuries: report of 102 cases and review of the literature. J Neurosurg 2000; 92(suppl 1):12–17.

22. Mulder DS, Wallace DH, Woolhouse FM. The use of the fiberoptic bronchoscope to facilitate endotracheal intubation following head and neck trauma. J Trauma 1975; 15(8):638–640.

23. Buhs C, Cullen M, Klein M, et al. The pediatric trauma C-spine: Is the "odontoid" view necessary? J Pediatr Surg 2000; 35(6):994–997.

24. Management of pediatric cervical spine and spinal cord injuries. Neurosurgery 2002; 50(suppl 3):S85–S99.

25. Shaffer MA, Doris PE. Limitation of the cross table lateral view in detecting cervical spine injuries: a retrospective analysis. Ann Emerg Med 1981; 10(10):508–13.

26. Swischuk LE. Emergency pediatric imaging: changes over the years (Part I). Emerg Radiol 2005; 11(4):193–198.

27. Scarrow AM, Levy EI, Resnick DK, et al. Cervical spine evaluation in obtunded or comatose pediatric trauma patients: a pilot study. Pediatr Neurosurg 1999; 30(4): 169–175.

28. Shen H, Tang Y, Huang L, et al. Applications of diffusion-weighted MRI in thoracic spinal cord injury without radiographic abnormality. Int Orthop 2007; 31(3):375–383.

29. Jagannathan J, Dumont AS, Prevedello DM, et al. Cervical spine injuries in pediatric athletes: mechanisms and management. Neurosurg Focus 2006; 21(4):E6.

30. Viccellio P, Simon H, Pressman BD, et al. A prospective multicenter study of cervical spine injury in children. Pediatrics 2001; 108(2):E20.

31. Anderson RC, Scaife ER, Fenton SJ, et al. Cervical spine clearance after trauma in children. Neurosurg Focus 2006; 20(2):E3.

32. Ware ML, Gupta N, Sun PP, et al. Clinical Biomechanics of the Pediatric Craniocervical Junction and Subaxial Spine. In: Brockmeyer DL, ed. Advanced Pediatric Craniocervical Surgery. New York: Thieme, 2005:27–42.

33. Patel JC, Tepas JJ 3rd, Mollitt DL, et al. Pediatric cervical spine injuries: defining the disease. J Pediatr Surg 2001; 36(2):373–376.

34. Cirak B, Ziegfeld S, Knight VM, et al. Spinal injuries in children. J Pediatr Surg 2004; 39(4):607–612.

35. Gilles FH, Bina M, Sotrel A. Infantile atlantooccipital instability. The potential danger of extreme extension. Am J Dis Child 1979; 133(1):30–37.

36. Wholey MH, Bruwer AJ, Baker HL Jr. The lateral roentgenogram of the neck; with comments on the atlanto-odontoid-basion relationship. Radiology 1958; 71(3):350–356.

37. Violas P, Ropars M, Doumbouya N, et al. Case reports: atlantooccipital and atlantoaxial traumatic dislocation in a child who survived. Clin Orthop Relat Res 2006; 446:286–290.

38. Ferrera PC, Bartfield JM. Traumatic atlanto-occipital dislocation: a potentially survivable injury. Am J Emerg Med 1996; 14(3):291–296.

39. Mikawa Y, Watanabe R, Yamano Y, et al. Fracture through a synchondrosis of the anterior arch of the atlas. J Bone Joint Surg Br 1987; 69(3):483.

40. Osenbach RK, Menezes AH. Spinal cord injury without radiographic abnormality in children. Pediatr Neurosci 1989; 15(4):168–174 (discussion 175).

41. Rahimi SY, Stevens EA, Yeh DJ, et al. Treatment of atlantoaxial instability in pediatric patients. Neurosurg Focus 2003; 15(6):ECP1.

42. Fielding JW, Hawkins RJ. Atlanto-axial rotatory fixation. (Fixed rotatory subluxation of the atlanto-axial joint). J Bone Joint Surg Am 1977; 59(1):37–44.

43. Pang D, Li V. Atlantoaxial rotatory fixation: part 3-a prospective study of the clinical manifestation, diagnosis, management, and outcome of children with alantoaxial rotatory fixation. Neurosurgery 2005; 57(5):954–972.

44. Pang D, Li V. Atlantoaxial rotatory fixation: part 1—Biomechanics of normal rotation at the atlantoaxial joint in children. Neurosurgery 2004; 55(3):614–625 (discussion 625–626).

45. Pang D, Li V. Atlantoaxial rotatory fixation: part 2—new diagnostic paradigm and a new classification based on motion analysis using computed tomographic imaging. Neurosurgery 2005; 57(5):941–953.

46. Subach BR, McLaughlin MR, Albright AL, et al. Current management of pediatric atlantoaxial rotatory subluxation. Spine 1998; 23(20):2174–2179.

47. Bonadio WA. Cervical spine trauma in children: part I. General concepts, normal anatomy, radiographic evaluation. Am J Emerg Med 1993; 11(2):158–165.

48. McCall T, Fassett D, Brockmeyer D. Cervical spine trauma in children: a review. Neurosurg Focus 2006; 20(2):E5.

49. Dogan S, Safavi-Abbasi S, Theodore N, et al. Pediatric subaxial cervical spine injuries: origins, management, and outcome in 51 patients. Neurosurg Focus 2006; 20(2):E1.

50. Roaf R. Instrumentation and fusion technique for lumbar spine. Guidelines according to underlying pathology. Orthop Rev 1986; 15(1):56–57.
51. Lalonde F, Letts M, Yang JP, et al. An analysis of burst fractures of the spine in adolescents. Am J Orthop 2001; 30(2):115–120.
52. Glassman SD, Johnson JR, Holt RT. Seatbelt injuries in children. J Trauma 1992; 33(6):882–886.
53. Crawford AH. Operative treatment of spine fractures in children. Orthop Clin North Am 1990; 21(2):325–339.
54. Gaufin LM, Goodman SJ. Cervical spine injuries in infants. Problems in management. J Neurosurg 1975; 42(2):179–184.
55. Leventhal HR. Birth injuries of the spinal cord. J Pediatr 1960; 56:447–453.
56. Pang D, Wilberger JE Jr. Spinal cord injury without radiographic abnormalities in children. J Neurosurg 1982; 57(1):114–129.
57. Launay F, Leet AI, Sponseller PD. Pediatric spinal cord injury without radiographic abnormality: a meta-analysis. Clin Orthop Relat Res 2005; 433:166–170.
58. Bosch PP, Vogt MT, Ward WT. Pediatric spinal cord injury without radiographic abnormality (SCIWORA): The absence of occult instability and lack of indication for bracing. Spine 2002; 27(24):2788–2800.
59. Pang D, Pollack IF. Spinal cord injury without radiographic abnormality in children— the SCIWORA syndrome. J Trauma 1989; 29(5):654–664.
60. Choi JU, Hoffman HJ, Hendrick EB, et al. Traumatic infarction of the spinal cord in children. J Neurosurg 1986; 65(5):608–610.
61. Grabb PA, Pang D. Magnetic resonance imaging in the evaluation of spinal cord injury without radiographic abnormality in children. Neurosurgery 1994; 35(3):406–414.
62. Dickman CA, Zabramski JM, Hadley MN, et al. Pediatric spinal cord injury without radiographic abnormalities: report of 26 cases and review of the literature. J Spinal Disord 1991; 4(3):296–305.
63. Kriss VM, Kriss TC. SCIWORA (spinal cord injury without radiographic abnormality) in infants and children. Clin Pediatr (Phila) 1996; 35(3):119–124.
64. Turgut M, Akpinar G, Akalan N, et al. Spinal injuries in the pediatric age group: a review of 82 cases of spinal cord and vertebral column injuries. Eur Spine J 1996; 5(3):148–152.
65. Kulkarni MV, McArdle CB, Kopanicky D, et al. Acute spinal cord injury: MR imaging at 1.5 T. Radiology 1987; 164(3):837–843.
66. Yamaguchi S, Hida K, Akino M, et al. A case of pediatric thoracic SCIWORA following minor trauma. Childs Nerv Syst 2002; 18(5):241–243.
67. Fesmire FM, Luten RC. The pediatric cervical spine: developmental anatomy and clinical aspects. J Emerg Med 1989; 7(2):133–142.
68. Marinier M, Rodts MF, Connolly M. Spinal cord injury without radiographic abnormality (SCIWORA). Orthop Nurs 1997; 16(5):57–63.
69. Pang D. Spinal cord injury without radiographic abnormality in children, 2 decades later. Neurosurgery 2004; 55(6):1325–1342.
70. Pollack IF, Pang D, Sclabassi R. Recurrent spinal cord injury without radiographic abnormalities in children. J Neurosurg 1988; 69(2):177–182.
71. Spinal cord injury without radiographic abnormality. Neurosurgery 2002; 50(suppl 3): S100–S104.
72. Vogel LC. Unique management needs of pediatric spinal cord injury patients: etiology and pathophysiology. J Spinal Cord Med 1997; 20(1):10–13.

73. Leventhal HR. Birth injuries of the spinal cord. J Pediatrics 1960; 56:447–453.
74. Norman MC, Wedderburn LC. Fetal spinal cord injury with cephalic delivery. Obstet Gynecol 1973; 42(3):355–358.
75. Burke DC. Traumatic spinal paralysis in children. Paraplegia 1974; 11(4):268–276.
76. Gordon N, Marsden B. Spinal cord injury at birth. Neuropadiatrie 1970; 2(1):112–118.
77. Abroms IF, Bresnan MJ, Zuckerman JE, et al. Cervical cord injuries secondary to hyperextension of the head in breech presentations. Obstet Gynecol 1973; 41(3):369–378.
78. Shulman ST, Madden JD, Esterly JR, et al. Transection of spinal cord. A rare obstetrical complication of cephalic delivery. Arch Dis Child 1971; 46(247):291–294.
79. Bracken MB, Holford TR. Effects of timing of methylprednisolone or naloxone administration on recovery of segmental and long-tract neurological function in NASCIS 2. J Neurosurg 1993; 79(4):500–507.
80. Dormans JP, Criscitiello AA, Drummond DS, et al. Complications in children managed with immobilization in a halo vest. J Bone Joint Surg Am 1995; 77(9): 1370–1373.
81. Anderson JM, Schutt AH. Spinal injury in children: a review of 156 cases seen from 1950 through 1978. Mayo Clin Proc 1980; 55(8):499–504.
82. Givens TG, Polley KA, Smith GF, et al. Pediatric cervical spine injury: a three-year experience. J Trauma 1996; 41(2):310–314.
83. Wang MY, Hoh DJ, Leary SP, et al. High rates of neurological improvement following severe traumatic pediatric spinal cord injury. Spine 2004; 29(13):1493–1497.
84. Kewalramani LS, Tori JA. Spinal cord trauma in children. Neurologic patterns, radiologic features, and pathomechanics of injury. Spine 1980; 5(1):11–18.
85. Aufdermaur M. Spinal injuries in juveniles. Necropsy findings in twelve cases. J Bone Joint Surg Br 1974; 56B(3):513–519.
86. McPhee IB. Spinal fractures and dislocations in children and adolescents. Spine 1981; 6(6):533–537.
87. Hubbard DD. Injuries of the spine in children and adolescents. Clin Orthop Relat Res 1974; 100:56–65.
88. Campbell J, Bonnett C. Spinal cord injury in children. Clin Orthop Relat Res 1975; 112:114–123.
89. Carreon LY, Glassman SD, Campbell MJ. Pediatric spine fractures: a review of 137 hospital admissions. J Spinal Disord Tech 2004; 17(6):477–482.
90. Brown RL, Brunn MA, Garcia VF. Cervical spine injuries in children: a review of 103 patients treated consecutively at a level 1 pediatric trauma center. J Pediatr Surg 2001; 36(8):1107–1114.
91. Manary MJ, Jaffe DM. Cervical spine injuries in children. Pediatr Ann 1996; 25(8): 423–428.
92. Bode KS, Newton PO. Pediatric nonaccidental trauma thoracolumbar fracture-dislocation: posterior spinal fusion with pedicle screw fixation in an 8-month-old boy. Spine 2007; 32(14):E388–E3893.
93. Vaccaro AR, Sahni D, Pahl MA, et al. Long-term magnetic resonance imaging evaluation of bioresorbable anterior cervical plate resorption following fusion for degenerative and traumatic disk disruption. Spine 2006; 31(18):2091–2094.
94. Aryan HE, Lu DC, Acosta FL Jr., et al. Bioabsorbable anterior cervical plating: initial multicenter clinical and radiographic experience. Spine 2007; 32(10):1084–1088.
95. Arikoski P, Silverwood B, Tillmann V, et al. Intravenous pamidronate treatment in children with moderate to severe osteogenesis imperfecta: assessment of indices of

dual-energy X-ray absorptiometry and bone metabolic markers during the first year of therapy. Bone 2004; 34(3):539–546.

96. DiMeglio LA, Ford L, McClintock C, et al. Intravenous pamidronate treatment of children under 36 months of age with osteogenesis imperfecta. Bone 2004; 35(5): 1038–1045.

97. Urdzikova L, Jendelová P, Glogarová K, et al. Transplantation of bone marrow stem cells as well as mobilization by granulocyte-colony stimulating factor promotes recovery after spinal cord injury in rats. J Neurotrauma 2006; 23(9):1379–1391.

98. Divani AA, Hussain MS, Magal E, et al. The use of stem cells' hematopoietic stimulating factors therapy following spinal cord injury. Ann Biomed Eng, 2007 July 20; [Epub ahead of print].

Index

Printed in the United States
by Baker & Taylor Publisher Services